Multimethod Clinical Assessment

N. Wardrop

Multimethod Clinical Assessment

by

W. Robert Nay, Ph.D.

University of Illinois

GARDNER PRESS, INC.

Distributed by Halsted Press

Division of John Wiley & Sons., Inc.

New York • Toronto • Sydney • London

GARDNER PRESS, INC.
19 Union Square West
New York 10003

Distributed solely by the Halsted Press Division
of John Wiley & Sons, Inc., New York

Library of Congress Cataloging in Publication Data

Nay, W Robert.
Multimethod clinical assessment.

Bibliography: p.
Includes indexes.
1. Personality assessment. I. Title.
BF698.4.N39   616.8'9'075   79-57
ISBN 0-470-26654-6
Printed in the United States of America

Designed by Raymond Solomon

To My Grandparents
John and Loretta Nay
Jonathan and Katherine Wright
James R. Bailey

Contents

PREFACE   xiii

OVERVIEW   1

**UNIT I: THE GOALS OF A COMPREHENSIVE
        CLINICAL ASSESSMENT**

Chapter I: The Comprehensive Clinical Assessment   5

Toward a Comprehensive View of the Client   12
  THE BASIC ID: A Multimodality assessment scheme   14
  Behavioral diagnosis   18

Chapter 2: Categories of Information   23

Current Behavior   25
Conditions   27
  Location   27
  Activities   29
  Times   29
  Antecedents and consequences   30
  Modeling influences   34
Historical Information   36
Client Resources   38
  Cognitive-intellectual abilities and deficits   38
  Physical abilities and handicaps   39
  Social skills and social-skill deficits   39
  Person support   40
  Physical surroundings   40
  Financial resources   41
Client Motivation   41

**UNIT II: THE METHODS OF A COMPREHENSIVE
        CLINICAL ASSESSMENT**

UNIT II-A: THE INTERVIEW

**Chapter 3: Self-Report within the Interview: Defining the
        Problem**   49

Major Categories of the Interview   49

vii

Intake-Orientation: Getting to Know the Client   51
    The introduction   52
    Confidentiality   54
    Physical setting of the interview   55
Orientation and Statement of the Problem   57
Definition of the Problem   68
    Focusing with questions   68
Behavioral Observations   73
    Physical appearance   74
    Voice and speech   74
    Nonverbal behavior   77

Chapter 4: The Case History   79

Categories of Historical-Developmental Information   82
    Description of birth   82
    Developmental history   82
    Medical history   83
    Characteristics of family and family history   84
    Interpersonal skills   84
    Educational history   85
    Sexual development   86
    Occupational history   87
Methodological Issues   87
    Organization of the history   88
    Questioning strategies   89
    The autobiographical approach   90

UNIT II-B: WRITTEN METHODS

Chapter 5: Written Self-Report Methods   95

Assessment Methods   96
    Free response measures   96
    Checklists   98
    Rating approaches   99
    The semantic differential   102
    Idiosyncratic rating schemes   104
Important Considerations in Selecting
  a Written Self-Report Instrument   107
    Norms   107
    Reliability   108
    Validity   110
    Response sets   115

UNIT II-C: OBSERVATION METHODS

Chapter 6: Self-Observation: Methods and Issues   119

Definition of the Problem   122
Recording Procedures   123
    Mechanical devices   124
    Product-related measures   125
    Written records   126
Setting   130
Sampling   130
Important Issues   133
    Reactivity   133
    Reliability of self-collected information   138

Chapter 7: Independent Observations: Description, Development, and Validation of Methods   143

Method Options   144
    Mechanical approaches   145
    Product-related measures   149
    Written methods   155
Selection, Definition, and Validation   165
    Selection of targets for clients   166
    Approaching validity in instrument construction   167

Chapter 8: The Setting   180

The "Natural" Setting   181
    Important issues   182
    *Methodological variant: Observation by setting
    "participants"*   186
    An ecological approach   189
The Clinical Natural Setting   193
The Clinical Contrived Setting   195

Chapter 9: Sampling   203

Event Sampling   204
Time Sampling   207
    Methodology   211
    Cueing devices   216

Chapter 10: Reliability Assessment: Strategies and Issues   219

Definition and Methodology   220

Interobserver agreement   221
Multifaceted Reliability Assessment   226
   A "generalizability" approach   231
The Quest for Reliability: Issues in Training
   and Assessment Methodology   236
   Selection and training of observers   236
   Complexity as a predictor of observer agreement   245
   Observer expectation and biases   246

UNIT II-D: PSYCHOPHYSIOLOGICAL ASSESSMENT

Chapter 11: Psychophysiological Methods   255

Psychophysiological Responses: Possibilities for
   Measurement   257
Major Modalities of Psychophysiological Assessment   261
   Heart functioning   261
   Electromyogram (EMG)   264
   Electroencephalography (EEG)   266
   Skin responses   267
Other Psychophysiological Methods   269

UNIT III: CLINICAL DECISION MAKING

**Chapter 12: Organizing the Assessment to Facilitate Clinical
   Decision Making**   273

The Tactics of Clinical Assessment: Some Potential
   Problems, Some Recommendations   278
   Clinical assessment errors   278
   Multimethod assessment of a child behavior problem   285
   Multimethod assessment of an adult male   295
Communicating Assessment Findings   299
   Formats for the written report   301
   Potential pitfalls   308

UNIT IV: CLINICAL ASSESSMENT FOR CASE EVALUATION

Chapter 13: Treatment Evaluation Strategies   313

(Philip C. Kendall and W. Robert Nay)

Significance: Clinical vs. Statistical   314
Group vs. Single-Subject Designs   315
The B Design   316
The A-B Design   316

The B-C Design 320
The A-B-A or A-B-A-B Design 321
The A-B-A-C-A or Successive Treatments Design 323
The Multiple-Baseline Design 324
  Methodological issues suggested by the
    multiple-baseline design 326
The Simultaneous Treatment Design 328
The Changing-Criterion Design 330
The Single-Case Designs: A Summary 332

REFERENCES 334

AUTHOR INDEX 353

SUBJECT INDEX 359

Preface

In recent years the clinical assessment of clients—their thoughts, feelings, sensations and overt actions—has been expanded to include information other than that obtained in the interview or via a psychometric instrument. Strategies for systematic observation conducted by the client himself or by others, as well as psychophysiological measures suitable to the practical needs of the clinical arena, increasingly augment the self-report. While the assessor is burdened with the task of selecting from among many methodological options for pretreatment assessment or case evaluation, few writers have provided him with a strategy for organizing this task and integrating information collected across diverse aspects of the client and his life situation.

Multimethod clinical assessment offers a strategy for assessment that provides such a schema, a schema that should be applicable to change agents of diverse theoretical orientations and methodological sophistication. Following a presentation of those aspects of the client and his life situation that might be selected as a focus for assessment, the reader is offered a variety of assessment options across interview, written, observation and psychophysiological method categories. Practical descriptions of methods are integrated with a discussion of current research findings and contemporary issues. Material describing important issues in the construction and evaluation of methods is also offered for the interested change agent or applied researcher.

In addition to being useful as a primary text or parallel reading for graduate courses in clinical assessment, this text could be employed in undergraduate courses that review tests and measures of clinically relevant phenomena. Also, courses involving program evaluation, single case evaluation or assessment methods suitable to the applied researcher might find the methodological and evaluation coverage to be of benefit to the student interested in clinical problems. The human services professional in academia, in an agency, or in private practice will find this information to be of use in planning, carrying out and evaluating efforts at client behavior change.

I wish to thank my publisher, Gardner Spungin, for his flexibility and good humor in permitting me to take the time necessary to write this book at a rather unique pace. I have learned much about clinical assessment from my efforts of training students. To those graduate students and undergraduate mental health workers at the University of Illinois who have asked difficult questions and raised issues with me I offer my appreciation. A special thanks goes to Dan Rybicki and Paul Turner. Having outstanding colleagues to call upon contributes in many ways to the completion of any book. I particularly wish to thank Fred Kanfer, Gordon Paul, Bill Redd, John Gottman and Doug Bernstein for the intellectual stimulation and support they provided as this project unfolded.

Yuki Llewellyn and Gail Hamel, who served as my secretaries over the last two years, were unusually good to work with. Cudos also to Rachel Dyal for serving as an outstanding copy editor.

Finally, I appreciate the support and, in some cases, sacrifices of my sons: Don, Greg, Jack and Christopher. I've learned a lot just from being with them and watching them develop. To my wife Joyce, I'll communicate my thanks in person.

Multimethod Clinical Assessment

AN OVERVIEW OF MULTIMETHOD CLINICAL ASSESSMENT

Sara seemed to respond well to our combined therapeutic strategy. After four weeks she began reporting an improvement in her mood and had her first week of full-time work at her place of employment. Her positive self-statements and demeanor improved remarkably about this time. After a total of eight weeks we reduced therapy sessions to twice monthly; we terminated her from regular contact after twelve weeks. Sara reported that she felt she could "stand on her own feet" for the first time in her adult life. We agreed with her assessment. Follow-up at one year after treatment showed Sara to be continuing to make progress. She had just been promoted to a new position of authority and was actively contemplating marriage for the first time.

This behavioral change agent (BCA) is obviously quite pleased with the outcome of intervention, and from this report we might be led to term it a success. We would, however, reasonably wish to know the ingredients of this success if we are students of behavior change. What was the decision-making process that led to a satisfactory selection of goals? How did the BCA come to select a successful therapeutic approach from the myriad of potential interventions available? Given this therapist's exuberance, we might also wish to know about the *specific* criteria and methods that were employed to evaluate therapeutic outcome. These questions are central to the task of the clinical assessment. In exploring possible ways of answering them, this book will provide the reader with a strategy; a way of thinking about the task of coming to understand the client, his problems and life situation, with an ultimate eye toward formulating intervention objectives that can reasonably be achieved. A first unit explores the *goals* of the clinical assessment, the kinds of questions

1

that the BCA might wish to ask to obtain a comprehensive view of the client and the situation within which that client lives as interdependent predictors of the client's behavior within a given point in time. *Behavior is construed broadly to include not only overt motor acts but also the client's thoughts, beliefs, values and any other aspects that help the BCA to understand the client's objectives.* In Chapter 1, we begin by exploring the schemes for comprehensive assessment devised by other authors. A detailed presentation of those "categories of information" that the present author would include in a comprehensive assessment are included in Chapter 2. Once the BCA has decided to focus upon specific aspects of person or situation in planning the assessment, it is obvious that methods must be selected that permit a comprehensive view of each of these "modalities" or information categories. Thus the second unit focuses upon the *methods* of the clinical assessment, with chapters providing a review of methodological variants and important issues suggested by each of four major methods categories: the interview, written methods, the use of observation as an assessment tool, and psychophysiological assessment.

Now that the reader has a grounding in potential goals and methods, the third unit presents the basic assumptions of a multimethod approach to assessment; a strategy for planning and organizing the assessment as a prelude to clinical decision-making. This unit also includes a review of methodological options and important issues suggested by communicating assessment findings in writing, and it underscores the value of organized record keeping.

The fourth unit emphasizes the importance of systematic case evaluation, particularly in this age of consumer enlightenment and humanistic values. A variety of single-case evaluation schemes that have emerged from the clinical-experimental literature will be offered as possibilities for the BCA who wishes to increase the certainty with which the processes of intervention can be related to therapeutic outcome. While this section may not be of interest to all readers, the author hopes that it will serve to stress the importance of case evaluation and the manner in which clinical assessment data can be employed to this end.

Chapters within each of the four units will integrate practical suggestions and explicit examples of methodology with a presentation of important issues suggested by the contemporary literature. In addition, issues suggested by the construction of assessment tools and their reliability and validity will be raised at appropriate points, and the author hopes they will provide the reader with a foundation for critically evaluating assessment methods. The reader will note the omission of certain psychometric instruments that are frequently included within the clinical assessment. Rather than duplicate this coverage the reader is referred to several excellent textbooks (e.g., Cronbach, 1970; Wiggins, 1973) for a description of tests of intellectual functioning, personality, aptitudes, interests and the like. This text offers a variety of methods that might be viewed as alternatives to or complements of a more formal psychometric assessment, depending upon the reader's theoretical biases.

UNIT I
The Goals of a Comprehensive Clinical Assessment

1

THE COMPREHENSIVE CLINICAL ASSESSMENT

The proliferation of therapeutic methods sometimes seems to outstrip the average BCA's ability to keep up with it all. Selections on the therapeutic menu include such possibilities as Primal Scream therapy, Reality therapy, Rational-Emotive therapy, Client-Centered therapy, variants of behavior modification, Gestalt therapy, Transactional Analysis, variants of psychoanalysis, existentialism, and the endless possibilities of phenomenology. Many BCAs identify themselves as being primarily associated with a particular method and indeed, when the BCA is asked his "orientation," the question usually means: "What kind of therapist are you?" As these therapeutic entities may focus on some specific aspect of the client's behavior (such as irrational beliefs, self-statements, recollections of events in the past, verbal statements within the interview), one might suppose that they restrict the scope of the assessment that precedes intervention. While it might be extreme to assume that this is the standard case, adherence to a particular therapeutic strategy does require that certain kinds of information be known about the client and may propel the BCA in the direction of a less than comprehensive assessment. Many BCAs seem to avail themselves of therapy methods in supermarket fashion, selecting a pound of therapy X and a container of treatment Y as if they were mutually exclusive ways of understanding the client, rather than methods directed toward separate aspects of the person which, taken together, form a comprehensive and rich understanding of the client-in-situation. Regardless of the validity of this author's fears and his general disdain for proselytizing for one or another "kind" of therapy, the reader may well ask at this point: How is a comprehensive view of the client obtained? This chapter will offer a review of the information categories that a BCA might decide to include in gaining a systematic view of the client. To provide a framework for this review we will begin by discussing major goals for the clinical assessment of common interest across BCAs. The foremost of these goals must be that of *description:* of the client, his problems and objectives, and his life situation.

Description holds a prominent place in the history of clinical assessment and suggests a variety of issues that are worth considering prior to turning to other assessment goals. The idea of attempting to describe, define, categorize or classify an individual's behavior, particularly a behavior that we term "abnormal," is not new. Virtually every textbook of abnormal psychology or psychopathology begins with an outline of the characteristics of normal versus abnormal behavior, usually expressed with much caution and reservation. The reader is no doubt familiar with such terms as "neurosis," "psychosis," "schizophrenia," and "personality disorder" as descriptive labels for certain behaviors. While a formal classification system was not developed until the middle of the twentieth century, descriptive labels have been employed for centuries and can be traced to the earliest of times. We do not have language records for primitive man; however, we assume that he must have been able to identify certain classes of unusual behavior, since we believe he used trephining, the drilling of holes in the skull, as a means of "treating" his fellows.

The first formal attempt to classify contranormative behavior was made by Hippocrates, the father of modern medicine, who might also be thought of as a precursor of modern psychiatry. He postulated that disturbances of thought were due to the relative balance of four body humors (or fluids): blood, phlegm, black bile, and yellow bile. Treatment involved a regimen for living to bring these humors into a more appropriate balance. At various other times the deviant individual was thought to be possessed by the devil or some other supernormal force, or may have been labeled a witch. Once the deviance was identified, "treatment" would be directed toward casting out the force that presumably caused the individual's aberrant behavior, and a shaman or other religious figure might be called on to perform the exorcism. In some instances, elaborately punitive methods were employed to make an "assessment." If the individual died while being tortured, it was evidence that he in fact was not possessed (a small comfort). We have evidence of such treatment in the religious trials that occurred in New England in the seventeenth century.

During the early and middle part of the nineteenth century, persons experiencing problems in living were viewed as being morally deficient and best served by family members within the extended family. It was perhaps only a matter of time before the sometimes highly unusual behavior displayed by such persons would provoke scientific interest. Advances in medical science during this period, most notably Pasteur's germ theory of disease, suggested that many physical ailments could be treated by locating and destroying the organisms responsible for the outward "symptoms" displayed by the patient. The finding that syphilis, which caused a variety of physical as well as mental disturbances (often including bizarre behavior), was caused by a microorganism lent credence to this idea. The outward or behavioral manifestations previously thought to be a sign of spiritual possession or moral laxitude would now be viewed as symptomatic of an underlying disease. It is important to realize that a major goal of medical science is to develop a classification scheme that enables the physician to diagnose disease or bodily insult based upon a systematic appraisal of a patient's outward symptoms. As might be imagined, it was not long until medicine attempted to include various "mental diseases" within such a classfication scheme. An early attempt was made by Kraepelin (1896) to provide a description of the syndrome (grouping of symptoms) occurring within certain major categories of abnormal behavior. Specifically, Kraepelin classified mental disturbance into two categories: *dementia praecox* (later termed "schizophrenia" by Joseph Bleuler) and *manic-depressive psychosis*; and postulated that both of these disorders could be traced to underlying physical causes. The early years of the twentieth century saw the introduction of a variety of classificatory labels. It is interesting to note that even theorists who postulated exclusively psychological or environmental causes for abnormal behavior continued to employ the labels of classification that had emerged from a medical perspective. The description of the hysterical personality by Freud, and the later writings of psychoanalytic personality theorists continued this trend, even though they considered the underlying disease process to be conflict between certain hypothesized components of the psyche (e.g., id, ego, superego, shadow).

Now that medical science had a language to describe various categories of abnormal behavior, a search for presumed etiologies to explain particular categories (which presumably would lead to a fixed course of treatment) became a logical pursuit for physicians who specialized in treating psychological abnormality (psychiatrists) as well as for experimental psychologists. Diagnosis and classification were furthered by the mental testing movement which began in the late nineteenth century with the work of Binet and others who attempted to categorize the intellectual functioning of school children so that suitable academic environments could be uniquely tailored to each child's abilities. The need for immediate classification of intellectual ability and aptitudes during World War II resulted in increased interest in developing paper and pencil tests to assist the assessor in placing a given individual into one of the classification categories. As might be imagined, the proliferation of diagnostic labels soon produced a good deal of confusion, and the necessity for a formal nomenclature that could be employed across mental health professionals soon became evident. For that reason, the American Psychiatric Association developed a Diagnostic and Statistical Manual that provided a listing of major categories of abnormal behavior, and for each, descriptions of subcategories to assist the BCA in making a diagnostic "impression." The revision of the DSM in 1968 (DSM II) defined six major categories of abnormal behavior: mental retardation, organic brain syndromes, psychoses not attributable to physical conditions listed previously, neuroses, personality disorders and certain other nonpsychotic mental disorders, and psychophysiological disorders. For each, subcategories are followed by a description of personality, behavioral or other characteristics that would assist the assessor in making a diagnosis. This diagnostic manual is revised from time to time (the latest revision is DSM III), and is employed by many BCAs today as a means of diagnostic description.

The popularity of the diagnostic and classification approach is perhaps attributable to its potentially ideal characteristics. A classification system provides diverse BCAs with a common language for describing abnormal behavior and should immediately suggest a course of intervention once a diagnosis has been made of the patient's symptoms. Unfortunately, this is often not the case. The use of a formal diagnostic system such as the DSM can be criticized on at least three grounds. First, we must ask whether or not different assessors will agree as to the major category as well as the subcategory to which the client's abnormal behavior is assigned. Second, the DSM assumes that psychological disorders can be uniquely placed in a particular category; that is, symptoms that clients display are mutually exclusive so that assignment to a particular category can be made. Finally, and at a somewhat different level, the question of the impact of labeling upon the client's behavior must be addressed; that is, if an indivdual is labeled using one of the more deviant of the classificatory categories, will this serve as a self-fulfilling prophecy? The first two questions are directed at the foundation of such a classification scheme, while the last has to do with a more humanistic concern, and might be asked *even if* the classification scheme should prove to be reliable and valid.

With regard to the first question, a number of investigators have compared agreements in diagnoses made by a wide variety of professionals. Some of the more frequently cited research will be briefly discussed. Schmidt and Fonda (1956) compared the diagnoses made by three "chief psychiatrists" with those made by members of a group of eight psychiatric residents for a population of 426 patients admitted to a state hospital in one six-month period. The authors employed the chief psychiatrists' diagnoses as criteria for agreement both for major categories (e.g., organic, psychotic, characterological) as well as for eleven subtypes (e.g., acute brain symdrome, chronic brain syndrome, mental deficiency, involutional, affective, schizophrenic, unclassified, neurosis, personality pattern, personality trait, sociopathic). As might be imagined, the authors found good agreement in assignment of patients to the major categories. For example, the residents agreed with the chief psychiatrists in 92 percent of the organic cases, 80 percent of the psychotic cases and 71 percent of the characterological cases. While this may seem to be rather excellent convergence of agreement, misdiagnoses ranging from 8 to 29 percent do suggest a good deal of variability and may be unacceptable if regimens of drug or other severe modes of treatments are assigned based upon these diagnoses. For the specific labels (subtypes) that were used, agreement ranged from zero to 80 percent with a mean of 55 percent across the subtypes. Generally, better agreement was found for disorders that had some organic (physical) basis, as opposed to psychotic and characterological disorders. Ward, Beck, Mendelson, Mock and Erbuagh (1962) criticized the Schmidt and Fonda findings because psychiatric residents assigned diagnoses. Beck et al. performed a similar investigation comparing the ratings of pairs of experienced, board-level psychiatrists who rated 153 psychiatric out-patients. Placement of the patient in one of six diagnostic categories showed agreements ranging from 38 to 63 percent. A variety of similar evaluations of diagnostic reliability have reported similar results (Sandifer, Pettus and Quade, 1964; Ullmann and Gurel, 1962; Zubin, 1966).

The second question addresses the homogenity of classification categories. Obviously, if the categories are to have any meaning at all, an individual's "symptoms" or behavior problems must be sufficiently distinct to permit an assignment to a particular category. A much cited study by Zigler and Phillips (1961) best illustrates the problems of any diagnostic scheme attempting to so compartmentalize human behavior. These authors reviewed the hospital records of 793 psychiatric patients, categorizing them into four major diagnostic groupings: manic-depressive, psychoneurotic, character disorder, and schizophrenic. The authors then noted the presence of one or more of 35 "symptoms" which the admitting psychiatrists or referral agencies found to be present at the patients' admission to the hospital. In only three cases did a particular symptom appear in any given category more than 50 percent of the time, which suggested that particular symptoms and categories are not highly correlated. To give an example, "tenseness" was displayed by 32 percent of those patients labeled manic-depressive, 46 percent of those labeled psychoneurotic, 33 percent of those labeled character disorders and 36 percent of those labeled schizophrenic, with "suspiciousness" shown for 25 percent of the manic-depressive clients, 16 percent of the psychoneurotics, 17 percent of the character disorders and 65 percent of the schizophrenics. Depression, hallucinations, suicide attempts, bodily complaints, emotional outbursts, assaultive behavior, and many others were similarly found *across* all four categories and not exclusively in any one. Similarly, Ullmann and Hunrichs (1958) found no significant differences between three diagnostic categories for three measures of anxiety and four concept-formation tasks. In summarizing their own findings as well as those of Zimet and Brackbill

(1959), the authors state:

Within the limits of psychological tests, then, the concept that the neurotic patient is highly anxious and the personality disorder patient is minimally anxious is not borne out. Even in the three major diagnostic groupings of psychosis, neurosis, and personality disorder, the most important criteria for classification in the particular category were not observed. (p. 230)

The third problem of classification is the potential impact of labeling on the way others behave toward the "patient," how they view him, and how the patient views himself. Many investigators have reported that our expectancy for an individual to behave in a particular fashion can greatly color our view of his behavior. This can be shown at the level of a researcher who is motivated to see particular results (Rosenthal, 1966; Rosenthal & Jacobsen, 1968), as well as at a more informal level within everyday social discourse. For example, when students were randomly assigned labels regarding their intellectual functioning (for instance, high vs. low intelligence), teachers tended to behave toward those children according to their expectations, which in turn affected the children's performance. Rosenhan (1973) studied the impact of diagnostic labeling upon the behavior of eight researchers who were admitted to psychiatric hospitals as "pseudo-patients" in order to study the workings of a psychiatric ward from within that setting. Each of the pseudo-patients feigned the symptom of "hearing voices" in order to be admitted to the hospital, but were instructed to behave normally once placed on the ward. Except for not taking medications, all of the pseudo-patients participated in ward activities just like any other patient, while making extensive notes of their experiences in the participant-observer role. All but one of the pseudo-patients were admitted with a diagnosis of schizophrenia, and interestingly enough, the label "stuck" even when they were released from the hospital ("schizophrenia in remission"). At no time did the staff members find out that the pseudo-patients were not "abnormal," although other patients quickly guessed their role. Thus, once the patients were labeled, the staff members saw them in terms of those labels even though each of them behaved in a normal fashion upon admittance. Rosenhan, (1973) states: "Once a person is designated abnormal, all of his other behaviors and characteristics are colored by that label. Indeed, that label is so powerful that many pseudo-patients' normal behaviors were overlooked entirely or profoundly misinterpreted" (p. 253). An analysis of the pseudo-patients' notes revealed that every aspect of their behavior was viewed as symptomatic of their psychological disorder. For example, note-taking itself was viewed as being "pathological" (supported by the reports of staff members in hospital charts). In most cases, the pseudo-patients were ignored when they asked questions of staff, treated almost as if they did not exist, and all experienced a great feeling of depersonalization and lowered self-esteem. Rosenhan concludes that persons who are labeled as being pathological are caught up in a Catch-22 cycle; once labeled, everything that the patient does is viewed as being further indication of his "problem." It is difficult or impossible to break out of this role to be viewed along more positive lines. In addition, Rosenhan believes that the labeled patient may come to view himself as being sick or disturbed, with obvious implications for his future behavior. Along these lines, the work of George Kelly (1955) suggests that the constructs an individual employs to evaluate his own behavior may change if that individual is forced to assume a divergent role. The person's behavior may now change to come into congruence with these cognitive changes. Meichenbaum (1975) and others have talked of the impact of one's self-instructions or self-statements as predictors of future behavior, while a variety of writers (Kanfer, 1975; Mahoney, 1975) have discussed how standards for self-evaluation can be instigated via the expectations that others (such as parents and peers) have for an individual's behavior.

Other researchers have criticized formal diagnostic labels for these as well as other reasons. For example, Fairweather, Sanders, Maynard and Cressler (1969) offer a series of principles necessary to the creation of a social system that would permit a psychiatric patient to readjust to the community. An important aspect of these principles is the flexibility of roles available to the patient; a tolerance for deviance. Labels that might hold continuing implications for the individual's behavioral possibilities would not be employed. McGee (1974) describes an idealized model of crisis intervention that would integrate the patient back into the community as quickly as possible. Central to this model is the absence of diagnostic labeling. The BCA is aided in helping the client by an analysis of each individual's resources and existing strengths. An excellent review of problems encountered in employing diagnostic labels as well as suggested alternatives to the labeling process may be found in Rappaport (1977).

While traditional diagnostic-labeling practices have been and can be criticized on a number of grounds, the reader must ask himself why such practices continue to flourish in many settings and across many categories of BCAs. It is almost trite to say that human behavior is multiply determined by a complex set of person and situation variables. Yet wouldn't it be lovely if we did have a battery of paper and pencil measures that could be quickly administered and interpreted in the clinical setting? A simple set of scores would provide a unique description of the client that suggest a recognized plan of treatment. Thus, if a client were provided with label "X," the BCA would only have to look up the treatment for "X" from among a menu of treatments available for various psychological disorders. Furthermore, wouldn't it be nice (or would it?) if people did behave consistently across situations? Regularity in behavior would make possible accurate predictions regarding appropriate treatment (once a person was labeled) for persons ranging from the mildly "neurotic" to the criminal or self-destructive individual, and would greatly improve the cost-effectiveness of intervention. Currently, it is obvious that diagnosis as it is applied in many settings seems to assume that one or more of these wishes are indeed true, when in fact we are far from seeing the fulfillment of any of them (even if all of us agreed that they are desirable goals).

This text assumes that it is premature to label an individual as falling into a particular diagnostic category given the lack of utility of all but the broadest of such categories in predicting an individual's behavior; indeed, it may be a disservice to so label him. The chapters to follow will present a variety of alternative methodological options useful in obtaining a rich description of the client's behavior-in-situation. *Description* is emphasized with behavior broadly defined to include a client's thoughts, imagery, feelings, attitudes, and any other aspects of the person that assist in understanding how best to meet the client's objectives.

Along with description, the BCA might have at least three additional objectives that can be achieved if a comprehensive assessment is carried out. The BCA might wish to understand the facets of person and situation that elicit and maintain the client's behavior or in some fashion delimit possibilities for behavior. *Causality* is the attempt to explain why an individual experiences discomfort in his life situation or behaves or fails to behave in some fashion. Intervention may take causal factors into account, capitalizing upon them whenever possible. The clinical assessment should also provide information regarding *methods* best suited to a client's individual requirements. The BCA will wish to select from among the array of available methods those which are most likely to meet the client's objectives, are acceptable to the client and are capable of being implemented in a practical and ethically sound fashion. Finally, the clinical assessment should provide a data base that may enable the BCA to *evaluate* the impact of intervention upon the client's behavior. Preintervention assessment provides a "baseline" that may be used to evaluate both the process and outcome of intervention when further assessments are made as intervention proceeds.

We will now explore assessment strategies offered by other writers which meet the criterion of a comprehensive description of the client and his life situation.

Toward a Comprehensive View of the Client

It is improbable that intervention goals which are likely to optimally meet the client's requirements will emerge from a single interview or the administration of a particular psychological test. The selection of certain aspects of the client and the client's life situation as the focus of the assessment and the suitability of particular assessment methods depend upon the nature of the client's problems and stated goals. Unfortunately, it is often difficult to know which aspects of the client or the life situation should be the *focus* of the assessment, particularly when the BCA has only the client's initial original statement of problems and concerns at hand. Some clients are artful self-observers and can competently pinpoint the phenomena that cause them to seek services. Unfortunately, this is not always the case, and the BCA who fails to obtain information beyond the client's verbal report may obtain an inaccurate or misleading view. Thus, a primary role of the clinical assessment must be to obtain an objective and comprehensive view of the client *as a prelude* to sifting out pertinent information and focusing upon particular bits and pieces of the client's life and behavior that shape intervention goals. As Goldfried and Davison (1976) point out, to do otherwise may lead to the selection of inappropriate goals which will restrict in advance the possibility of meeting the client's needs. This leads to the question: are there certain kinds of information that, across clients, maximize the likelihood of detecting important aspects of the client's behavior-in-situation? It is worth noting that the standard psychometric assessment battery includes an intake interview, case history, intelligence test, and objective personality test, as well as some category of projective measure. While it is beyond the scope of this text to review the various psychometric instruments that are available to the BCA in organizing such a battery, it is obvious that the client's verbal and written self-report are emphasized if this approach is adopted. While incidental behavior displayed by the client during the interview or while responding to a test might be observed and noted by the BCA, direct assessments of the client's behavior in ordinary life situations as well as an evaluation of psychophysiological response channels are excluded. Direct assessments may be useful in providing a comprehensive view of the client, particularly when a verbal or written self-report is contrasted with the client's actual behavior. Recently the emergence of behavioral intervention approaches has prompted increased attention to assessing more than the client's self-report. An extensive literature specifically addresses the area of "behavioral assessment" (Hersen and Bellack, 1976; Ciminero, Calhoun, and Adams, 1977; Cone and Hawkins, 1977). While behaviorists may disagree regarding the specific aspects of the client's behavior that should be the focus of intervention, all include some variant of the three response systems originally discussed by Lang (1968; 1971): verbal-cognitive, motoric, and physiological. In addition, any assessment scheme that does not address aspects of the environment within which the client functions—the ecological milieu that may determine the appropriateness of particular thoughts, feelings or actions—is necessarily limited. Distinctions between normal and abnormal behavior frequently rest upon subcultural norms; indeed, the fabric of our society is a mosaic of normative variants that cluster around some rather central beliefs (codified in law and religion) about how each individual ought to treat his fellows.

A comprehensive assessment thus expands an evaluation of major channels (systems) of the client's behavior to include a look at the situation, the *context* within which the behavior occurs. The remainder of this chapter reviews two assessment schemes that are of interest because of their comprehensiveness. Each of the systems offers explicit alternatives that the BCA can evaluate in selecting or excluding certain categories of information for a particular assessment task.

THE BASIC ID: A Multimodality Assessment Scheme

In his book *Multimodal behavior therapy*, Lazarus (1976) suggests that the aspects of person and situation explored by BCAs in the assessment frequently depend on a limited theoretical point of view. If BCAs identify with a particular theoretical framework, they may develop "vested interests in strengthening and confirming that system's basic theoretical underpinnings" (p. 3). In contrast, Lazarus takes the position that all of us are beings who "move, feel, sense, imagine, think, and relate" (p. 4), and that neurological and biochemical factors obviously influence all aspects of an individual's functioning. A multimodal approach is based on the assumption that each of these major domains should be a routine part of preintervention assessment. An introductory comment by Lazarus provides an overview of this approach.

The content of each diagnostic inquiry depends upon the vicissitudes of the individual case; nonetheless, there is an overall structural framework that has general applicability. We are interested in discovering the client's intrusive behavior patterns (tics, compulsions, habits, mannerisms, etc.), negative emotions (times, places, and situations that elicit anger, anxiety, depression, etc.), unpleasant sensations (aches and pains, dizziness, flushing, etc.), intrusive images (disturbing recollections of unpleasant events or scenes), faulty cognitions (self-defeating values, attitudes, and beliefs), and interpersonal shortcomings (overcompetitive strivings, aggressive responses, childish demands, etc.). In addition to these maladaptive responses, we are also concerned with the client's deficits across each modality—the *absence* of useful behaviors, pleasant feelings, good sensations. Thus, the major assessment framework defines responses within each modality that are best *decreased*, as well as those that are best *increased*. (p. 5)

Lazarus employs the term BASIC ID as a mnemonic device to guide the BCA in exploring the major domains already mentioned: *behavior, affect, sensation, imagery, cognition* and *interpersonal*, with *drugs* a category that subsumes organic and physiological processes. Lazarus assumes that faulty problem identification is probably the "greatest impediment to successful therapy" (p. 14), and emphasizes that *each* of these modalities must be explored as a part of the comprehensive assessment. In addition, he hypothesizes that the more modalities that are "deliberately invoked" by any approach to intervention, the better the likelihood that durable results will be obtained. Each modality will now be presented in more detail.

Behavior. This category has to do with overt verbal or motor behaviors that may "undermine effective living" if they occur to excess or fail to occur. Lazarus suggests that the BCA evaluate the *characteristics* of the behavior, focusing upon its frequency, intensity, and duration. Major questions involve asking "when, what, how, who and where, rather than why" (p. 32). In line with the functional analytic point of view espoused by many behaviorists, Lazarus would have the BCA explore antecedents of the behavior as well as consequences applied by the client or some aspect of the environment following the behavior. He emphasizes that this modality is unique in that the BCA can directly observe what the client does or says, whereas modalities having to do with sensation, imagery, and the like can only be assessed via the client's self-report. For this reason, self-reports of internal events should be contrasted with behavioral concomitants or referents, if present. He states: "We will not belabor the point that therapy remains incomplete until verbal self-reports coupled with objective observations have been carefully scrutinized across each modality of the basic id." (p. 33)

Affect. Lazarus suggests that while clearcut aberrations in affective responses (e.g., violent rage, severe depression) are easy to detect when displayed by the client, the stimuli in his daily life that provoke anger, anxiety, and other emotions demand careful identification. He would have the BCA begin by inquiring as to the feelings that might be provoked by behavioral excesses or deficits (for instance: When you are unable to do X, how does that make you feel? When X occurs, what does that feel like?). In addition, the BCA should obtain a "profile" of situations that tend to elicit negative as well as positive feelings (e.g., "What makes you cry ... glad ... happy ... scared?"), and attempt to explore precisely what the client experiences that would cause him to label it happy, sad, and so forth.

Sensation. Lazarus makes the point that some individuals are not able to experience sensations; they seem to be "switched off below the head" (p. 35). In other cases, an exaggerated experiencing of sensations may be the problem (e.g., the hypochondriac who reports intense pain when no medical reason can be found). Many clients present physical complaints involving bodily sensations (headaches, nausea, dizziness, aches and pains). The BCA should carefully explore the precise characteristics of such sensations with the client. In addition, Lazarus would encourage the BCA to inquire as to the client's experiencing within each of the different sensory channels (touch, smell, taste, hearing, sight). Thus the BCA might inquire about the client's appetite, pleasant sights, smells, sounds, and so forth.

Imagery. Lazarus defines imagery as the various "mental pictures" that may influence a client's life. Imagery might be a primary problem (e.g., repetitive unpleasant imagery) or imagery may occur with other modalities (e.g., imagery associated with an avoidance of heights). Lazarus requires each client to obtain certain images with an instruction such as: "Please picture your childhood home." He inquires about the client's parents, requiring the client to "take a tour in imagination" throughout the rooms of the home, focusing upon each sensory modality within the imagery (e.g., smells, tastes that the client experiences), followed by asking the client to picture a particularly "safe" place within the home. Lazarus reports that these images were selected from among hundreds because they yield important clinical material, particularly when they are discussed in detail and related to the various cognitive and affective elements that they evoke.

Cognition. In exploring the client's thinking, a major goal is to identify misconceptions causing illogical thinking. Derived from Lazarus and Fay's (1975) twenty most common mistaken beliefs as well as the irrational beliefs outlined by Ellis (1962), Lazarus attempts to discover which of these illogical philosophies the client subscribes to. Lazarus is also interested in evaluating the "shoulds": the set of self-statements that define a client's expectations for himself and for others around him ("I should succeed at everything I do"; "Everyone should like me and I should like them"; "Hard work should pay off"). Lazarus is particularly sensitive to perfectionistic standards that the client may have adopted which inevitably lead to self-defeating behavior. Finally, Lazarus would have the BCA pay close attention to the client's attributions regarding his or her behavior. That is, to what persons, objects, or other phenomena does the client attribute some aspect of his behavior (e.g., "I can't succeed because *my family holds me back*"; "*I'm not smart enough* to do X"; "I'm the way I am *because of X, Y, or Z*"). Lazarus points out such faulty cognitions to the client at the first appropriate opportunity. Such insights "usually open up other areas for discussion, and many attitudes, values and beliefs are thus available for exploration" (p. 40).

Interpersonal relationships. Interpersonal assessment, according to Lazarus, involves two levels of discourse. First, the BCA listens to the client's report of interactions with others (such as, "I really told X off the other day"; "I know Mr. Edwards likes me because he consistently pays more attention to me than the other guys"; "My wife always ignores me"). Second, the BCA should *observe* the way the client responds in actual interpersonal situations. Lazarus suggests that the group (e.g., family, therapy group) is a useful medium for observing the client's interactions with others. In addition, the client's responses to the BCA may be observed in the individual therapy situaion. Lazarus suggests that it is "a serious mistake to insist that the client-therapist dyad is necessarily pivotal, or that the client's feelings toward the therapist are identical to those elicited in other important relationships. They may or may not be, and it is incumbent upon the therapist to determine which facets are unique or specific to the ongoing dyad, and which reveal the client's general interpersonal feelings" (p. 42). In addition, Lazarus emphasizes that the self-reports of many clients are inaccurate, and it is important to carry out various validity checks (by direct observation of the client, assessment of contradictions or inconsistencies in the client's self-report, interviews with significant others in the client's life, and so on). Finally, Lazarus would have the BCA pay attention not only to the client's direct verbal messages (denotative content), but also to paralinguistic (characteristics of speech) and kinesic (body language, facial expression) communications (to be discussed in detail in Chapter 3). In comparing verbal content with paralanguage and body language the BCA may frequently note inconsistencies which can then be followed up by further questioning.

Drugs. Lazarus employs the label "drugs" to represent much more than substances an individual ingests, although an assessment of possible alcohol or other substance abuse may be in order in some cases.

In this modality, the first assessment consideration concerns the person's overall physical appearance, mode of attire, signs of intoxication, noticeable skin disorders, speech disturbances, tics or psychomotor disorders. The client is asked about physiological complaints—aches, cramps, headaches, asthma, tachycardia, dizziness, shortness of breath, and so forth. Consultation with a physician is often essential. Chemotherapy is usually required when clients appear to be suffering from physiological depression, or when mood swings from high to low occur for no apparent reason, or when irrational thoughts and feelings seem to be racing out of control. The multi-modal therapist does not see drug treatment as both necessary and sufficient, but when florid symptoms are medically well-controlled, all the other modalities need to be carefully assessed and any problems that emerge must receive specific treatment." (p. 43)

In addition, the BCA might inquire about the client's physical fitness, exercise, diet, and general well-being. The idea is to obtain a complete picture of the client's physical status and physical response to the environment.

Lazarus underscores the *interdependent* nature of the seven modalities and encourages the BCA to employ information collected in any one modality in posing questions and constructing assessments in other categories. For example, the BCA might wish to understand the specific relationship between two or more modalities. Questions such as "When X *behavior* occurs, how does that make you *feel?*"; or "When you experience that *sensation* of tightness, what do you *do* in response?" are obvious examples of combining modalities in the assessment-questioning process.

The BASIC ID seems to focus heavily upon the person; aspects of the client which may assist the BCA in understanding current problems and potential objectives for change. The "interpersonal" categories of this approach explore the response of other persons to the client, but there is little emphasis upon the subcultural milieu and physical setting in which the client functions. Kanfer and Saslow (1969) have developed a comprehensive assessment strategy that gives more equal weighting to the *situation* and *person* as interdependent predictors of the client's functioning. Their behavioral diagnostic scheme will now be presented.

Behavioral diagnosis

Kanfer and Saslow (1969) have developed a comprehensive approach to viewing the client's behavior-in-situation, emphasizing the client's ability to exert control over his own life. While adopting a learning theory point of view, the authors point out that their diagnostic scheme is "consistent with earlier formulations of the principles of comprehensive medicine... which emphasize the joint operation of biological, social, and psychological factors in psychiatric disorders" (p. 429). In agreement with Lazarus's BASIC ID model already presented, Kanfer and Saslow focus upon carefully *describing* the client's behavior in a manner that would provide information necessary for developing an intervention plan. Following an initial *definition* of the problem, the authors suggest that the BCA explore the client's *motivation* to exert changes in his life, the client's *physical-biological resources* and the *sociocultural milieu* within which the client functions (which may set up expectations or provide limitations for the client's behavior) as well as the client's *past behavior* and changes in that behavior over time. In addition, the authors suggest that the client's ability to exert *self-control* over his behavior, the *social relationships* ordinarily present, as well as the *social-cultural-physical environment*, also be appraised. While certain categories of information may not seem applicable to a given client, analysis of all the categories contributes "to the better understanding of what the patient needs to learn to become an autonomous person [as well as] an inventory of his existing socially effective behavioral repertoire which can be put in the service of any treatment procedure" (p. 437). Each of the categories of the behavioral diagnosis will now be presented in more detail. This author will attempt to paraphrase major points; the reader is referred to Kanfer and Saslow (1969) for a more extensive presentation.

Initial analysis of the problem situation. As a preliminary step, the authors suggest that the BCA assign the client's problematic behavior to one of two major categories of change goals. First, the problem may be a behavior that occurs *to excess*. By "to excess" the authors mean that the behavior occurs at too great a *frequency*, for too long a *duration*, or at a *level of intensity* that is discomforting to the client or others around him. In addition, an excess would include behaviors that occur *under conditions where any occurrence at all is socially unacceptable* (e.g., sexual exhibitionism, physical assaults, stealing).

In contrast, a *behavioral deficit* is a class of behavior that causes discomfort or promotes inefficiency because it *fails to occur at some socially expected level or at a level commensurate with a client's expectations.* Specifically, the behavior (e.g., eye contact; eating; certain hygiene behaviors; use of social approach behavior) either *fails to occur with sufficient frequency,* occurs for *too brief a duration,* or *does not occur in an appropriate form or under socially expected conditions.* Kanfer and Saslow (1969) cite examples of this last category: social withdrawl, amnesia, fatigue syndrome, and the lack of certain sexual responses (e.g., impotence). It is implicit that the lack of occurrence of a certain class of behavior might be variously labeled as normal or abnormal depending on the subcultural group to which the client belongs. For example, the set of social behaviors that we term "table manners" would be expected to occur only in certain settings.

In addition to focusing upon the problem, Kanfer and Saslow (1969) think it important for the BCA to assess a client's *strengths:* the special talents, assets, and other resources that the client brings to bear upon his life situation. The authors urge the BCA to survey major domains of the client's behavior and interests, as well as the immediate surroundings in which the client lives to evaluate assets. The authors state:

Any segment of the patient's activities can be used as an arena for building up new behaviors. In fact, his natural work and play activities provide a better starting point for behavior changes than can ever be provided in a synthetic activity or relationship. For example, a person with musical talent, skill in a craft, physical skill or social appeal can be helped to use his strengths as vehicles for changing behavior relationships and for acquiring new behaviors in areas in which some successful outcomes are highly probable. While a therapeutic goal may ultimately be the acquisition of specific social or self-evaluated behaviors, the learning can be programmed with many different tasks and in areas in which the patient has already acquired competence (pp. 431–432).

Clarification of problem situation. Once the BCA has classified the client's behavior as excessive or deficient, Kanfer and Saslow (1969) recommend that further information be obtained regarding the consequences of the behavior for the individual, in the *context* of the occurrence of the behavior. This process is typified by such questions as: what does this behavioral excess or deficit do for the individual? or, how does the behavior in some way restrict the client's opportunities? If the current situation were changed, how would that affect these outcomes? Thus, a client who is behaving in a deviant fashion may be receiving positive social support for that behavior from other persons who themselves receive some benefit from the client's behavior.

Next, the authors explore both the client's current and potential motivation for enacting changes in his life and an exploration of potential ways of motivating the client.

Motivational analysis. The BCA should first explore the incentives that currently motivate the client. The authors recommend surveying activities and their potential satisfactions, such as achievement of recognition, sympathy, social relationships, financial rewards, success in vocational or avocational tasks, securing dependency, maintaining good health, sexual satisfaction, or money and material rewards. They suggest that the BCA can obtain clues by looking at the amount of time the client engages in these activities or seeks them out. From a practical standpoint, the authors wonder how frequently the client has been successful in attaining these incentives, as well as the probability of their availability in the future. The BCA should also explore classes of aversive events that the client may seek to avoid. In addition, the authors believe the BCA should explore the attributions the client makes about his behavior (e.g., caused by fate, self, or others) and determine whether the client tends to naturally consequate appropriate and inappropriate behavior using the incentives listed. Finally, the BCA should evaluate whether or not the client is willing to give up certain gains currently associated with problematic behavior or submit to aversive consequences associated with new but more desirable behavior.

Developmental analysis. Biological changes: In this category the BCA is asked to explore the client's past and current physical status to determine handicaps, bodily insults or other physical-medical factors that may interfere with the achievement of goals. The BCA should explore how the client has dealt with such phenomena in the past as well as current adjustment.

Sociological changes: The BCA should define the client's sociocultural milieu (urban vs. rural environment, religious affiliation, level of socioeconomic achievement, level of education, etc.), and evaluate whether the client's current behavior, attitudes and beliefs are congruent with sociocultural norms. Kanfer and Saslow provide the following examples: "How is a college orientation of an adolescent accepted by his peer group in a poor neighborhood? How does the home and neighborhood environment respond to a patient's religious, social and sexual activities and fantasies?" (p. 434). In addition, the BCA should explore possible recent changes in the client's sociocultural milieu and the extent to which those changes may be related to the client's current problems or goals (e.g., the impact of moving to a new community or changing jobs). Finally, the BCA should explore role conflicts impinging upon the client. For example, is there congruence between the client's role in job, family, and community? Obviously, incongruities should be carefully explored and may provide a useful perspective for understanding the client's current dissatisfactions and objectives.

Behavior changes: The BCA should explore the history of the client's problems, evaluating behavioral excesses or deficits from their inception to the present, trying to note factors that may be functionally related to that behavior (e.g., specific conditions under which the behavior was first noted). The BCA should also explore how biological, social, or sociological events in the client's life seem to be related to behavior changes.

Analysis of self-control. The BCA is asked to explore whether or not the client is able to exert control over problematic behavior and under what conditions the client is able to do so. Strategies that the client employs for self-control may be usefully employed within intervention, while strategies that have been unsuccessful in the past should also be known to the BCA. The BCA should learn how the client goes about *acting upon* his environment (e.g., actively manipulating persons or physical settings versus passively responding). Does the client tend to emphasize positive or aversive control in providing consequences to himself (e.g., withdrawing from desirable activities as a consequence of negative behavior; rewarding himself via positve self-statements, dinner in a restaurant, etc., for appropriate behavior)? Any conditions limiting the client's possibilities for self-control should be defined.

Analysis of social relationships. The BCA should define the cast of characters in the client's life: persons currently present and significantly involved in the client's family, vocational, or other life settings. Persons who in some way maintain the client's current behavior by providing incentives for appropriate or inappropriate behaviors, or who punish or restrict possibilities for desirable behavior or model inappropriate behavior, must be identified. The BCA should explore whether or not such persons could be effectively employed in a treatment program to facilitate the client's goals. In some cases, the primary problem may be some aspect of a client's relationship with someone else (e.g., communication within a marital dyad; parent-child interaction), in which case a comprehensive analysis of all parties involved is necessary. Finally, Kanfer and Saslow (1969) would have the BCA determine the expectations for behavior that others have for the client as well as the client's expectations, since these expectations may indeed shape and perhaps delimit the client's behavior.

Analysis of the social-cultural-physical environment. This category overlaps with the previous "developmental analysis" in defining the norms for behavior in the client's social environment. It is important to evaluate how the environment is likely to respond to a client's excesses and deficits, as well as how the environment will respond to the behavior the client learns as intervention proceeds. If social norms are consonant with intervention goals, the environment may well facilitate the client's objectives. If they are not, persons within the client's environment may subtly or actively punish the client for contranormative behavior, even if the BCA and client decide that such behavior is of value to the client. In addition, Kanfer and Saslow (1969) inquire about social, intellectual, sexual, vocational, economic, religious, moral, or physical restrictions imposed by the environment which may place limitations upon the client's behavioral possibilities. Finally, the BCA should determine the extent to which the client's milieu is supportive of the client's seeking intervention services. If such services are not valued, members of the client's environment may fail to support the client's behavior change efforts or actively sabotage possibilities for change.

Kanfer and Saslow (1969) emphasize that each category should "call attention to important variables affecting the patient's current behavior" (p. 437), and emphasize that the BCA should attempt to obtain information *across* categories in clearcut, explicit language that does not call for high-level abstraction. In addition, they emphasize the importance of augmenting the client's verbal report with other methods of data gathering (such as reports of others, observations) and the concept that no data relating to the patient's past or present experiences be viewed as irrelevant. Finally, Kanfer and Saslow (1969) do not intend to "infinitely" expand the scope of the clinical diagnosis, but encourage the BCA to "make a selection from the numerous investigative avenues explicitly opened by the present conceptual model" (p. 438) in deciding which modalities of information are to be the focus for the assessment. While the method of inquiry may vary, the authors emphasize that each major area be examined whenever the clinical assessment is performed.

Kanfer and Saslow (1969) have proposed an extensive and detailed model for data gathering as a prelude to intervention. This author doubts that many BCAs even approach the comprehensiveness of this model in performing clinical assessments. However, focusing on a restricted number of the categories that they present might result in a distorted picture of the client-in-situation.

The next chapter will present a detailed review of major categories of information that the present author would include in a comprehensive clinical assessment. The reader will immediately notice the overlap between the author's assessment model and these comprehensive approaches of Lazarus (1976) and Kanfer and Saslow (1969). The assessment schemes of other authors could also have been included within this chapter. Those presented were offered because they varied in approach, while still offering a comprehensive view of the client. The material in Chapters 1 and 2 should not be thought of as being exhaustive, but merely as one step in reviewing the possibilities available to the BCA for looking at something other than the presenting complaint offered by the client's verbal self-report. It is this author's contention that only after a comprehensive clinical assessment is performed can the BCA be in a position to know which elements of the client's life situation and current behavior are logical foci for intervention. The author believes too that intervention methods logically follow from the assessment picture that emerges. . When intervention methodology, *in advance*, predicts modalities of information that are to be the potential targets for an assessment, it is possible that the BCA and client may select goals which will not promote maximally desirable change in the client's life. A comprehensive clinical assessment should be thought of as emerging from a systems view of human behavior similar to that proposed for the natural sciences (Bertalanfly, 1968). In this conceptualization, major domains of the client's behavior (e.g., overt motor behavior, affective responses, cognitions, imagery, physiological responses, and so forth) as well as the physical-interpersonal-cultural environment, are interdependent elements, each of which influence the other in ways that hold major implications for the client. In taking this systems approach, the BCA is often presented with many optional targets for change (e.g., changing the environment, which then instigates change in the client, or vice versa). If carried out properly, the comprehensive clinical assessment should provide sufficient and detailed information to best determine the specific element toward which intervention should be directed.

2

CATEGORIES OF INFORMATION

The various assessment formats and classification schemes described in Chapter 1 all aim to provide information regarding potential goals for client behavior change. These goals fall into one of the following categories (Nay, 1976).

First, an increase in the frequency of some behavior or group of behaviors the client currently exhibits may be in order. A client may engage in a desirable behavior only on rare occasions and perhaps even at inappropriate times. A depressed client, for example, may think positive thoughts about himself or say positive things to other persons very infrequently, which may be distressing both to the client and to those who interact with him. A goal of intervention here might be to increase the frequency of positive thoughts or verbalizations to some level agreed on by client and therapist. As another example, a child who is perfectly able to dress himself and engage in certain hygenic behaviors may fail to do so on a regular basis. An increase in the frequency of such behaviors might be considered important by a parent, teacher, or staff member who supervises the child and is concerned with the child's health and physical appearance.

A second goal of intervention might be to incorporate some new behavior within a client's repertoire, to remove a "deficit" (Kanfer and Saslow, 1969). We all begin life without a vocabulary. To acquire new behaviors or information, we learn from persons (models) who employ "new" words and perhaps provide encouragement for our initial attempts at mastery of these skills. In some cases, even adults lack skills that might permit them to function more comfortably and efficiently in their social interactions or job. Thus, learning certain social skills may permit an individual to take advantage of opportunities requiring the instigation and maintenance of social relationships. It is important that the client's *current* behavioral repertoire be thoroughly assessed to define a starting point for the instigation of new behavior. A teacher, for example, cannot expect a child to spell "cat" if the child has not yet learned the letters of the alphabet.

Finally, a goal of intervention might be *to reduce the frequency of a repertoire behavior* because of its current or potential ill effects on the individual himself and/or those who interact with him. Frequent tantrums of a young child, smoking cigarettes or excessive eating, or, as an extreme example, self-destructive acts of a suicidal adult or self-mutilating child are all behaviors that might be chosen to reduce in frequency.

The foregoing all focus upon problems or concerns that might be raised by the individual client or that might be individual goals for one or more persons who happen to be a part of a larger social system (e.g., a marriage or family). It is important to note that intervention goals may also be directed toward *changing the system itself* as is frequently the case in marital or family therapy (Haley, 1976; Gurman and Kniskern, 1978). Frequently, it is only possible to understand personal concerns by assessing aspects of the significant relationship(s) in the (referred) client's life. Often, intervention becomes redirected from the initial client and targets to aspects of these relationships (e.g., improving communication, altering family roles). In some cases individualized goals for significant others augment or replace targets initially labeled as a problem. For this reason, it should be noted that the term "client" will be employed in a broad sense in this chapter. The client could be an individual, a couple, or a family. While some of the assessment categories to follow obviously focus exclusively on the individual client, many would be relevant toward assessing some system of persons. Also, the material to be presented on observing persons-in-settings (Chapters 7, 8, and 9) and the review of ecological assessment (Chapter 8) is of particular relevance to a systems-level assessment.

Because of the complexity of human behavior, some combination of the above goals often becomes desirable within intervention, and quite divergent intervention strategies may be employed in each case. In addition, to accomplish client behavior change, intervention goals may be directed at changing some aspect of the environment that influences the client's behavior in some fashion.

Given these potential goals of intervention, this chapter will explore those *categories of information* that might serve as a focus for clinical assessment. While not pretending to be exhaustive, these categories provide the BCA with a comprehensive view of the client's goals in the context of his life environment. The potential usefulness of information in each category will be described, along with references to the methods chapters that follow.

Current Behavior

The BCA's interaction with the client usually begins with an initial description of problems or concerns. Whether the client is self-referred or is referred by others, the BCA must employ this initial "problem description" as a starting point in the process of deciding on intervention goals. These goals must be well-defined and stated clearly to ensure appropriate selection of intervention strategies, and must be explicit enough to permit an evaluation of therapeutic success. It would be difficult for a BCA to design an intervention approach to improve a client's "attitude" or to assist a client in "feeling better" if the BCA had no idea of what these terms meant to the client. Following an open-ended interview (Chapter 3) permitting the client to state his reasons for seeking therapeutic services, the BCA then attempts to ensure that he understands the client's descriptive language. As many clients may initially be unable to state their goals clearly, the transaction between the client and BCA must continue as a process of definition until therapeutic goals can be stated by both parties with some degree of certainty. Often the definition of the problem itself becomes an initial goal of the interchange, and the client is encouraged to speak freely, with the BCA assisting the client in clarifying feelings about behavior or life situations that are of current concern.

One way of understanding the client's self-description of his life is to focus on the *referents* of the phenomena described. First, the BCA should discover whether or not there are observable referents that might assist both BCA and client in detecting the problematic phenomena. If the behavior involves *verbal and/or motor components*, it may be possible for the BCA or others (e.g., setting participants, such as the client's spouse or a staff member) to provide a description of its characteristics or even to assess its frequency using one of the observational methods described in Chapter 7. When problematic behavior occurs in more than one locale, such as a child misbehaving both in school and at home, it is advantageous to observe it in all relevant settings to determine where interventions might optimally take place. Chapter 8 discusses the methods and issues related to the setting in which a client is observed.

While many social behaviors are "overt" and thus detectable by others, some potential targets, such as discomforting feelings of anger or sadness, are exclusively "covert" and unobservable to others, or have covert components (e.g., a client's anxiety is indicated by body tremor, while concomitant nausea is not observable, and hence considered covert). A client complaining of "nervousness" or of being "upset" may be able to localize certain physical sensations as part of the potential target. Feelings of "lightness in my stomach," "a hot feeling across my forehead," "a tingling sensation at the base of my spine," or certain muscular tensions are among the physical referents that frequently occur as a part of the client's anxiety. Certain of these physical sensations may evoke a good deal of discomfort for the client and may themselves become a focus of intervention.

Just as a client's behavior or feelings may have physical referents, the client may report specific *cognitive or imaginal referents* that reliably occur and perhaps evoke discomfort. While it is impossible to know precisely what is going on in a client's mind (Nelson and McReynolds, 1971; Simkins, 1971), it is important that the BCA take steps to assist the client to define such phenomena verbally. Thoughts themselves may provoke discomfort or inefficiency (e.g., the repetitive unpleasant thoughts of the obsessive client, the frequent negative self-statements of the depressed individual), or they may control other aspects of the client's behavior targeted for change. Thus, individuals may cognitively review what they are about to do, or "self-instruct" prior to engaging in a particular behavior (Meichenbaum, 1975). Obviously much of our overt behavior is either preceded by some thought or image or occurs simultaneously with a cognitive event.

Chapter 3 shows how the BCA might focus the client's attention on both physical and cognitive or imaginal phenomena so that they may be carefully defined, while Chapter 6 illustrates how either event category might be systematically monitored by the client himself. Client record-keeping permits the client to become attuned to the onset and characteristics of such events as they occur. In many cases, self-monitoring itself leads to desirable behavioral change, which is perhaps due to increased self-awareness and the observational skills the client develops.

It is important that the BCA learn about *temporal* features of the potential target; its current or desirable *frequency* as well as *duration.* A person, for example, is seen as having a very negative view of himself, not exclusively because of the statements he makes, but because of the frequency of such events. If negative self-statements are made with great frequency, we conclude that the individual in fact holds this negative self-evaluation. Similarly, a child's scholastic ability, an accountant's contribution to a business, or the current status of a marriage are defined by the frequency with which certain phenomena do or do not occur, and probably not exclusively by the characteristics of any one event. When a client states that he wants to "quit smoking," "gain control of his anger" or "become more efficient in getting work done," he is obviously employing a frequency criterion not only to evaluate his current behavior (event does not occur frequently enough), but to set goals for himself. Thus, our client would probably be pleased if the frequency of his smoking was reduced significantly from the current fifty cigarettes per day, or if the frequency of anger episodes were reduced. It may be important to know that a problem event described as "most discomforting" occurs only rarely or for very abbreviated periods of time. As the client reviews potential targets, some priorities of goals must be set, since it is usually impossible to "change everything" at once. It may be costly and inefficient to encourage the client to invest an extensive amount of time to alter a problem event that occurs only on rare occasions and may be elicited by the very special characteristics of a particular situation. A determination of current frequency also permits the BCA and the client to evaluate whether or not a target has changed as a result of intervention. In some cases frequency may not change, and duration first shows the effects of intervention (e.g., the duration of a client's anxiety attacks is reduced although no change in their frequency is noted). Both frequency and duration assessments provide useful descriptive information regarding the characteristics of the client's current behavior and serve as primary criteria for evaluating the efficacy of intervention.

Conditions

Once the BCA has a clear idea of precisely which aspects of the client's current life situation might be the focus for intervention, and client and BCA can discuss these phenomena in words understood by both, the potential targeted phenomena must be placed in the context of the client's life situation. Virtually no aspect of our behavior occurs in a vacuum—that is, outside of the situations, other persons, and objects that come to be a part of our environment. We could, for example, spend considerable time teaching a youngster a language to communicate his needs. However, regardless of the extent to which the child mastered this language, it could not be funtionally employed if other persons in the child's environment could not use it. However, we would expect the child to try to employ some collection of sounds that would in fact enable him to communicate with others to meet certain of his social and other needs. Although this is an extreme example, it illustrates the importance of one's environment as a potential delimiter as well as controller of one's behavior. While virtually no one would argue that one's behavior is solely a product of "nurture," one's immediate surroundings obviously have much to do with the classes and characteristics of the behavior that one displays.

Location

One condition that must be ascertained is the *location* or set of locations in which the problem phenomena occur (or desirable behavior does not occur). A review of these locations may indicate that the client's environment fails to encourage or permit some desirable event or actively elicits or encourages an undesirable event because of the physical characteristics of the setting. For example, it may be difficult or impossible for the "shy" and socially unskilled male undergraduate to meet and develop relationships with females if he attends a predominately male university or chooses a part-time job where his only colleagues are men. His current living situation obviously does little to facilitate encounters with females and in fact inhibits such events. Similarly, a teacher may notice that it is singularly difficult to control his students if rather noisy physical education classes are conducted in an adjoining room. This location clearly makes it difficult for students to pay attention and actively distracts them at times.

Along these lines, the "failing" student who studies while listening to the radio or while talking with others in the room, and the obese person who fills the apartment with boxes and bags of snack foods, may find that their environments are constructed to interfere with their goals. Regardless of whether the stated goal is to increase or decrease a particular event, the BCA should carefully evaluate the characteristics of those locations both where the behavior seems currently to occur at *high rate* and at *low rate.* Returning to the poor student, it may be important to know about places where the student finds it *easier* to study and does so with greater frequency. An intervention strategy might capitalize on the characteristics of this high-rate setting by limiting the client's studying to such noninterfering locations. Not only should the BCA, using one of the interview approaches presented in Chapter 3, encourage the client to describe these locations at the outset, but it may also be useful to have the client self-monitor locations where the desired behavior occurs for some period of time prior to intervention (see Chapter 6). In addition, an independent observational assessment of the setting by the BCA (see Chapter 7) may reveal characteristics of the client's living space that the client is not aware of.

Another important reason for defining the location of the targeted behavior is the possibility that certain phenomena in the client's environment may "control" its frequency. The term "stimulus control" has been used by some investigators (Ferster, Nurnberger, and Levitt, 1962; Goldiamond, 1965) to describe how environmental stimuli come to elicit behavior through their contiguous association in time. Goldiamond (1965) describes the use of stimulus control as a treatment approach to slimming a young obese male. Because his client had previously consumed large quantities of food while talking on the telephone, watching TV, reading in bed, or engaging in various other activities, Goldiamond assumed that many locations and activities had come to elicit the urge to eat. Treatment required the client to limit his eating to one location in the home; gradually the other locations ceased to serve as controlling stimuli because they were no longer associated with the positive act of eating. The person who automatically lights a cigarette on picking up the telephone or finds that sitting at his desk at the office brings forth thoughts related to academic pursuits or his job may be responding to such "controlling" stimuli. A thorough evaluation of the settings where some behavior occurs at a high rate, along the lines suggested above, may permit the BCA to identify controlling stimuli and either systematically reduce their controlling properties or employ them to advantage in an intervention strategy.

Activities

While the physical location of a target may limit its occurrence or exert controls, the activity engaged in may be similarly important. For example, if the target seems to occur at roughly equal frequency across a variety of the client's ordinary activities, we might assume that the characteristics of such activities are not predictors of the target, and we can look for other possibilities. However, if the frequency of the problematic event seems to be related to certain activities engaged in, a careful analysis of the activities may assist the client and BCA to better understand the behavior. Certain activities may require skills that the client does not currently possess, force the client to interact with persons who fail to encourage appropriate behavior and in fact encourage inappropriate behavior, or tend to be negatively self-valued or hold negative consequences for the client because of his previous experience with them. If a young child, for instance, becomes "fearful" and "nervous" when asked to engage in athletic activities, the BCA may be assisted in understanding the child's discomfort by viewing this behavior in the context of previous experiences (e.g., being ridiculed for a lack of athletic skills). It is impossible to catalog all the ways that particular activities could come to inhibit desirable behavior or encourage inappropriate behavior.

Times

For reasons similar to those for identifying locations and activities, it may be important to identify the specific *times*, within and across days, when the target occurs. If certain times are reliably associated with the occurrence or nonoccurrence of the target, a careful evaluation of events occurring at these times may assist the BCA in better understanding the factors controlling the behavior. Thus, the parent who finds his child to be particularly noncompliant and verbally abusive late in the afternoon should consider the possibility that the child is fatigued and may require an afternoon nap, or perhaps is hungry because it is just before dinner time. While time does not usually in itself control behavior, one can think of examples of the time of day serving as a direct instigator of certain events. The disruptive behavior of students in a classroom immediately prior to the final bell, for instance, is predictable not only by the students' general fatigue and readiness to leave school, but by their clock-watching which serves to cue the gathering of books and other preparations for leaving.

Antecedents and Consequences

Behaviorists have long been interested in the relationships between certain stimuli[S] that, when presented, consistently elicit a particular response[R]. As applied to human behavior in natural settings, the BCA is encouraged to explore possible functional relationships (Bijou, Peterson, and Ault, 1968) between the "conditions" already mentioned, the behavior of other persons or certain internal/covert events experienced by the client (e.g., thoughts, imagery, sensations) *and* the target. Such events may occur as antecedents to the target, serving to cue or instigate its occurrence, or as consequences that follow occurrence and which serve to maintain the target at some level of frequency. It is worth noting that overt acts (e.g., compulsive eye blinks, ritualistic hand-washing) may be maintained by thoughts or physiological sensations (e.g., they are performed in order to reduce "anxiety"), while events occurring exclusively at a covert level (e.g., excessive thoughts and ruminations, depressive ideation) may be triggered and maintained by external events in the individual's environment (e.g., negative social sanctions delivered by others). It is difficult to conceive of any behavior that is exclusively instigated or maintained by either covert or overt antecedents or consequences. This should be kept in mind in the discussion that follows. After a presentation of the nature of antecedent events that might serve to cue or to trigger some problematic behavior, a review of overt as well as covert categories of consequences will be provided. The potential role of persons in the client's environment who may serve to instigate behavior via social learning or "modeling" mechanisms (Bandura, 1969; Bandura and Walters, 1963) will also be addressed.

Regarding environmental antecedents, the BCA should explore conditions of location, activities and time already described to evaluate whether one or more of these phenomena reliably precede the occurrence of the target. Their role as possible instigators of the target already has been reviewed.

Those persons who interact with the client and seem to be consistently present just prior to and/or during instances of the target should be noted. Given the interdependent nature of behavior displayed by members of a dyad or small group (such as a family), it may be useful to evaluate whether certain acts on the part of others seem to be reliably related to certain acts on the part of the client. BCAs who would view the client from a "systems" perspective (Haley, 1963; Watzlawick, Beavin, & Jackson, 1967) would find it impossible to evaluate the client's behavior in isolation; that is, without also exploring the behavior of others who may have instigated or responded to it once it occurs. In this context, it may be impossible (and rather meaningless) to know whose behavior within the system is serving as antecedent or consequence for the client, given the impact of *all* members of this system upon each other. Along similar lines, social psychologists have emphasized the way certain classes of positive or negative behavior may be exchanged to achieve a homeostatic level that is valenced in a positive or negative direction. Thus, the problem behavior of a child may not only involve the child behaving in a negative fashion towards others, but also in the child *receiving negative communications.* Others can influence the client's behavior via instructions they provide, positive or negative consequences they can potentially dispense and/or via behavior they display.

To discover covert antecedents serving to instigate or maintain a behavior, the assessor must obviously rely on the client's self-report in defining the thoughts, feelings, images, or perhaps physiological sensations (e.g., discomfort, dizziness, anxiety, or nausea) that seem to reliably occur prior to or following the onset of the target. Chapter 6 will present suggestions for assisting the client to self-monitor and keep a written record of such antecedent or consequent events. After some period of pretreatment self-gathered data collection, both the BCA and client may be in a better position to define systematically the internal events that hold instigating or maintaining value for the targeted behavior.

When we engage in certain behaviors, there are often positive or negative consequences that may affect the probability of our engaging in that behavior at some future time. A brief review of classes of consequences may be useful. Terminology employed is from Skinner (1953, 1957). Consequences may come from the external environment, and may assume many forms. When a one-year-old knocks a bowl of soup onto the floor and older children laugh and make much of the infant's behavior, this laughter and attention are considered a *positive reinforcement* if the probability of the infant's pushing the bowl onto the floor is *increased* in the future. In fact, any event that follows behavior is termed a positive reinforcement if it increases the probability of the target's future occurrence. In the present example there is a good chance that the infant may engage in the "mess-making" again to gain his older sibling's attention.

Negative reinforcement defines the situation in which *the removal of aversive consequences is contingent on some desirable targeted behavior.* For example, a child sent to his room for "being bad" begins to make a great ruckus, tossing objects about the room, crying, and generally making noise. The mother may say to the child, "As soon as you stop all that racket, you may leave your room" (the consequence will be terminated), and when the child quiets down, the mother goes to him and tells him to come back outside and play. Thus, the termination of aversive consequences is contingent on a targeted behavior (being "quiet").

When negative consequences are employed, they are most frequently presented within a punishment paradigm. A *punishment* or *punisher* is any event that *follows* some behavior and that *decreases* the probability of the behavior at some future time.

Examples of consequences fall into three general categories: material, social, and activity (obviously overlap is possible). A *material consequence is a tangible object that is either provided to a client for some appropriate behavior or removed following some inappropriate behavior.* Thus, a material consequence must have some physical properties. Examples of positive material consequences are: food, cigarettes, toys or craft items, as well as that "great American standby," money. Negative material consequences most often involve the removal of some material incentive contingent on undesirable behavior. Behavior modification programs have often been criticized for introducing material consequences into settings (such as home or classroom) that will not be present to maintain behavior once the "program" is terminated (see Nay, 1976). A *social consequence is any verbal or physical behavior on the part of one person*—for example, a staff member of parent—*that either increases or decreases the probability of a client engaging in a behavior.* Obviously, this is a very broad definition; however, it is extremely difficult to categorize the possible social consequences that might influence a client's behavior. Often social consequences are very subtle. A smile, a glance, a touch on the shoulder, a word stated with a certain inflection, even the person's body stance, may define whether a communication is viewed as being positive or negative by the recipient and predict its subsequent effect on behavior.

Of course, there are a number of easily observable social consequences, including such verbal statements as "Good job," "I like the way you ———," or any other statement that provides positive feedback to the recipient. Then there are physical behaviors: a pat on the back, a kiss, a hug, a smile, a nod of the head; in fact, any nonverbal gesture the recipient finds positive.

Negative social consequences include verbal criticisms such as "Poor job," "I'm very unhappy with the way that you———," or any other remark that provides negative feedback to the recipient about his behavior. There are also physical negative consequences, including a shove, slap, hit, shake of the head, frown, failure of the initiator to maintain eye contact with the recipient, or any other physical gesture that communicates to the recipient that the initiator is displeased with his behavior.

In summary, social consequences are often difficult to define, and their value depends completely on how the recipient evaluates them. Sometimes what an independent observer might think is a negative social communication (e.g., a push or a shove) might be viewed positively by the recipient. I remember one family whose members used physical raps and hits as signs of affection. Rather than tell his son verbally that he approved of his performance in a baseball game, the father reached over and lightly slugged him on the arm during a therapy session. This was obviously viewed by the son as a positive communication. Within this family, past experiences had made it very clear what kinds of social communication were positive and what kinds were negative.

Finally, *activity consequences provide access to some desired activity or event contingent on some behavior of interest.*

Any event that occurs *within the individual* (not directly observable by others) and *increases or decreases* the probability of some behavior that it follows is an *intrinsic consequence.* This category of "covert" or "intrinsic" behaviors may include an array of cognitive events (thoughts, imagery, fantasy), as well as physiological states (feelings, sensations, pain). Kanfer and Marston (1963) were among the first to emphasize the manner in which an individual develops internal standards for judging his own behavior and accordingly reinforces himself (e.g., positive and negative self-statements) for performance. Bandura and Kupers (1964) and Mischel and Liebert (1966) are among investigators who have shown that the self-reinforcement standards adopted by individuals are influenced by the standards observed in others. Thus, standards for self-reinforcement may be learned without any direct contact with an event, merely by watching someone of influence (a model) demonstrate such standards. In fact, Bandura and Perloff (1967) have shown that internal self-reinforcement is as effective at controlling children's behavior as are externally administered rewards such as candy or toys. Thus, the task of the BCA is not so simple as to merely define material and social consequences delivered by other "extrinsic" agents.

A couple of examples of the importance of these private or "covert" events may be in order. Let us assume that as a youngster you are paid $3.50 to cut Mr. Brown's lawn. You have been paid $3.50 for cutting the lawn for the last two years and have come to count on this income to buy necessary items (gum, candy, etc.). The material reinforcement of $3.50, contingent on lawn cutting, thus increases the probility that you will mow his lawn on a regular basis (a "positive" reinforcement), and you view this as a fair wage and an appropriate consequence of your efforts. Say that two months ago Mr. Brown began paying you $6.00 for the same lawn cutting, and you have received this consequence on four occasions since that last time. If Mr. Brown now again offers you $3.50, you may view this formerly positive consequence as negative in the light of your current level of pay, and in fact you may view this lower figure as a punishment. Your current cognitive set is that $6.00 is appropriate pay for your performance, and $3.50 may be viewed as signifying a poor job. Thus, the way that you cognitively view the financial consequence is the important determiner of its reinforcing properties.

A father's harsh words when his son spills the paint are only a negative consequence in that they provoke unpleasant cognitions in the child ("My daddy doesn't love me," "He won't let me work with him again") or physiological responses (stomach tightness, rapid breathing, a slight feeling of nausea, or any of a number of possible physical sensations that we might label "anxiety").

Perhaps the real value of taking a complete case history, of developing rapport within a positve relationship, and in carefully evaluating the verbal and nonverbal communications that a client emits is in understanding the way that a client labels those events that may come to control his behavior.

In collecting information regarding antecedents and consequences, the BCA will wish to rely heavily on the client's self-report in the interview situation (Chapter 3), perhaps on observational data collected by the client himself (Chapter 6), as well as on information collected by the BCA, trained observers (Chapter 7), or indigenous others who have occasion to observe the client on a regular basis. In addition, if it becomes relevant to assess the client's physiological responses to stimuli in the natural setting, the methods and procedures outlined in Chapter 11 should be of use to the BCA and add a dimension of assessment to the self-report and observational data already obtained.

Modeling Influences

While behavior may be influenced by the consequences the client receives from his environment, many investigators have shown that a wide variety of behaviors may be instigated or eliminated via persons who serve as models within the client's environment (Bandura, 1976; Bandura and Walters, 1963; Kanfer and Phillips, 1970). A number of terms, such as "social facilitation," "copying," and "imitation," have been used to describe this process; we will employ the term "modeling" to describe those novel behaviors that are initially learned or those repertoire behaviors that are either increased or decreased in frequency by exposing a client (observer) to some person (model) within his environment. Research has shown that an observer must actively and discriminately attend to the model for behavior change to occur. A variety of observer as well as model characteristics (such as age, intelligence, level of status, level of power, etc.) may affect the probability that the observer will actively attend and thus imitate some model. In addition, while it is not necessary to provide reinforcement to either the model or the observer for the modeling effect to occur, such reinforcement often elicits active attention to the model and thus increases the probability of modeling. Bandura and Walters (1963) and Bandura (1969) describe three major categories of modeling effects. It may be important for the BCA to keep each of these in mind in defining persons in the client's environment who might serve as models in instigating appropriate and desirable behavior.

First, *observational learning* accounts for the learning of novel or nonrepertoire behavior via exposure to a model. Children presumably learn to communicate with others via the presence of parental models who use certain words and language, often reinforcing their children for appropriate imitation. Peers may also serve as important models of language and social-skill behaviors. In fact, most of what we learn is certainly acquired via the process of modeling and not by a trial-and-error or successive approximation process (wouldn't this be an inefficient and costly way to learn?).

Second, *inhibitory and disinhibitory* effects have to do with increasing or decreasing the frequency of certain previously learned behaviors via association with punishment. As an example of inhibitory effects, an observer's behavior may be reduced in frequency following his exposure to a model who is punished for engaging in the same behavior. For example, a child who was previously unafraid of the water may avoid even stepping into the surf (inhibition) following exposure to a parent who displays fear and discomfort while at the water's edge. Here the parent has inhibited the child's behavior via modeling, as the child has never directly experienced any punitive effects associated with water activities. Similarly, a child who has previously learned to "fear" the water, perhaps due to a previous experience involving ingestion of water (or exposure to an inhibiting model), might approach the water and begin to play at the water's edge on exposure to a similarly-aged model who fearlessly and happily swims and generally enjoys the waterfront area (a disinhibition effect). In this case, the child has been disinhibited by a model who shows fearless approach behavior in the situation. The notion of disinhibitory effects has been employed quite successfully in the therapeutic situation, where the fearful client is exposed to models who approach the feared stimulus in a fearless or gradually coping fashion (Bandura, Blanchard and Ritter, 1969; Meichenbaum, 1975).

Third, a category of *social facilitation effects* applies to the increase in frequency of repertoire behavior not previously associated with punishment. For instance, a group of strangers standing on a street corner look up in response to an individual who is gazing up at some unseen point. All the strangers have been socially facilitated by this model. That is, the model's behavior facilitated or increased the frequency of the repertoire behavior of looking up. Another example might be the smoker who immediately lights up a cigarette on observing some similar person (model) lighting up in person or in a movie. Models presented via film or videotape have been called "symbolic models" (Bandura and Walters, 1963) and seem to evoke behavioral change in a manner similar to that of live models.

The BCA should carefully evaluate the behavior of persons present in the client's life situation to determine whether or not an inhibitory or disinhibitory effect or social facilitation is in any way responsible for the incidence or lack of incidence of some potential target. In addition, the BCA should carefully evaluate persons who might serve as models for instigating nonrepertoire, novel behavior desired by the client. Such models might be family members or peers in the natural setting. Or other clients or staff in institutional settings who already display appropriate behaviors could be made available to the client to increase the probability that desirable modeling effects would occur. In discussing the role of models in an institutional setting, I have stated (Nay, 1976):

> Within the institutional setting the BCA must carefully evaluate potential models of influence to the client. While such models may well display behaviors in opposition to treatment goals, they may be trained to model behaviors that promote desired behavioral change. Models might be other clients. For example, it would make little sense to provide praise and other positive reinforcement for reduced comsumption of food for an obese client if the client is permitted to eat in the presence of other clients who typically consume great quantities of food. Perhaps until the client alters his eating habits within a setting where such facilitating models are not present, exposure to this group of "energetic" eaters should not be permitted.
>
> It is interesting to consider that many institutions segregate clients with certain problem behaviors because of convenience to staff members providing supervision and care. Thus, a group of hyperactive, retarded children might be separated from the ordinary classroom setting because of their disruptive influence and placed together in another class setting. Or a group of very aggressive delinquents might be segregated from more appropriate peer models because of their disruptive and destructive impact upon less aggressive members of a living cottage. In ordinary academic programs students exhibiting behavior-management problems are often separated from other class members within "special" classes. While this may be justifiable on many grounds (e.g., makes behavioral control easier, allows for specialized training, reduces disruptive effects of the clients upon others) such procedures certainly limit client exposure to appropriate models. In fact such homogeneous groupings increase the likelihood that inappropriate behaviors will be modeled and supported by other clients exhibiting similar behaviors. Such segregation drastically limits the array of social and other behaviors that each member may be exposed to. Regardless of the treatment applied to such a homogeny of "problem" clients, the BCA is necessarily working against the negative effects of the grouping.
>
> There is little data to suggest how particular problem behavior clients might optimally be grouped for most effective treatment. It does seem likely, however, that more heterogeneous groupings increase the array of models exhibiting appropriate behaviors as well as providing more appropriate groups of potentially reinforcing agents. The BCA may very well be faced with constructing a change program for such homogeneously grouped clients, or may be obligated to segregate certain clients for the protection of other clients as well as staff. The problems of negative models and inappropriate peer agents of reinforcement just discussed should be weighed against the gains inherent in such homogeneous groupings (pp. 33–34).

Historical Information

While the primary focus for clinical assessment is on the client's current behavior as it is instigated and maintained in the natural environment, many writers have suggested that contemporary behavior may best be viewed in the context of the client's past behavior and developmental history. Although the collection of a comprehensive case history detailing the client's behavior in his environment at each developmental level is of primary importance in therapeutic orientations focusing exclusively on the role of early events in the shaping of one's "personality," most BCAs would not compile such a comprehensive history, while others might not collect any historical information at all. Regardless of one's theoretical orientation, it is obvious that a client's previous experiences may have much to do with the nature and characteristics of his current behavior via learning processes, and the study of these past events may provide information with important implications for the client's present and future functioning. In reviewing a variety of oft-employed predictors of a person's future behavior (e.g., structured and unstructured psychological tests, the interview, behavioral observations), Mischel (1968) points out that an evaluation of "demographic indices" of a person's past behavior and social competence may be a better predictor of the individual's future responses than the "best test-based personality statements or clinical judgments" (p. 135). Thus, the individual's previous occupational pursuits, marital history, educational attainment, and socioeconomic status are among indicators of social competence and adaptability that may yield excellent predictions of that individual's future behavior. Gough, Wenk, and Rozynko (1965), for example, found that the summary of parolees' past behavior (including occurrence of prior commitment and frequency of previous delinquencies, type of offense, age at first admission), called the "base expectancy," was a better predictor of parole violations than such traditional personality measures as the Minnesota Multiphasic Personality Inventory and the California Psychological Inventory. Along similar lines, both previous institutional adjustment and pre-institutionalization patterns of behavior have been found to be the best predictors of future behavior on the part of psychiatric residents (e.g., Fairweather et al., 1969; Lasky et al., 1959; Lorei, 1967; Zigler and Phillips, 1961), and previous academic performance has proved the best predictor of future academic grades (e.g., Kelly, 1966).

Mischel (1968) points out that it is most important to consider the relative cost of obtaining various categories of assessment information; when this is done, an assessment of past history is usually much more economical than batteries of tests or professional interviewing time. He notes that predictions should be most accurate when the past situations that are sampled are *most similar* to the specific future situations toward which predictions are aimed. Thus, future job success would be predicted best by past job performance, future motivation to attend therapy sessions and carry out agreed-upon behavior-change methods would be best predicted by past attempts at engaging in therapeutic change, and so forth. This latter point of Mischel's is perhaps best exemplified by the selective way in which many writers suggest the case history be employed. For example, Morganstern (1976) points out that a behavioral assessment "rarely" includes a complete life history since the past is considered relevant "only to the extent that it affects the present" (p. 72). He indicates that "background information must have some relevance to either the client's present behavior or the treatment intervention being planned, to warrant much time and exploration or to ethically justify the clinician's interest" (pp. 72–73). Unfortunately, it is often difficult for the assessor to decide during the initial assessment precisely which categories of behavior may prove to be most relevant to meeting the client's ultimate goals. Some standard, yet abbreviated screening of major categories of past life events is recommended by many writers (e.g., Kanfer and Saslow, 1969; Lazarus, 1971; Wolpe, 1973) to ensure a comprehensive context within which to view the client's current behavior. Chapter 4 will illustrate a variety of formats for assessing major categories of life history information, some of which do not involve interview time (e.g., Lazarus, 1971).

Client Resources

While the previous informational categories are frequently a part of a thorough "workup," "intake," or "behavioral assessment," few writers pay systematic attention to evaluating the resources that the client brings to the therapeutic situation. "Resources" is defined here rather broadly to include both external (to the client) phenomena in the client's life environment and personal strengths that might be capitalized on within a treatment plan, or personal deficits or handicaps that limit treatment possibilities in some fashion, or both. An assessment of resources permits the BCA to develop a realistic intervention plan that is practically suited to the everyday demands the environment places on the client. Specific categories of resources that might be evaluated include the following.

Cognitive-Intellectual Abilities and Deficits

Both the goals and methods of therapeutic change must be geared to the client's level of intellectual functioning. The reader familiar with popular individual tests of intelligence (the Wechsler Adult Intelligence Scale, Wechsler, 1958; the Stanford-Binet, Terman and Merrill, 1960) will recall that an intelligence score is the product of a variety of specific assessments of both verbal (e.g., vocabulary, information, social comprehension) and motor performance (e.g., motor speed, psychomotor coordination) abilities. A treatment plan that expects or demands client behavior well beyond these repertoire abilities will certainly fail; hence an individualized assessment of intelligence is frequently employed as a part of an assessment "battery" with clients.[1]

Often, instead of employing a structured examination, intellectual functioning is assessed "clinically," typically by evaluating a client's vocabulary level and fund of information in terms of intelligence test norms. While reducing the cost of such an assessment, clinical judgments may be confounded by the subcultural experiences to which the client has been exposed (e.g., the client may not have mastered certain words due to limited learning or modeling experiences in his current living situation), and do not take into account performance abilities that are a major part of a formal assessment of intellectual functioning. In any event, the relevance of an intellectual assessment obviously depends on the skills and abilities required by a potential intervention plan.

Physical Abilities and Handicaps

Along with considering intellectual functioning, a program of intervention must take into account the client's physical condition as well as basic physical abilities and any deficits or handicaps. When a plan of intervention specifically requires the use of certain motor behaviors (e.g., walking, coordinated finger movements), the BCA must be certain that the client's physical development will permit the desired response, and that no disease process or physical insult inhibits or precludes the performance of this behavior.

Social Skills and Social-Skills Deficits

Frequently the instigation or enhancement of social skills necessary to initiate and maintain social relationships are themselves the targets of intervention (Goldstein, 1973; McFall and Lillesand, 1971; Sarason and Ganzer, 1973). It may also be important to obtain a rough assessment of the client's social functioning when other classes of behavior are targets. Because most persons function within some kind of social system (e.g., family, occupation, schoolroom, ward), an evaluation of a person's social skills permits the BCA to ensure that a treatment plan does not call for social behaviors not in the client's repertoire. In addition, the client who is socially adept may in fact be able to call on the persons around him for support in carrying out a program of intervention.

Many investigators have developed assessment as well as therapeutic intervention programs relating to social-skills behavior beyond what the assessor may be able to observe within the limits of an interview (Chapters 3 and 4). Chapter 7 provides a series of methods that may be useful for behaviorally observing a client's skills in the natural setting or in analogue situations created in the clinical environment (specifically discussed in Chapter 8).

Person Support

It is useful to identify persons available and ordinarily present in the client's environment who may have some impact on the goals and processes of intervention. The client's spouse, children, relatives, or a friend might be helpful in assisting the client to carry out a program of intervention, in collecting data as a means of assessment, in providing consequences within a behavior-change program, or in modeling some targeted behavior whose frequency the BCA wishes to increase. On the other hand, some persons in the environment may interfere with the goals of intervention by modeling inappropriate behavior or providing little support or even discouragement for the client. In addition, certain persons may actively provide positive consequences for the client's inappropriate behavior, contrary to the goals of intervention. Thus, persons in the environment should be evaluated in terms of what they might potentially offer in carrying out a program of intervention, as well as the manner in which they might detract from a client's goals. Similarly, in an institutional setting the BCA should evaluate staff members who work directly with the client to determine those persons who might optimally be trained as direct agents of treatment or serve in support roles as intervention is carried out.

Physical Surroundings

It has already been pointed out that assessment of "controlling stimuli" or other aspects of the environment that may facilitate or inhibit a client's behavioral goals is most desirable. The BCA would do well to assess the manner in which the client's home or living setting supports or detracts from potential treatment goals (e.g., it may be very difficult for a parent to reduce quarreling among siblings if the children do not have adequate bedroom or play space). Ideally, the BCA traverses the natural environment and evaluates the client's physical surroundings. Often, desirable behavioral change can come about merely by changing some aspect of the physical environment that restricts the client's movement, access to objects or persons, or in some other way detracts from the client's behavioral goals. This strategy is certainly an economical way to effect behavioral change whenever it is possible. Unfortunately, many BCAs ignore the client's living environment and de-emphasize the potential controls the environment might exert on behavior in their exclusive focus on client verbal behavior in the clinical setting. Obviously if the client's verbal report suggests the possibility of controlling stimuli or functional relations between some targeted behavior and a specific location in the environment, it becomes increasingly important for the BCA to directly assess that setting.

Financial Resources

While not directly germane to many goals and methods of intervention, a client's ability to pay for things may have an important bearing on the options available to him. Restricted finances often impose a complex array of hardships on a client. These may create a good deal of discomfort and interfere with the time a client has and his motivation for changing his behavior. A client may need to obtain a second job, which may remove the client from the home and thus reduce interactions with other family members during waking hours. Finances may limit the client's avenues of transportation to employment or other opportunities, and may even impede the seeking out of medical or psychological services. Many agencies, for example, require clients to pay for intervention services, and limited financial resources may restrict a client's options in obtaining such services. While many BCAs are uncomfortable when inquiring about financial resources, it is certainly advisable to probe this category when one has reason to believe that a client's finances restrict certain life options or when monetary resources or the services they buy (e.g., transportation, day-care services, medical services) may be necessary for achieving a client's intervention goals.

Assessment of these and other categories of client resources, particularly those specifically relevant to a client's goals and/or the proposed methods of intervention, should be undertaken in the first meetings between client and BCA. Resources can frequently be assessed via the behavioral observation of the client, particularly when interviews or other meetings take place in the client's natural environment and form a context—a comprehensive picture of the client and his possibilities for behavioral change. By being alert to each of these categories during initial interviews, the BCA is in an excellent position to construct, with the client's help, a program of intervention that capitalizes on the client's resources and takes into account any limitations imposed by one or more of the above categories. This ensures a treatment program specifically tailored to the client, which would seem to enhance the probability of desirable behavioral change.

Client Motivation

If each of the previously described categories of information is adequately assessed, the BCA is likely to avoid an inadequate or limited definition of the problem (e.g., Lazarus, 1976; Morganstern, 1976). It is also important to ascertain the relative significance *for the client* of each of the stated goals, as well as the client's motivation to exert sufficient effort to bring about changes in his own behavior, the environment, or both.

While the BCA may wish to assess categories of incentives that might be employed as a part of a treatment program, some determination of the client's preintervention motivation should be undertaken. The best treatment plan may not be successful if the client is not sufficiently motivated to assume responsibility for certain aspects of the program (e.g., record keeping; practice or homework assignments, etc.). This initial motivation might be assessed by evaluating the client's self-statements regarding his rationale for seeking services and adopting certain goals (Chapter 3), as well as his past efforts (past attempts) at behavior change (Chapter 4). Keeping appointments at assigned times (presuming that a mutually satisfactory time is worked out in advance for meetings between BCA and client), carrying out "homework" assignments, as well as the degree of investment the client shows in discussing and defining goals and in the delineation and carrying out of initial client responsibilities within the therapeutic contract, are among categories of evidence that might be evaluated by the assessor as indicants of motivation. Obviously, examining any one criterion in isolation may be misleading and may lead the BCA to adopt unrealistically high or low expectations regarding client motivation. The BCA should be very sensitive to questions and concerns raised by the client regarding goals or methods—particularly any reservations the client may express in agreeing to perform some task or to participate in an intervention strategy. The "failure" of many well-designed intervention strategies is often blamed on client "resistance," but may be due to inadequate evaluation of client motivation in the light of potential intervention goals and the corresponding ordering of these goals. While a variety of strategies may be employed to enhance and maintain client motivation to change some aspect of his behavior-in-situation, it is the BCA's ethical responsibility to ensure that the goals and methods chosen are in fact acceptable to the client and represent the client's best interest to the greatest possible extent (Morganstern, 1976; Nay, 1976). The ethical and legal issues suggested by the selection of goals and methods have been discussed at length elsewhere (Craighead, Kazdin and Mahoney, 1976; Martin, 1975; Nay, 1976).

The following is an outline that should assist the BCA in formulating assessment questions across each of the categories of information presented in this chapter. This outline might be used as a reference in employing the methods described in Chapters 3–11; that is, as a guide to what information should be collected.

I. **Description of Target**
    A. *Client's Self-Statement of Problem/Concern*
        1. *Client attribution(s).* To what persons or life events does the client attribute the targeted behavior (e.g., self, specific others, forces beyond control, job)?

B. *Referents of Target*
  1. *Overt.* Does the target involve motor or verbal behavior that an *independent observer could detect?* Describe in detail.
  2. *Covert.*
      a. Is there a cognitive-imaginal event that occurs as part of the target or as the target proper? Describe content in detail.
      b. Is there a physical sensation (e.g., muscle tension, fatigue, pain) that occurs as part of the target or as the target proper?
          (1) Define body locus (e.g., chest, stomach).
          (2) Define nature of sensation along dimensions such as temperature (hot vs. cold), pain (sharp vs. dull intensity), muscle tone (tight vs. loose), mobility (fixed vs. varied locus), others.
      c. *Current frequency.* Over the past 3–4 weeks, what is the approximate frequency/day or frequency/hour (with very high-rate events)?
          (1) What is client-stated ideal frequency for the target?
      d. *Current duration.* Over the past 3–4 weeks, what is approximate duration of each instance of the target?
          (1) What is ideal duration (if relevant)?
      e. *Current intensity.* How would client rate intensity of the event along some dimension of relevance (e.g., degree of anxiety)?
          (1) What is ideal intensity?

II. **Conditions of Occurrence**
  A. *Location(s).* Describe specific locations where the target occurs at its highest rate.
      1. At which locations does the behavior occur at its lowest rate?
  B. *Activities.* Describe activities engaged in when the target occurs at its highest rate.
      1. For which activities does the behavior occur at its lowest rate?
  C. *Time.* Does the occurrence of the target seem to be related to specific times or time blocks (e.g., morning vs. afternoon)?
      1. Describe *high-rate* times. What activities does the client engage in during these times?
      2. Describe *low-rate* times. What activities does the client engage in during these times?
  D. *Antecedents to Target.* What events, persons, or other phenomena reliably (consistently) occur immediately proir to the target or seem to elicit target?
      1. Review locations, activities, and times to focus client's (and assessor's) attention on possible *environmental antecedents*.
      2. Define *covert events* (e.g., thoughts, images, physical sensations) that are antecedent to the target.
  E. *Consequences for Target.* How do persons within the client's environ-

ment respond to occurrences of the target? How does the client respond?

1. Define *environmental consequences.*
   a. Positive consequences (material or social feedback; i.e., attention).
   b. Negative consequences (loss of valued material items, loss of valued social support, verbal or physical punishment).
2. Define *self-mediated consequences.*
   a. Pleasant or positive thoughts or imagery, pleasant physical sensations or relief from aversive sensations (e.g., reduction in anxiety).
   b. Unpleasant or negative thoughts or imagery, unpleasant physical sensations.
   c. Self-determined material or activity consequences; positive or negative (e.g., client rewards himself with "time off," a restaurant meal; client restricts himself from a desired activity).

(*Note:* It is most important to define the relative strength of each consequence noted in terms of its impact on the client's behavior. These consequences may also be usefully employed to increase desirable behavior and/or decrease undesirable behavior.)

III. **Historical Information**
   A. Use case history format (presented in Chapter 4) to obtain *general* case history information, if relevant to presenting problem and assessor's orientation.
   B. Trace the *history of the target* from the client's earliest recollection of its occurrence (or nonoccurrence, if relevant). Define:
      1. Specific events, persons, or other stimuli associated with the earliest occurrence of the target (e.g., "can you recall anything that seemed to bring on the ...?").
      2. Frequency and characteristics of the target over time.
         a. Try to relate increases or decreases in frequency to life events or client attempts at handling the target.
      3. Client's previous attempts at changing the frequency of the target (e.g., "When Billy first wet his bed, how did you handle it? What did you do?").
         a. Success of previous change attempts.

      (*Note:* This may provide clues to the client's expectations and skills as well as strategies that might be tried in the client's contemporary environment.)
   C. Combine II-A and II-B so that comprehensive life history information is integrated with obtaining a history of the target. Thus, following client description of a life history category (e.g., grammar school education), inquire as to any occurrence of the target during this period as suggested in II-B.

IV. **Client Resources.** Via questioning in the interview as well as observations of the client, attempt to define resources in the client's environment as well as the client's abilities and skills that should be considered in planning treatment. Specific categories to evaluate might include:

A. *Cognitive-Intellectual Abilities and Deficits.*

B. *Physical Abilities and Handicaps.*

C. *Social Skills and Social-Skills Deficits.*

D. *Person Support.* Persons (e.g., spouse, children, relatives, friends) that might be usefully employed in intervention (e.g., as record keepers, appropriate models, consequators); persons whose availability to the client might interfere with the goals of intervention (e.g., inappropriate models, spouse hostile to the client's seeking intervention, relatives who provide positive consequences for inappropriate behavior).

　　1. In institutional settings the assessor should evaluate *staff members* in a similar fashion.

E. *Physical Surroundings.* Does the client's home or living setting in any way support or detract from potential treatment goals (e.g., it may be very difficult for a parent to reduce quarreling among siblings if the children do not have adequate bedroom and play space)? (*Note:* A home visit is most useful to obtain valid assessment of living conditions.)

F. *Financial Resources.* Does client's current financial status permit the client to pay for intervention services (many agencies require this)? Do finances detract from potential intervention goals (e.g., restrict client transportation, require client to work, promote client concerns)?

G. *Task and Vocational Skills.* Does client possess skills to seek and maintain desired employment? Define strengths and deficits.

　　1. *Academic skills.* Does school-aged client display skills necessary for desired academic achievement? Define strengths and deficits.

H. Other resources of specific relevance to potential intervention goals.

V. **Client Motivation.** Do client self-statements, past attempts at behavior change, keeping of appointments, carrying out homework assignments (e.g., to self-monitor a behavior), and client activity and nonverbal behavior in the interview suggest that the client is sufficiently motivated to carry out some proposed treatment strategy? If not, this should be discussed with the client prior to undertaking intervention.

Footnote

[1]It should be noted that subtest and total scores on these structured tests have been shown to depend on the respondent's learning history and can often be im-

proved by further learning experiences. One or more of these "abilities" may in fact be chosen as a target for change in some instances, with a treatment plan devised that provides for a gradual and systematic mastery of the skill.

UNIT II
The Methods of a Comprehensive Clinical Assessment
UNIT II-A The Interview

SELF-REPORT WITHIN THE INTERVIEW:
Defining the Problem

The statements a person makes about himself or his life situation constitute a major source of information within assessment. However, the manner in which self-statements are assessed in interview formats, as well as the manner in which such data are employed in treatment and/or research, has varied considerably. While many BCAs have viewed the interview as the primary medium for understanding the client (e.g., Carkhuff, 1969a, 1969b; Rogers, 1951), multimethod assessment employs the self-report as one of a series of sources of information that, taken together, describe an individual's functioning. In fact, the self-report often constitutes the first category of information available to the BCA and frequently directs further assessment efforts.

Major Categories of the Interview

Cannell and Kahn (1968) have defined two major categories of interviewing: the therapeutic interview and the research interview. "Therapeutic" suggests that the interview has been initiated by the respondent (or client), and that the respondent is motivated to "obtain relief" from certain life problems. They emphasize that the therapeutic interview is traditionally considered a source of information as well as "a direct and powerful source of help" (p. 526). They conclude: "Therapeutic interviewing is thus a highly specialized form of information and interpersonal transaction, and it has become the subject of an equally specialized literature" (p. 526). In contrast, the research interview is defined as a two-person conversation, "initiated by the interviewer for the specific purpose of obtaining research-relevant information, and focused by him on contents specified by research objectives of systematic description, prediction, or explanation" (p. 527). Here the interviewer's role is markedly different from the respondent's in that the interviewer not only initiates the conversation, but structures the respondent's interactions around topics defined by specific questions. While the therapeutic interview is guided by information and ongoing behavior presented by the client, the research interview is often predicted by a predetermined series of topic goals determined by the interviewer *prior to* any interchange.

As might be imagined, the importance of building rapport within a positive relationship is much less important in the research interview, given the abbreviated occasions of interaction between interviewer and respondent. In contrast, regardless of one's theoretical orientation or methods, the therapeutic interview, with its focus on very personal information, is limited by the degree to which the client will trust the BCA and actively participate in the assessment and/or therapeutic transactions. Obviously, a poorly or clumsily handled interview, which in some way fails to meet the client's expectations or needs, may result in client resistance or outright termination. While this chapter will focus on the therapeutic interview, many of the methods and issues to be discussed are applicable to the researcher as well.

There are many different kinds of interviews that fall within the "therapeutic" designation suggested by Cannell and Kahn. One could arbitrarily discriminate between interviews where the collection of information prior to treatment planning is a major goal and those where intervention strategies are mutually agreed on, carried out, or monitored in some fashion. While conceptually neat, this differentiation between "assessment" and "intervention" assumes a dichotomy that may be illusory. In fact, even though the first interviews between BCA and client will logically focus on an initial statement of the problem and definition of intervention goals, desirable behavioral change may occur merely as a function of these initial transactions. For example, the client's behavior may be a function of (reaction to) the interactions that take place *in* the interview (called "reactivity") as well as of a host of nonspecific variables (e.g., placebo effects, expectancies or demands for behavior change provided by the interviewer). While this chapter will focus on the interview situation where *assessment* of the client is of major interest, the potential for reactivity effects as a function of the interview should be kept in mind. Later chapters dealing with observational assessment methods will focus on reactivity as well as certain nonspecific factors in more detail.

It may first be useful to define specific interview formats in terms of the goals of data collection. The *intake-orientation interview* provides the BCA with an initial statement of the problem as well as the first opportunity to observe and get to know the client. In succeeding interviews the client is encouraged to *focus* his problems and concerns in clear and explicit language in terms of behavioral referents that both client and BCA can understand. Client problems, of course, do not occur in a vacuum, and it is often useful to obtain information about the development of the client as well as the problem behavior over time. The *case history interview* permits the interviewer to obtain a detailed chronology of the client's life history, with special emphasis on a developmental history of problems and concerns defined in the intake and focusing process. Following the collection of this information and its integration with information gathered by other methods, a final interview might best be described as the *pinpointing interview*. In pinpointing, the BCA reviews the information already obtained with the client and may attach certain interpretations to the findings. This presentation becomes elaborated into a mutual discussion and categorization of potential goals for behavior change, resulting in a series of priorities explicitly and clearly stated (often in the form of a verbal or written contract). This definition of specific goals is important in that it determines the criteria by which the client as well as the change agent can evaluate the success of intervention. The assessment of historical-developmental information in the case history interview will be presented in Chapter 4. The presentation and discussion of the pinpointing interview will be postponed until Chapter 12, which presents guidelines and a rationale for integrating and summarizing data collected across self-report, observational, physiological, and other assessment methods for each of the categories of information discussed in Chapter 2.

The topics that follow are organized sequentially from the issues and methodological options that the BCA might be faced with on first meeting the client to those occurring further along in the interview process. In addition, information the BCA should obtain in these first interviews, both in terms of content and categories of observational data, will be discussed. This presentation will draw on a variety of therapeutic orientations, as the methods and issues relevant to the competently handled interview are quite similar, regardless of the BCA's orientation.

Intake-Orientation: Getting to Know the Client

As a frame of reference for the material that follows, the reader should attempt to recall what it's like to meet another person. For many, the situation is a bit awkward and leads to some degree of anxiety and discomfort as two persons begin to share information about one another and establish some measure of rapport. The BCA's initial meeting with the client may be thought of similarly. The task becomes: How can BCA and client establish rapport so that both feel comfortable in speaking freely? The following is a summary of suggestions made by various writers.

The Introduction

Clients come to be referred to the BCA in a variety of ways, and the mode of this assignment may well predict the degree of care needed in introducing the client to the assessment setting. In some cases, the client will be fully familiar with the methods and procedures of the referral agency (e.g., an inpatient client referred for a psychological workup), and may even be familiar with the BCA. In most cases, however, the client is unfamiliar with both the agency and BCA to whom he is assigned, and this unfamiliarity may instigate some questions in the client's mind that should be clarified before proceeding. In addition, the client may have some expectations about what the assessment or therapeutic process is to be like or about the BCA or agency in particular. To the extent that these expectations are faulty, they may interfere with the process of establishing rapport and collecting information. Wallen (1956) has attempted to categorize the kinds of expectations a client might have for a BCA and some of the problems these may cause. First, the BCA may be viewed as a "threat." The client may view a decision to seek psychological services as an admission of weakness, and only seek such services because of certain negative consequences of his behavior which seem beyond his control.

If a person is proud of independence and detachment from others, he is likely to steer clear of professional helpers. But the imminent loss of his job or the breakup of his marriage may motivate him sufficiently to visit a [BCA]. After arriving, however, he may be defensive because he feels he has given up some control over his own life. . . . Attitudes of this kind are quite likely to occur in men who have achieved high status and have authority over others [p. 95].

Another view of the BCA as a "threat" relates to persons who are coerced into seeking services by certain external forces (e.g., the courts, parents or important others), and this may result in some level of defensiveness or poor cooperation. As Farber (1941) points out:

. . . if an investigator is a staff [BCA] he is often seen by the inmates as the dreaded "bug doctor" who might, by an interview or test, find a man insane or feebleminded and commit him to a stigmatized institution. The fear and apprehension engendered in the inmate by a summons from the "bug doctor" will profoundly influence the experimental or interview situation. Finally, it must be kept in mind that in any situation where an inmate is faced by an official who has it in his power, or is thought to have it in his power, to help or hurt that inmate, then the inmate will be on his best behavior, his responses shaped and colored by his desire to make a favorable impression [p. 298].

Second, the client may attribute certain supernatural powers to the BCA and view him as a "miracle worker"—the assumption being that long-term patterns of behavior can be rapidly changed by intercession on this "super-human's" part. This attitude obviously predicts the degree to which the client will view himself as responsible for his own behavior. Perhaps the emphasis in the popular media on brief and miraculous cures, often resulting from "truth serum," or episodes of catharsis or "insight" is responsible for this expectation.

Some people overvalue psychological help; they assume that the [BCA] can change them by some subtle means so that they will be successful, happy, or lovable. This attitude is often not openly expressed in the first contact of clinician and client, but therapists find evidence of it in comments made during therapy [Wallen, 1956, p. 96].

Wallen also points out that this attitude can frequently be seen as a pattern of turning to others for help, justification, or protection.

People who regard the [BCA] as a miracle worker easily come to see him as a threat. Indeed, the great power which must be attributed to him if he is to perform wonders is in itself threatening. The possession of unusual abilities is no guarantee that they will be used to help instead of hurt; this guarantee must come from the client's faith in the kindness and good intentions of the clinician. Consequently, clients who endow clinicians with magical powers must also reassure themselves of his kindness. They will be alert to signs that he likes them and will be oversensitive to any indications of the clinician's possible insincerity or lack of sympathy. Unrealistic vigilance of this kind can easily lead them to misinterpret the clinician's speech and behavior [p. 97].

Third, Wallen indicates that the BCA may be viewed as an "intercessor," as a sort of accomplice of the client in manipulating some aspect of his life environment or the persons therein.

Sometimes people seek [behavior change] services in order to manipulate a specific person in their environment. In these instances, the [BCA] is seen as an authority whose pronouncements can change opinions that the client has been unable to alter. For example, a young man wishing to dissuade his parents from sending him to medical school may request vocational guidance. Actually he is not interested in guidance; he hopes that the [BCA's] findings will alter his parents' attitude. He may want copies of the test score sent to his parents or may ask the [BCA] to see them personally after the test is finished. Under these conditions, the vocational counselor will probably doubt the validity of the test scores. The client's special interest in the outcome introduces an unknown amount of distortion into the results [p. 97].

Further, the BCA may be employed as a pawn in certain legal proceedings, such as the altercations between spouses prior to divorce; as a means of justifying settlements involving children or property; or as a means for the client to avoid certain responsibilities in his life situation. Obviously, this phenomenon can severely bias the information the client is willing to reveal. In response to this third category of expectation, Wallen suggests:

When the relationship is largely for diagnostic purposes or when it is confined to a single interview, the [BCA] needs a clear conception of his role in the ways in which he can give help. In general, it is wise to follow the rule that the [BCA] is a consultant, and that the client must assume responsibility for his own actions. This principle does not prevent the [BCA] from reporting his findings to other specialists of concern, nor from preparing special reports setting forth his judgments about the client [p. 98].

In order to provide the client with information that may dispel certain unrealistic expectations of either the setting or the change agent, the BCA would do well to begin with a statement introducing himself and then the agency. A self-introduction should include a brief statement giving the BCA's name, specific role within the agency, and importantly, how the referral to him was made if the client did not refer himself. This might go as follows:

Hello, my name is Robert Jeffers and I'm a (psychologist or counselor etc.) here at the center. My job typically involves helping clients to learn skills that will enable them to obtain employment and that's why you were referred to me. I understand that you are interested in working with people. Maybe in a few minutes we can talk about some of the possibilities for you.

Next, any methods the client ought to be aware of should be presented.

The way (I) usually go about things is to first get to know you and to answer any questions you might have about our agency—then, to find out exactly what brought you here. After we have this information we will know better if we (I) can be of help—and if so, how. So you can expect that the first three or four sessions we have will involve this "getting to know" process and gathering information.

The BCA should be sure to ask the client if he has any questions about the BCA or the agency. If the client's expectations seem inappropriate, the BCA should take whatever time is necessary to define clearly how the agency (or BCA) can and cannot meet the client's goals, and if necessary, refer the client elsewhere. A careful evaluation of expectations prior to the onset of assessment ensures that the client's major questions are answered and that any (revealed) client concerns about the nature of treatment or the agency are dealt with.

Confidentiality

Many BCAs inform the client of procedures for confidentiality *prior to* collecting personal information. This verbal (or written) statement informs the client of the way information collected will be employed by the BCA and agency, persons who will have access to the information, and the agency's general policies regarding the storage of such information. It is most important that procedures for confidentiality be reviewed with a client during this initial period. The client has a right to know how personal data will be used before revealing any information (see Martin, 1975, for an excellent review of court decisions relating to confidentiality). This becomes especially important in agencies that have a dual role of clinical service and teaching and/or research. If client records are to be shared with other members of a treatment team, practicum group, supervisors, other colleagues, or in clinical staffings, all this should be included in the statement of confidentiality provided to the client. The client should also be made aware of his rights to exclude certain information from the formal (written) record-keeping process if and when he decides to do so.

If the BCA plans to audio- or videotape the client's behavior during the interview or if observations are to be performed by other colleagues and/or students via one-way mirrors or concealed microphones, the client must be informed of the precise nature of these activities and should certainly be informed of his right to refuse participation. Failure to obtain consent from the client may constitute ethical as well as legal violation of the client's privacy and certain civil rights. For the protection of all concerned, the BCA and client should specifically agree on how often recording procedures will be employed (perhaps on forms provided by the agency). Particularly when audio- or videotape recordings are made, it is good practice from both an ethical and legal standpoint to obtain verbal consent for each recording session following the first (at which time written consent is given). Even if the BCA's agency does not employ formal consent procedures for audio/video/observing procedures, the BCA might do well to protect himself by having an appropriate consent form typed up and used in the manner suggested. In addition, some other persons (e.g., another staff person, a family member) should witness the client's signature on both of these forms.

Physical Setting of the Interview

Ideally, the BCA will interview the client in a comfortable agency setting or office. Another option is to interview the client in his ordinary life situation (e.g., his home), perhaps as a prelude to a series of behavioral observations, which will be described in the chapters that follow. When the interview does take place in the agency, the BCA must ensure that the setting does not in any way distract the client from the task at hand (e.g., a highly public setting, accessible to other clients and staff members, or noisy, disruptive locations should be avoided) and will make the client as relaxed and comfortable as possible. Houck and Hansen (1972) have made a number of recommendations that the BCA would do well to approximate whenever possible.

We should recognize that the physical setting may have some influence on the patient's precontact attitude. The physical surroundings, indeed, may become extensions of the [BCA] in the patient's eyes. A shabby, uncomfortable office may be occasion for the patient to project these attributes to the [BCA]. The waiting room and office should be kept at a comfortable temperature; carpeting on the floor often helps to quell extraneous sounds. If there is a secretary in the office, she should be unobtrusive but available to the patient, if necessary. . . .

In the [BCA's] office itself, the chairs should be comfortable, and the [client's] chair should be preferably at the side of the [BCA's] desk rather than across from the desk, if room arrangement allows this. It is preferable that nothing be on the desk between the [client] and the interviewer. Such an arrangement will tend to reduce psychological distance as well as geographical distance. This arrangement also allows the individual to look away from the [BCA] if necessary but still permits the [BCA] to observe facial expressions.

No section on physical settings is complete without comments on the presence of the telephone. If it is at all possible, the telephone bell should be dampened or shut off during therapy sessions. . . . Even if time lost through telephone calls is made up at the end of the session, the patient may become annoyed with the interruptions and the therapist's lack of attention [pp. 151–152].

In crowded, noisy ward or cottage environments that did not provide formally designated space for such interviews, I have employed such settings as the client's room or a walk to a comfortable outdoor location *when the client's status and institutional regulations permitted it.* Obviously, clients in correctional or locked-ward settings should never be taken from those environments without the express approval of those directly and legally responsible.

If the foregoing recommendations are followed, the client ought to be aware of the nature of the agency, its methods and goals, and how the process of collecting information prior to treatment planning will proceed. If all goes well, this initial period of introduction may succeed in substantially reducing any anxiety or discomfort that the client (and perhaps the BCA) might experience in the initial encounter. The sections that follow will review major kinds of information the BCA might gather as well as strategies for facilitating data gathering while maintaining and building on the rapport already established. Information gathered would seem to fall into one of two major categories: the specific *content* (verbal report) that the client freely provides or offers in response to the BCA's questions and certain *behavioral observations* the BCA makes regarding the client's characteristics and behavior during the course of the interview. Each of these categories of data is uniquely important, and the BCA will wish to assess carefully the degree of correspondence between data gathered across the two modalities to see where agreements and disagreements exist. This checking-reliability process generates questions for further exploration in later interviews and provides the BCA with a more comprehensive view of the client.

Orientation and Statement of the Problem

Many writers recommend that the BCA begin by obtaining an overview of client-defining characteristics and "orientation" information as a means of getting to know the client. Houck and Hansen (1972) justify such data gathering as a further means of building rapport in a structured format.

The [BCA] should be cognizant of the [client's] emotional status and recognize that he is faced with a human being who, in all likelihood, does not want to be in the interviewing situation. After the [client] is seated and comfortable, we can begin to put him more at ease by requesting routine kinds of information. Such facts as the [client's] full name, his address, telephone number, age, marital status, number of children, place of employment, type of job would be included under this heading. We may do this even though we are in full possession of the information. Then, we go over it by asking the patient to corroborate the information which we have to correct any of it which may be wrong. Such a tactic is neutral, allows the [client] to begin to settle down and at the same time, allows the [BCA] a little more time for observation and assessment. From this point we may lead into the next phase [statement of problem], inasmuch as the flow of conversation has already begun [p. 153].

Sullivan (1954) has called this initial period of orientation the "reconnaissance" in that it permits the BCA to obtain a "rough social sketch of the patient, which is to be brief, and not an extended life history" (p. 73). Sullivan emphasizes that the reconnaissance provides information regarding the relative ease or difficulty with which the client can establish a relationship, his concentration on the procedure, his sensitivity to the other person—in this instance the interviewer—and his "attitudes" described by such terms as reserved, guarded, suspicious, hostile, defensive, or conciliatory. The reconnaissance also provides information regarding the client's attitude toward his own memory—whether he seems to trust it or not, as well as his attitude about "answering questions." Finally information is obtained regarding the client's need for reassurance. A wealth of other gross impressions may result from this orientation period which the interviewer can repeatedly test and evaluate as the interview process proceeds.

Alternatively, orientation data may be obtained via a brief written questionnaire which the client completes prior to the interview. This information could then serve as a foundation for becoming acquainted with the client in the initial interview, with the BCA employing the client's written responses as an entree to conversation (e.g., I see that you work for General Telephone. Could you tell me what you do for them?).

It should be noted at this point that strict adherence to any standardized greeting or orientation should be avoided. The BCA should attempt to tailor his approach to the client based on his evaluation of the client's agenda for the interview. Extensive probing of orientation information or filling out forms may provide a nice transition for the hesitant client while it may be viewed as rather cold and "standoffish" by the client eager to reveal personal information, ask a question, or clarify the nature of the dialogue to come. In a sense, the BCA must carefully follow or "track" with the client's verbal and nonverbal communications for clues as to discomfort, irritation, anxiety, or other signs that may assist in regulating the pace at which the interchange moves from the impersonal to personal level. Many researchers have suggested that this ability to "track" *with* the client is a major predictor of success in the interview (e.g., Carkhuff, 1969a, 1969b; Goldstein, 1975; Truax and Carkhuff, 1967). A later section will describe categories of behavior that the BCA might be sensitive to in this "tracking" process.

Once the client's agenda of questions, concerns, and expectations has been dealt with and the BCA has an initial description of the client, the interview should proceed to a description of the events that brought the client to the BCA. The client's agenda typically involves telling the BCA his own perception of what the problem is, often in language that is rather imprecise or even disorganized. The BCA's agenda should be to clarify the client's statements so that a comprehensive and explicit description of problems or client concerns is obtained. While these two agendas lead to the same end, it may be difficult to satisfy both, particularly in the first or second interview. If the BCA is overly controlling of the client's verbal report, requiring complete and explicit descriptions of each client statement in terms of the *BCA's language*, this systematized effort may occur at the expense of rapport (Morganstern, 1976). Clients who are repeatedly placed "on the spot", who have to categorize, quantify, and seemingly defend every verbal statement made in terms of how, what, where, or why, may become defensive and uncomfortable. Alternatively, the BCA does not want to be in the position of not knowing what the client means by certain global or nonspecific statements as encounters between client and therapist proceed. Giving the client complete control of the process of the interview may not provide sufficiently detailed information for the goals of intervention to be systematically considered. Thus, the BCA has an obligation to the client to fully understand what is said, yet to do so in a manner that meets the client's needs. Goldfried and Davison (1976) summarize this point very nicely in describing guidelines for intake orientation interviews.

Although there are a number of similarities between behaviorally and traditionally oriented interviews, behavior therapists tend to focus more on concrete details as relevant to the client's problem than on current maintaining variables. The reasons for this focus should be obvious when we consider what is involved in conducting a behavioral analysis. What may not be so apparent, however, are the potential negative side effects associated with getting details from clients. One potential problem is that pressing for specifics may interfere with the establishment of rapport. By continually having to use concrete examples to illustrate what he means, the client may get the feeling that he is not understood, either because of his own inability to communicate or the therapist's insensitivity... A second drawback to focusing on details is that it may blind the therapist to other significant problems not yet discussed [pp. 39–40].

Perhaps the best way to proceed is to first encourage the client to provide information to the BCA about his life situation in his own language and at his own pace. The BCA might begin by asking open-ended questions that do not require the client to focus on one or another problem—for example, "Mr. ———, now that we've gotten to know each other a bit, I wonder if you might tell me what brings you here today?" or "I notice here on this intake sheet [a form filled out by the client prior to the interview which asks for a listing of problems] that you're having some difficulties in dealing with your son, Billy. Could you tell me about this, please?" In conducting this initial, open-ended phase of the interview, the BCA must be sure that he actively attends to what the client says, mentally storing pertinent information and questions suggested by the client's statements that may be followed up as the client is gradually asked to focus and be more specific. While I tend to avoid taking notes while a client is speaking, it frequently helps to be able to jot down certain key words or statements so that they can be recalled as a basis for a follow-up later in the interview. The BCA might say to the client: "I want to be sure that I remember things that you tell me, and from time to time, if you don't mind, I'll make a note or two here on this pad." As an alternative, the interview can be audio-recorded.

To facilitate a client's "opening up" about his problems and revealing personal information, the BCA may employ certain communicative strategies that serve to indicate his understanding of and empathy with regard to the client's statements. Many investigators have suggested that the interview process will be enhanced to the extent that the therapist can actively and accurately "tune into" (or empathize with) what the client is communicating both verbally and nonverbally (e.g., Carkhuff, 1969a, 1969b; Truax and Carkhuff, 1967). Along similar lines, Raush and Bordin (1957) emphasize the role of "therapist warmth" in fostering a positive relationship in which therapeutic goals may be attained. They state that therapist warmth has three components. The first is commitment—the therapist's commitment to be of assistance to the client expressed both verbally and nonverbally. These authors emphasize that the commitment of a specified period of time to the client as well as the therapist's skills and efforts in understanding and aiding the client facilitate warmth. Second, they suggest that the therapist's methods may facilitate warmth. The therapist should ask questions that permit the client to tell about himself and how he views his world. In response to the client's personal views, the therapist should indicate his interest and understanding of the client by actively listening and attending, nodding, and showing other verbal and nonverbal signs of interest. Lastly, the therapist's *spontaneity* may communicate warmth. Formalism, stiffness, or lack of spontaneity in responding to the client may communicate rigidity and coldness, while extreme impulsivity (very quick responses, responses that do not permit the client to finish a sentence or interrupt the client, etc.) may on the other hand, communicate a compulsive, unnatural quality on the BCA's part. If the BCA is carefully and accurately tracking with the client, the kind of response called for in a particular situation should be suggested. The BCA is encouraged to act naturally and to respond to the client's communications *not* according to a preprogrammed schedule or preconceived norms, but in terms of the thoughts and feelings elicited by the client's verbal and nonverbal communications which quite naturally become translated into behavior. This is often referred to as the *evocative message* that the therapist feels or experiences in response to a client's statements.

Benjamin (1969) and Ivey (1971) are among writers who have categorized a number of potential responses of the interviewer to the interviewee, ranging from no response or silence to interpretation of the client's statements or nonverbal behavior. *Silence* can communicate many things to the interviewee, depending on its context. Brief silences accompanied by nonverbal gestures that indicate "go on, I'm listening" often permit the interviewee to provide a complete and comprehensive statement of his feelings or concerns without interviewer interruption. Benjamin points out:

> As a deliberate response, silence implies that the interviewer has decided to say nothing, regarding this as the most helpful thing he can offer at this point. He decides not to interfere verbally, but he's there in the interview, and his presence is felt by the interviewee. It is as if the interviewer were saying: "You know I am listening. The best way in which I can be of help right now, I believe, is to keep quiet" [p. 111].

Alternatively, a lack of verbal and/or nonverbal responses to client questions, expressions of intense feelings, or verbal or nonverbal behaviors communicating: "Should I go on; is what I'm saying okay?", might have a devastating impact on rapport in the interview. Certainly, very lengthy silences should have a justifiable purpose. The interviewer should carefully observe how the client reponds to initial brief periods of silence (does it facilitate client responding, cause anxiety or concern?), and adjust the use of silence in later stages of the interview accordingly. In fact, *this process of testing out interviewer responses by evaluating their effects on the interviewee should occur on a continuous basis within the interview,* with such "process" data employed to regulate and adjust, include and exclude response categories.

The category of response most similar to silence might be called the *minimal verbal response* (e.g., "Mm-hm," "Right", "Yes," "I see")—a minimal communication indicating that the interviewer is listening and wishes the interviewee to proceed. Many interviewers who take a "nondirective" therapeutic approach (Rogers, 1952) are often caricatured (wrongly) as employing this category of response to *any* client statement. Obviously, a minimal response permits the interviewee to learn very little about what the interviewer actually *does* understand. As such, it should be employed judiciously. If overused, it may lead to client misinterpretation (e.g., "Am I boring him?", "Maybe I'm not telling him what he wants," etc.).

Among the more active interviewer responses, *restatement* or *summarization* permits the interviewee to learn precisely what the interviewer has listened to and received (Ivey, 1971). Benjamin (1969) suggests that restatement can be accomplished in a number of ways, each with the same rationale: "to serve as an echo, to let the interviewee hear what he has said on the assumption that this may help him, encourage him to go on speaking, examining, looking deeper" (p. 113). At a minimal level, the interviewer may restate part of the communication that seems to be most worth having the interviewee hear again. The following is an example of a partial restatement.

Interviewee: Every night, I don't know why it is, but when we're getting ready for bed my husband and I tend to argue about things . . . silly things, but we argue.
Interviewer: You argue each night.
Interviewee: It all seems so silly, the little things we argue about . . . I mean you'd think we would fight over the big things like money, but no . . .
Interviewer: It's the little things.
Interviewee: Yes, and I just can't understand why we do it . . . I mean . . .

In contrast, a summarization does not attempt to restate the interviewee's exact words or even a part of his verbal communication, but instead integrates the content into a summary statement. This approach is particularly useful when the interviewee offers a number of divergent examples of a very similar phenomenon.

Interviewee: This week has really been something. Every night, literally every night Bill and I argued about something . . . it seemed like one long argument all week. Two nights ago, he came in late for dinner and, I don't know, I just couldn't help myself . . . I mean he does this all the time . . . so I asked him where he was, why he was so late. He just kind of flew off the handle, told me I was always on his back, never let up, the usual thing. I probably shouldn't have said anything else, but I couldn't leave it alone, I kept asking him why it was he was late all the time. He got so mad I thought he was going to hit me. Then last night, he got home on time, but it just didn't seem right . . . so artificial, like he was saying "okay, what are you going to say to me now?" . . . we ended up arguing again.
Interviewer: You argue most nights, even though the reasons are often different.
Interviewee: Yeah, I mean it just doesn't matter . . . we argue over everything.

The next, and more active interviewer response category is that of *reflection*. Benjamin (1969) nicely contrasts the restatement and summarizing responses with reflecting statements.

> To reflect the feelings and attitudes of the interviewee demands deeply empathic listening and understanding. To serve as a mirror in which the interviewee can see his feelings and attitudes reflected requires a facility in recognizing and verbalizing those feelings and attitudes. When restating, the interviewer tells the interviewee what he has said. When reflecting, he verbalizes what the interviewee feels. . . . Reflection consists of bringing to the surface and expressing in words those feelings and attitudes that lie behind the interviewee's words. The interviewer echos feelings not expressed as such by the interviewee but clearly sensed by the interviewer by what the other has said [p. 117].

Thus, reflection indicates that the interviewer has not only actively listened and understood what the interviewee has said, but is also attending to feelings expressed verbally as well as nonverbally by the interviewee. In addition, if the interviewer is accurate in his observation of the client, he may be able to express feelings that have so far been unrecognized, perhaps assisting the interviewee in putting such feelings into words for the first time. An example of reflection follows.

Interviewee: It's been this way since I married Bill . . . his son just won't . . . he won't accept me. It seems like no matter what I do I can't please him. Like last night for example I fixed his favorite dish and he merely sat there at the table looking blankly ahead. He didn't even say thank you. I mean I don't expect him to treat me like his real mother but the least he could do is be civil.

Interviewer: You can't seem to get through to him and it really hurts.

Interviewee: I guess it shouldn't but it really does. I mean, even though he isn't my son, I just want things to work out and I don't understand why they can't. I mean, what does he want from me . . . I can't ever be his real mom, but why won't he just accept me?

Interviewer: You feel kind of frustrated . . . what do I do next?, I mean I've tried almost everything.

A final and most active-directive category of interviewer response involves something more than restating or summarizing the interviewee's verbal content or reflecting his feelings. In this mode, the interviewer integrates previous interviewee responses and makes an *interpretation* of their meaning. The interpretation clearly adds something to the information already provided by the interviewee. It attempts to prompt the interviewee to experience a new perspective of his behavior, to see how another person (the interviewer) might interpret his responses. It is obvious that interpretation moves the interviewer into a much more directive role, and frequent interpretations can certainly alter the interviewee's frame of reference from that of tale-teller to active listener. Benjamin (1969) points out the possible pitfalls of interpretation.

We move slowly but surely from responses to leads. Ws are bringing ourselves on stage. The danger is obvious/that we take over at the expense of the interviewee; that we perform instead of him. We may end up enjoying this role so much we do not realize that we have turned him off; that we have put him in the audience, so to speak; that we have made of the interviewee subject a spectator object [p. 120].

Obviously the nature of an interpretation varies considerably depending on the theoretical orientation of the interviewer. Regardless, an interpretation typically attempts to provide some rationale for the inteviewee's behavior; that is, a statement regarding hypothesized motives or events that have influenced the interviewee's behavior in the interview or in his life situation (see Chapter 2). The interviewee is encouraged to consider the interpretation and evaluate its accuracy. Obviously, the potential pitfalls are numerous and an interpretation should be made only after the interviewer has sufficient data with which to back up his remarks. It should be pointed out that the emphasis on interpretation may vary considerably depending on the degree to which the BCA wishes to provide active direction. In addition, the role of interpretation must vary with the particular client. Many clients are perfectly able to interpret the rationale for certain behaviors they engage in or phenomena they experience (e.g., "I know that I always tend to feel down when I compete with Bob"); however, they may not be able to actively change the way in which they behave. For this category of clients, interpretation becomes less relevant. Alternatively, for the client who tends to have an inadequate understanding of his own behavior, has difficulty discriminating the antecedents and consequences of his acts, and is generally a poor self-observer, interpretation may be an important first step in assisting the client to decide on goals for intervention. The following is an example of an interpretation given to a parent experiencing difficulty in managing his adolescent son's behavior.

Interviewee: Well I don't know what else to say, I've told you all I can . . . I just cannot seem to get his attention. He just doesn't respond to me . . . I ask him to do things and it's the same . . . he just ignores me. We go round and round, and nothing seems to change.

Interviewer: I've been struck by the way you respond to Billy. Sounds like you've been very consistent, in that when you ask him to do something you try to *convince* him that it's the right thing to do, and when he doesn't agree with your explanation, you argue with him and try to convince him even more. It also sounds like that hasn't worked out very well so far. I wonder if you can think of some other possible ways you might respond, given that you're unhappy with how effective you've been so far.

Interviewee: I . . . I think I see what you mean. It's like he knows he can get an argument out of me . . . keep trying to explain.

Interviewer: And what's the end result for Billy, in terms of doing what you've asked him to do?

Interviewee: He ends up getting out of it, and I end up getting frustrated!

Interviewer: So trying to explain and reason each time hasn't worked out very well for you.

Interviewee: It really hasn't. I guess I've never really thought of it that way before, but how else can I respond to him?

(The interview might now proceed to a review of possible alternative approaches the client might make to his son to determine which approach he is most comfortable with.)

As an example of how the BCA might actively listen to the client using a compendium of the response categories just reviewed to enhance rapport, the responses of a low-empathic as well as high-empathic interviewer to the same client will be presented. The reader should note differences in the client's responses to the two interviewers in terms of personal concerns and information revealed. Both of these interviews are reprinted with permission from Goldstein (1973). The material in brackets is added by the present author.

Low Empathy

P: My family. Well, you know sometimes—sometimes I think my family could do—just as well without me. You know—like I'm a useless sort of object that just sort of sits around the house. When I—come home from work it's like—like there's nothing there.

T: I don't understand. [Query]

P: Sometimes it—sometimes it seems that they don't even know when I'm home. Kids'll be running around and—my wife—well sometimes the way she acts it would be better if I just stayed out. Some of the things she gets into—hmm. . . .

T: You mean she gets into a lot of trouble. [Restatement]

P: Yeah. She's always yelling and screaming—wants me to do things when I come inside—always telling me I have this to do and that to do. She dosn't realize I just wanna come home and I wanna relax a bit. Nah—I don't know how she can push me all the time—do this—do that—all the time.

T: You must really cause her a lot of trouble. [Interpretation]

P: Yeah—yeah. It was really different before. When we first got married it was—it was nice. We went out and saw different people, did—did some things together. Got along pretty good, too. Didn't have all this that's going on now.

T: Things might be better now if you hadn't changed. [Interpretation]

P: No—my wife changed. She got—she got different. Things started—you know—she started not to care about things. We couldn't go out as much. Then—then the babies came and then—wow—feeding them and taking care of them and doing all those things. Never had any time to do the things we used to do together. You know, it's usually hard for me to talk about things like this, but it's easy talking to you. Like—you know when I'd come home from work—my wife—she'd be running around the house after the kids—and when I'd come in the door I'd get ignored you know. No one says hello—no one asks you how you are.

T: Seems like your wife has her hands full with the kids without having to worry about you, too. [Interpretation]

P: It seems that way. Before we had the kids we didn't have these problems. Now it—it's just not the same. Now it seems like I'm either ignored or it's nag, nag, nag—all the time.

P: Take my father, for instance. He could down drinks with the best of them. My old lady will tell you that. Yeah, he really knew how to drink. Used to get into some terrible fights with my old lady though. Boy—he'd come home with a little too much in him—she'd really let him have it. I'd have to—pull the pillow over my head so I wouldn't hear the noise. Couldn't get to sleep.

T: Sounds like you're following in your father's footsteps. [Interpretation]

P: Yeah. She really used to get mad at him. You know, for drinking and all that. She used to yell at him. On his back all the time. Really be nasty to him. Maybe that's one of the reasons he's six feet under right now.

T: Your mother used to yell at him [Restatement]—so what's that matter now? [Query]

P: I think my wife's trying to do the same thing to me that my mother did to my father. There's a lot of things about the two that are kind of the same. Yell and fight—the yelling and carrying on. They'll both do it. Scream at you and call you a drunk. Telling me I can't take on any responsibility. [Pause] You know, you really understand what's going on. You seem to know how I feel. But my wife—always yelling about something. Money. Why don't you have more of it? Why can't we buy this? Why can't we buy that? I'm working—as hard as I can—and she does—she doesn't realize that. She thinks all I have to do is work—all the time. She thinks it's—it's easy for me to—to work every day. Always pushing me—I don't like to be pushed. I get—I'll get things done. But I have to work—at my own pace, otherwise—it just doesn't matter if I work or not if I can't work at my own pace.

T: Couldn't you try to speed up a little? [Suggestion based on interpretation]

P: Try her way? Uh—[pause]—she's in her own world. She doesn't care about anything that I do—or say. She doesn't care about me or anyone else. Sometimes I just feel like getting up and leaving. There's nothing there any more.

T: Why don't you just go away—it might help. [Suggestion based on interpretation]

P: Um, hmm.

T: Have you ever done this? [Query]

P: Um, hmm. Used to—get away for a couple of days by myself. But I always ended up coming back because I had no one else to go to.

T: There must be someone you could visit. Everyone has at least one friend [Suggestion based on interpretation] [pp. 389–371].

High Empathy

P: My family. Well, you know sometimes—sometimes I think my family could do—just as well without me. You know. Like I'm a—useless sort of object that sort of sits around the house. When I—come home from work it's like—like there's nothing there.

T: Your family doesn't seem to look forward to your coming home at night. [Restatement] You feel as though they don't really care about you. [Reflection]

P: Sometimes it—sometimes it seems that they don't even know when I'm home. Kids'll be running around and—my wife—well sometimes the way she acts it would be better if I just stayed out. Some of the things that she gets into—hmm . . .

T: She lights into you the minute you step in tired from work. [Summarization] Like she doesn't appreciate you and this hurts you. [Reflection]

P: Yeah—she's always yelling and screaming—wants me to do things when I come inside—always telling me I have to do this and that to do. She doesn't realize I just wanna come home and I wanna relax a little bit. Nah—I don't know how she can push me all the time—do this—do that—all the time.

T: Sounds like marriage has been a lot of trouble for you—worse than before? [Query based on interpretation]

P: Yeah. Yeah—really it—it was different before. When we first got married it was—it was nice. We went out and saw different people, did—did some things together. Got along pretty good, too. Didn't have all this that's going on now.

T: Those days were better [Restatement], but now?

P: Now—my wife changed. She got—she got different. Things started—you know—she started not to care about things. We couldn't go out as much. Then—then the babies came and then—wow—feeding them and taking care of them and doing all those things. Never had any time to do the things we used to do together. You know, it's usually hard for me to talk about things like this, but it's easy talking to you. Like—you know, when I'd come home from work—my wife—she'd be running around the house after the kids—and when I'd come in the door I'd get ignored, you know. No one says hello—no one asks you how you are.

T: You feel that the babies were more important to your wife than you. [Reflection]

P: It—seems that way. Before we had the kids we didn't have these problems. Now it—it's just not the same. Now it seems like I'm either ignored or it's nag, nag, nag—all the time.

P: Take my father for instance. He could down them with the best of them. My old lady will tell you that. Yeah, he really knew how to drink. Used to get into some terrible fights with my old lady though. Boy—he'd come home with a little too much in him—she'd really let him have it. I'd have to—pull the pillow up over my head so I wouldn't hear the noise. Couldn't get to sleep.

T: Your mother was very hard on your father then. [Summarization] Kinda upsetting to a young kid to hear all that fighting. [Reflection]

P: Yeah. She really used to get mad at him. You know for drinking and all that. She used to yell at him. Get on his back all the time. Really be nasty to him. Maybe that's one of the reasons why he's six feet under right now.

T: Sort of like the same thing your wife is doing to you? [Query based on interpretation]

P: Yeah. You're right. You really hit the nail on the head. You really understand what's going on. There's a lot of things about the two that are kind of the same. I think she's trying to do the same thing to me that my mother did to my father. Yell and fight—and call you a drunk. Telling me I can't take on any responsibility. Always yelling about something. Money. Why don't you have more of it? Why can't we buy this? Why can't we buy that? I'm working—as hard as I can—and she does—she doesn't realize that. She thinks all I have to do is work—all the time. She thinks it's—it's easy for me to—to work every day. Always pushing me. I don't like to be pushed. I get—I'll get things done. But I have to work—at my own pace, otherwise—it just doesn't matter if I work or not if I can't work at my own pace.

T: She just sees you as someone to bring home the dough—like she doesn't really care about you. [Summarization]

P: Yeah—she's in her own world. She doesn't care about anything that I do—or say. She doesn't care about me or anyone else. Sometimes I just feel like getting up and leaving. There's nothing there any more.

T: You just want to go—get out—leave all the problems behind. [Restatement]

P: Um, hmm.

T: It's probably always been easier to leave problems behind. [Interpretation]

P: Um, hmm. Used to—get away for a couple of days by myself. But I always ended up coming back because I had no one else to go to.

T: Getting away didn't really solve the problem, though. [Restatement] You felt kinda lost without your wife and family, huh? [Reflection]

P: Oh—it's hard when you're alone. It's—I have no place to go. Haven't any friends or—or close family. Except for my—my wife and kids. You know I—the way they treat me I know they don't want me. At least though when I'm home I have a roof over my head. I know I can sleep—I don't have to be wandering around in the streets for something to do. Someone to feed me [pp. 361–363].

The reader may note that in the low-empathy example, the interviewer's responses were dominated by seemingly premature interpretations and suggestions, with little use of restatement, summarization, or reflection categories. The reader should also note how the interviewer's interpretations quite dramatically affected the course of the interview, in particular provision of information, particularly regarding feelings. In fact, the low-empathy interview is characterized by the client's gradual diminution of responding as the interviewer takes on a very directive and active role.

In contrast, the high-empathy interviewer elicited much more extensive information regarding the client's concerns and feelings as well as specific data regarding the life situation. In contrast to the low-empathy interview, few interpretations are made, and those that are seem to facilitate the client's offering of information and expression of feelings. In addition, much more reliance on summarization and reflectiive response categories seems to set a tone in the interview that encourages the client to talk about *himself* and to share his personal perspective. Considerations of rapport aside (it's not hard to guess which of the interview styles would generate maximum rapport), it is obvious that the high-empathy interviewer employed a variety of responding approaches that showed his "tracking" with the informational and feeling statements offered by the client, leading to much more extensive data that might be useful in both understanding the client's concerns and in ultimately generating an intervention strategy. The reader is particularly discouraged from employing interpretation at the outset of a transaction. Early interpretation can only be based on a poor data base and may well inhibit the spontaneity and open-endedness of the client's responses.

Reviews of research evaluating the effects of these and other similar communicative approaches, as well as further practical examples, may be found in Goldstein (1973), Ivey (1971), Benjamin (1969), Carkhuff (1969a, 1969b), and Goldstein (1975).[1] It should be noted that while different writers have suggested that active listening and empathic communications facilitate the establishment of rapport, the role of empathy as a *primary* therapeutic strategy has been questioned (e.g., Mash and Terdal, 1976; Morganstern, 1976; Nay, 1976).

Definition of the Problem

Once a comprehensive self-report of the problem is obtained, as well as other relevant information about the life situation that the client wishes to offer, the BCA should make it clear to the client that it is important to review each of the problem areas so that: (1) the BCA can obtain a more precise description of each problem area in language both BCA and client comprehend, and (2) information may be obtained regarding the characteristics of the problem that might help the BCA to understand how undesirable behavior is maintained or why desirable behavior fails to occur at optimum frequency. Following a careful description of current concerns or problem behaviors the client wishes to reveal to the BCA, follow-up questions can determine specific conditions (e.g., location, activity, time, antecedents, and consequences) that may serve to instigate, maintain, or limit the behavior in some fashion, as well as client resources and motivation to actively pursue behavior change. The rationale for each of these categories of information was presented in Chapters 1 and 2. The collection of case history information permitting the BCA to place the client's problem(s) and concern(s) within a historical-developmental content will be addressed in Chapter 4. Chapter 2 presented a detailed outline of each of the categories of information the BCA will wish to assess as the client is encouraged to carefully focus the problem in the context of his life situation.[2]

The BCA should be aware of a number of methodological options that may assist in this focusing process. First, though, I should caution that any "technique" must follow from careful appraisal of the client by the BCA, to ensure that the method chosen has in fact a *purpose* in the information-gathering process and serves to maintain and build on rapport. With this in mind, the next section will present some of the issues related to *focusing* the client's statements using questions.

Focusing with Questions

If the interview has gone according to plan, the BCA at this point will have begun to establish rapport in providing the client with an opportunity to state his problems and concerns to an empathic and actively attending interviewer. In return, the BCA has made mental and perhaps written notes regarding the problem areas described by the client and now has the task of obtaining further information necessary for goal setting and treatment planning. The interview situation shifts its focus at this point, with the BCA taking the lead and serving in a more directorial capacity. The client's initial agenda of "telling you my problem" has presumably been at least partially achieved; the BCA must now provide a rationale to the client for *his* agenda of obtaining focused and understandable information about each potential target for intervention. The role change from active listener to questioner would seem to require some introduction. Cannell and Kahn (1968) cite the importance of providing a *frame of reference* for the questions asked. The very nature of the BCA's role suggests an initial frame of reference; it is supposed that the meaning of the question "How are you feeling today?" will be quite different when that question is posed by the BCA than by a friend, a colleague, or some other person. As the BCA adopts a more directive role, the client's frame of reference should change from providing information quite freely in his "own words" to providing information that "clarifies" questions provoked by the client's initial statement of the problem. If the BCA adopts the latter frame of reference while the client still holds the former (and no rationale for a change had been provided), one would expect the BCA's questions will only serve to generate concern in the client's mind (e.g., "Why is he asking all these questions?"). The BCA might present a rationale for this transition by explaining to the client, in clear and understandable language, why it is important to have more detailed information. This might be accomplished as follows.

Interviewer: I think I'm beginning to understand some of the things that concern you, and wonder if there is anything further that you would like to say?

Client: Well, I really don't know if I've been very clear, but somehow it's better just to talk about it.

Interviewer: I can appreciate that and want to be sure that I *do* understand each of the concerns that you talked about. I would like to ask you some questions that may help us to clarify some of the things that you said and also to understand how the concerns you raised fit in with other aspects of your life. In some cases, I'm going to ask you to be very specific and to give me as much detail as possible. Also, it sometimes helps me if you can provide an example, let's say from the last week or so that best describes a concern. Please feel free to let me know if I fail to ask you something that you would like to tell me about or if you have any questions generally.

Client: Okay.

The BCA must ensure that this rationale is understood by the client, and that any questions that the client has are answered prior to proceeding to the focusing process. In all cases, the interviewer should avoid preprogrammed responses. As Cannell and Kahn (1968) state:

The canned heartiness of programmed explanations, delivered irrespective of the respondent's mood or need for explanation, are poor substitutes for spontaneous interaction in which a skilled and sensitive interviewer provides explanations when the respondent is puzzled or hesitant, and does so in terms that fit the respondent's level of sophistication. A highly educated and sophisticated respondent may bear with an oversimple question in an interview, but he will not be satisfied with an oversimple explanation. Kinsey's classic phrase of assurance that the requested information "will help the doctors" constitutes neither explanation nor assurance for educated and analyical respondents [p. 575].

Once the frame of reference for focusing has been established, there are a number of issues that should be kept in mind in formulating questions. First, the BCA should ensure that the question is *clearly* stated at a level of vocabulary consonant with the client's verbal skills and instructs the client as to precisely what bit of information is sought. Thus a question such as: "What do you make of your husband's behavior?" forces the client to make a decision as to precisely what the BCA means by "make of." In this case, the client has no frame of reference for making a response. If the BCA is interested in exploring what the client thinks her husband's attitude is, or why she thinks that he behaves in a particular way, this should be stated directly within the question, "Can you tell me, why do you think he (then describes the act)?" Next, the question should be *well organized* and require a *single response*. A poorly organized, "double-barreled" question such as: "Will you please tell me about the kinds of arguments you and your husband have, why you argue and how things usually end?" forces the client to consider three questions simultaneously. Even if the first part of the question is dealt with first, the second and third parts may intrude upon the client's response. In addition, double-barreled questions are often incompletely answered and the BCA is forced to go back and re-present a specific part of the question to obtain a complete response.

Another issue to be considered is whether or not the question is relatively *open* or *closed*. An open question is one that forces the respondent to supply information necessary to satisfying the demands of the question, whereas a closed question requires the respondent to provide relatively little information, perhaps merely indicating agreement or disagreement with the interviewer's statement. While both categories of questions are frequently employed in the interview, the open question obviously provides information stated in the client's own language and should be emphasized over the closed-question format. Examples of *closed* questions are:

"Did Billy do well in first grade?"
"Are you feeling anxious right now?"
"Is your marriage a happy one?"
"Do the pains occur often?"

Here the respondent is forced to guess what the interviewer means by "doing well" or "feeling anxious" and to self-determine the criteria the BCA holds for the answer. Even though the client is not very happy with certain sexual aspects of his marriage, he may answer the BCA's question, "Is your marriage a happy one?", with a "Yes," feeling that "unhappy" signifies severe problems or contemplation of divorce. Thus, the criteria the respondent employs in deciding on a yes or no response may be different from the BCA's criteria. A much more *open* way of asking the preceding questions would be:

"What were Billy's grades in first grade?" or "How did Billy do academically in first grade?"

"What are you experiencing right now—could you describe the feeling?"

"What aspects of your marriage are most (least) satisfying?"

"How frequently do the pains occur?"

An open question forces the respondent to provide more extensive information in response to the BCA's query, and then permits the BCA to determine whether or not the information gathered is of sufficient importance to be followed up. In addition, by requiring the client to "fill in the gaps" in response to an open question, the BCA has a better opportunity to observe the client's behavior as the question is handled along the lines suggested below. Cannell and Kahn (1968) point out that definitive research on the advantages of open versus closed questions has yet to be done. In demanding less respondent effort and less revelation, the closed question is probably less threatening. On the other hand, the closed question may also invite an easy invalid response rather than a more difficult "don't know." The authors point out that the closed form is most appropriate "when the interviewer knows in advance the likely range of responses and has reason to minimize the demand on the respondent" (p. 567).

There are a variety of additional questioning strategies that the BCA may wish to employ. Each of these may meet certain goals that might arise within the focusing process.

Problem: The interviewee is likely to be threatened and/or readily deny concern with a topic area that the BCA has reason to believe is of importance in the client's life situation.

Response Options: Wallen (1956) suggests that the interviewer employ progressive questions that begin with a matter near the topic area of interest, followed by questions that lead progressively to the most specific query. Questions thus progress from less intimate to more intimate content areas.

Suppose that the clinician wishes to learn whether an 18-year-old boy has had sexual intercourse, and he believes that a direct question on this matter would meet with resistance. He arranges his questions in a progression:

"About how many dates do you have a week?"

"Where do you like to go on dates?"

"What kinds of girls do you like to go with?"

"Do many of the girls object to necking or petting?"

"Have you ever worried about getting the syph or the clap from any of them?"

"Why," or "Why not?"

In this illustration the final question is an indirect one which is ostensibly about worries. The progression prepared the way for a possibly threatening question by starting with a relatively nonthreatening series. Progression serves to introduce questions which would otherwise appear too blunt and perhaps shocking [p. 156].

Another approach is to embed a significant question within a series of seemingly "routine" questions. The significant question appears to be only an additional matter to be explored. Wallen (1956) provides an example in which the BCA was interested in the interviewee's sexual life but did not want to emphasize this interest by exclusively focusing upon that area.

"Have you ever had trouble with your eyes or vision?"
"What about eating, appetite, or stomach trouble?"
"Anything connected with sex organs or sex activity?"
"How about trouble sleeping or getting to sleep?"
"Any skin trouble?"
"How about your legs and back?"
Here the questions are asked in such a way as to give the impression of a routine examination in which one item is about as important as any other [p. 156].

Problem: A question asked within an initial context (e.g., questions about school, job) provokes nonresponding and/or discomfort on the interviewee's part.
Response Option: Wallen (1956) recommends that the question be reintroduced in another context, later in the interview process. His example of such a *held-over question* is provided below.

Early in an interview a client reports that he got into trouble and left school in the tenth grade. He shows no inclination to talk about the nature of the trouble, so the clinician holds the question until later. During the section of the interview devoted to discussing family relationships the clinician says: "You mentioned a little while ago that you left school because you got into trouble. What did your parents say about that?" If this question does not reveal the details of the trouble, the clinician may now inquire about it directly. The topic has been moved from the area of education into the area of home background in the hope that it will seem less threatening there [p.157].

Problem: The interviewee uses a term that the BCA is unfamiliar with or employs a global label (e.g., "aggressive," "neurotic," "nervous") that the BCA wishes to define more specifically. Frequently the interviewee will offer a term in an unusual or highly idiosyncratic fashion; it is most important that the BCA understand precisely what the word means to the client.
Response Option: Morganstern (1976) provides an excellent example of using a *narrowing* procedure to increasingly focus the client's responses in terms of mutually understood behavioral referents.

Client: When I'm in such "heavy," situations, I just get real "uptight." You know, I just can't make it, so I kind of drop out.
Therapist: I think I have some idea of what you are saying, but everyone has slightly different interpretations. So I wonder if you can help me get a better understanding of what you mean. For example, when you say that you're uptight in these situations, what does that mean for you?

Client: Well, uptight, you know. Tense.
Therapist: You mean your muscles get tense?
Client: My neck gets very sore—and I get a headache lots of times.
Therapist: Anything else happen that you notice?
Client: Well, either because of my neck or my headache, I start sweating a lot.
Therapist: So when you say you're uptight you are really experiencing physically. What kinds of things are you saying to yourself when this happens?
Client: I'm thinking, Man you are really paranoid. You just can't relax in any situation. You really are a loser. And then I want to get out of there fast . . . [p. 68].

Beginning with an open-ended question that permits the client broad latitude in first referencing his meaning of "uptight," the therapist becomes much more specific in directing his questions to particular phenomena the client has experienced that define this term.

Problem: In some cases it is useful to explore the interviewee's philosophy, conceptualization or evaluation of some phenomenon when this information does not clearly emerge from his account of personal matters. Thus, it might be advantageous to know that a teacher considers any form of positive feedback to students "bribery" or that a husband's and wife's views of an "ideal" marriage are quite divergent.

Response Option: The interviewee might be asked to respond to a hypothetical situation constructed by the BCA to explore the client's views. Thus, a teacher might be asked: "If you could be in charge of setting up the 'ideal' classroom, what would it be like?" or "What do you think causes children to misbehave?" Or, the client who has had difficulty holding a job might be asked: "What kind of work would you most like to do if you had your choice?" or "What is your definition of a good boss?"

It may be revealing to compare the client's responses to such hypothetical situations with his everyday response to the phenomena of interest. Also, the BCA is in a better position to suggest therapeutic alternatives consonant with the client's attitudes or values, or may, in some cases, suggest that the client consider an alternative conceptualization more compatible with the achievement of his goals.

Behavioral Observations

The second major category of information to be collected in the interview is the interviewee's observed behavior. Because the content of the self-report may be unreliable, biased by an array of possible expectations that the client holds or by the demand characteristics of the interview situation, observational data provide an additional source of information for the BCA to compare with verbal content. The extent to which the client's verbal report and other behavior categories correlate (e.g., the client reports that he is anxious, and is showing behavioral signs of anxiety) or do not correlate provides useful information regarding the reliability of the client's report—the degree to which the client is a good self-observer and has insight into his own behavior.

Physical Appearance

The BCA should carefully observe the client as he walks in and sits down. Wallen (1956) points out that the client's height, weight, and body structure create a global impression which may be summed up with such words as "petite," "frail," "hulking," etc. He indicates that the impression the client makes on the interviewer may be quite similar to the impression he makes on others, which is important information. Houck and Hansen (1972) recommend an appraisal of the individual's carriage, walk, and facial expression, as well as any special mannerisms. The client's clothing, hairstyle, and grooming may also be important indicators of his view of himself and certainly reveal the manner in which he attempts to portray himself to others. For example, if a 35-year-old lawyer were to present himself in a clinical setting with his shirt unbuttoned, without a belt, with stains or other marks on his clothing, this would certainly be considered atypical behavior for a person of his reference group. This bit of information, *in combination with other information collected in the interview,* may corroborate the BCA's findings that the client is expressing the way he feels about himself with his dress. It is important that the BCA *not go too far in generalizing from any one bit of information,* but employ every piece of information as part of a general picture of the client which can be pulled together following each interview session. Across interview sessions, a unified picture of the client begins to emerge which can be defended by the data collected. In summary, then, the BCA should look for any unusual aspects of the client's appearance, and evaluate it in terms of the sexual-social grouping to which the client belongs. Any marked deviations from the norm become parts of a clinical impression which must be stored, compared with other data collected, and contribute to an integrated picture of the client. However, as Wallen states: "A . . . limitation on inferences based on dress comes from the difficulty of knowing the norms of the client and his social group" (p. 121). Also, since it is fairly common for people to "dress up" for visits to a clinical setting, the BCA may be seeing the client as the client thinks he should appear for such an encounter, rather than as he ordinarily presents himself.

Voice and Speech

The client may communicate a good deal to the BCA in the style and manner of his speaking beyond the mere contents of his words. While the content may be important, a careful consideration of manner of speaking (or paralanguage) should be undertaken. For each of the categories to be mentioned, the BCA should try to obtain some approximate idea of its *frequency* as well as *intensity*, if relevant. If some speech-related behavior or mannerism becomes highly relevant to the client's problem behavior, then systematic observations might be undertaken using a formal coding system (see Chapter 7). Among the categories that should be considered by the interviewer are the following.

1. *Loudness of Speech or Intensity*. Was the client's voice excessively loud or excessively soft, and how does this relate to the specific topic being covered? Were there any changes in intensity of voice throughout the interview, and if so, what seemed to bring them about (e.g., coverage of a particular topic, gradual dissipation of anxiety, etc.)?

2. *Pitch of Voice*. The pitch of a client's voice (e.g., bass versus high-pitched) is often an indication of level of anxiety and mood state, particularly if the BCA has information regarding the client's ordinary pitch. If changes of pitch are noted in the interview, the BCA should attempt to relate these changes to the content the client is presenting or other events in the therapist-client transaction. In addition, if the client's voice is pitched in such a way that it is unpleasant to the BCA, this may be important, as others may respond in a similarly negative fashion to the client's voice. This may be of particular relevance when the client reports difficulty in the social situation.

3. *Speed*. Any marked deviation (e.g., very slow, very rapid) from the client's normal rate of speaking may provide useful information. Very slow talking is often associated with depression when displayed with other signs. Very rapid speech may be associated with elated, manic states. Of course it is important that the BCA (and others!) be able to understand what the client is saying, and if the client speaks too rapidly it may be useful to employ verbal and nonverbal prompts (e.g., raising the hand toward the client) to attempt to slow down the client's rate of speaking so that it is understandable. Often this can be handled by prompting the client: "I didn't quite get what you just said, could you say it again for me a bit more slowly?"

4. *Ease of Speech*. To what extent does the BCA have to probe or prompt the client to obtain a response to questions? Does the client hesitate, pause, or block prior to or within a communication?

5. *Spontaneity and Reaction Time*. Does the client speak without being prompted, offer information to the BCA, or remain quite guarded and nonspontaneous? In addition, when a question is asked, how quickly is the client able to process the question and make a response? Delayed reaction time often suggests that the client is carefully thinking over what will be said prior to speaking—perhaps a sign of overguardedness. In some cases, slow reaction time may be indicative of anxiety or of disorganized thought processes.

6. *Relevance*. Are the client's productions relevant to the questions—on target? If the BCA finds himself asking a question and receiving a response to

some other question or a disorganized response, this may be indicative of disorganized thinking on the client's part, or that perhaps the client is not actively listening to the BCA's questions and prompts. Also, is the client easily distractible when external sounds or other events occur, and if so, is this related to the area being discussed?

7. *Manner of Speaking.* Is the client's manner of speaking highly pedantic, excessively formal and intellectualized, relaxed, or inappropriately familiar? Obviously there are many ways that client speech can be categorized along these dimensions, but often the BCA experiences some reaction to the client's speaking (e.g., an *evocative message* where the client's behavior evokes a thought or feeling on the BCA's part), and these evocative messages may be of assistance in evaluating the relevance and appropriateness of the client's manner.

8. *Marked Deviations.* Is there any evidence of neologisms (made-up words, highly idiosyncratic language), echolalia (echolike repetitions of what has been stated), clang associations (phrases or sentences which repeat a particular sound), or word salad (mixtures of nouns and verbs that make no sense). The BCA should be sensitive to marked deviations in the client's speech from the social norms appropriate to the client's reference group. Highly unusual slang, phrases, or words may indicate disorganization of the client's thought processes must be carefully evaluated in the light of other data.

9. *Organization.* To what extent do the client's replies to questions or statements seem to be organized around a common goal or theme? Does the client have a topic he wishes to present to the BCA and, if so, can he stick to the topic without rambling on? Often the term "flight of ideas" is employed to describe the client who continuously changes the topic and whose ideas seem to be quite confused. While many severely disturbed clients show speech disorganization, the less disturbed but highly anxious individual may often become confused in presenting information. It is important for the BCA to begin gradually and systematically to let the client know that what was said was not understood; however, this should be done in a nonthreatening fashion. Statements such as: "I'm not sure I follow what you just said, could you tell me that again?" or "I really want to understand what you're telling me, and I had trouble on that last one, would you mind repeating that for me again please?" may be used. A lack of organization may be something that is generalized to other situations, leading other persons to respond to the client in a negative fashion. Thus, the organization of speech may itself become a target for change.

10. *Vocabulary and Diction.* One of the best predictors of full-scale intelligence for most individual tests of intelligence is the client's vocabulary, and level of vocabulary is a means of crudely approximating level of intellectual functioning. Of course there may be many problems introduced by this generalization, particularly when the BCA is interviewing a client from a

subcultural group which diverges from the norms on which a given intelligence test is based. Persons with poor vocabularies often perform well on nonverbal tests of intelligence, so it is important that vocabulary be evaluated in the light of the client's social and subcultural situation. However, it is useful to know whether or not the client's vocabulary is appropriate to his age, educational status, and occupational situation, since many clients are forced to function in social and cultural groups beyond their own subculture. One way of getting a rough idea of level of vocabulary appropriate to age is to evaluate the vocabulary subtest norms of an individual test of intelligence such as Wechsler Adult Intelligence Scale (Wechsler, 1958) or the Stanford Binet (Terman and Merrill, 1960) for adults or the Wechsler Intelligence Scale for Children (Wechsler, 1949) for younger clients. The BCA *must* place vocabulary and the client's fund of general information in the context of the client's current life situation and *not* employ such assessment in a vacuum.

Nonverbal Behavior

Many behaviors fall under this designation, and the following should be thought of as representing major categories.

1. *Motor Behavior.* Concerning client motor behavior within the interview from a psychiatric point of view, Sands (1967) states:

Here the [BCA] presents a picture of the patient's overall motor behavior during the interview. Were his motor acts appropriate to the situation? Were they smoothly coordinated, jerky, or awkward? Was there hyperactivity? (or underactivity?) If so, give a careful description. Was his motor behavior purposeful or seemingly aimless? Was any motor act self-injurious or self-destructive of objects in the room? Was the patient willing to shake hands in greeting? Was his handshake of normal firmness or was it abnormally limp? Was there evidence of cogwheel rigidity or waxy flexibility? Did the patient display wringing of hands, tics (stereotyped, repetitive motor behaviors like repeated face touching, scratching, etc.), twitching, or a tremor? If so, was it constant or "on intention" only? If the examiner suspects that the patient is abnormally slow, he may time the patient's reactions by giving him simple commands, such as asking him to walk across the room, to untie and tie his shoelaces, or to write out a dictated sentence. In the report, the examiner should give the time it took the patient to respond. The patient should be given a simple explanation for the test, such as "I want to see how long it takes you to do certain things" [p. 505].

Obviously the frequency of certain motor acts, particularly highly idiosyncratic or disruptive ones, gives the BCA some notion of over- or underactivity. Either category may be important as an indicator of affect and mood. Any highly stylized or idiosyncratic motoric mannerisms should be noted, and some assessment of frequency should be recorded.

2. *Posture.* The BCA should assess the manner in which the client is seated in the chair. Is his posture slouched, relaxed, highly rigid, slumped over the chair, etc., and does posture seem to change as a function of content

or other events in the interview? Many interviewers assess the client's gait (e.g., brisk, slow, unsteady, or poorly coordinated) and carriage (e.g., erect or slouched over).

3. *Facial Expression.* The BCA might assess the appropriateness of facial expression to the subject matter. discussed. For example, if the client is relating some positive personal experience, his facial expression should be appropriate to this, and not drawn, frowning, or in other ways negative. Correspondingly, discussions of personal problems should not typically be accompanied by a smile or similar expression. In sum, is the facial expression appropriate to the content offered by the client? Does facial expression *change* appropriately with change of content? Might the patient' face be characterized as expressive or unexpressive and flat? Does the client appear to be normally attentive, apathetic, or indifferent as indicated by facial cues? Does the patient at any point show elation (degree: mild pleasure, smiling, uncontrolled laughter), fear or anxiety (facial tremor, crying, frowning, poor eye contact, etc.), or anger (changes in facial color, obvious rage, scornful expression, etc.)? It is most difficult to interpret facial expressions and *the BCA should proceed with caution, attempting to correlate this information with other indicators of the client's current state.* However, if facial expression or other body language is not correlated with the content of the client's statements, the BCA must explore further in attempting to determine the accuracy of the client's verbal communications.

4. *Eye Contact.* Eye contact may be viewed along a dimension ranging from low frequency of eye contact with the BCA (or others present) to continuous eye contact. Either end of that continuum may provoke an uncomfortable response. Client eye contact is often an excellent nonverbal indicator of the client's current state. One could construct a variety of hypotheses regarding poor client contact (e.g., client disinterest, fear of BCA or interview situation, poor social skills, etc.), but these can only be checked by integrating this information with other data.

Footnotes

[1]The reader is referred to the training formats of Ivey (1971), Danish, D'Augelli, and Brock (1975), and Nay (1977) for a presentation of didactic and experiential strategies for training novice interviewers.

[2]A re-reading of Chapter 2 is encouraged. It should be noted that this outline merely suggests specific informational categories that the BCA might wish to address to ensure a comprehensive assessment of the problem. The interviewer's style as well as the client's approach to the interview will determine focusing methods and the order in which each category is explored.

4

THE CASE HISTORY

While the intake-orientation interview format focuses on determining the client's problems and/or concerns in the contemporary environment, many writers have suggested the importance of collecting comprehensive life history information to place this current behavior in the context of past experiences. In reviewing a variety of literature reporting psychiatric and psychological-clinical assessment methods, I was struck by the frequency with which the "case history" is described and underscored as a valuable assessment method. Perhaps the prominence of the case history results from the important role of early life events in certain theoretical formulations of psychopathology (e.g., Freud, 1922, 1933; Sullivan, 1953) and certainly the extensive emphasis on a gathering of historical information in the psychiatric-medical context.

For example, during the initial period of orientation to the interview or "reconnaissance," Harry Stack Sullivan (1954)[1] emphasizes the importance of obtaining a "rough social sketch of the patient, which is to be brief, and not an extended life history" (p. 73). Many of the categories Sullivan surveys are similar to those included within the case history formats of other investigators. Following a description of the client's age, place of birth, and current status of parents, Sullivan asks about the client's siblings (number, order, and characteristics), and inquires about family members comprising the home constellation during the client's first seven years. Sullivan states: "Sorting out such data is truly impressive to a great many people. They may have actually forgotten that grandma was the one bright spot in the home in their first seven years, and are glad to be reminded of it." (p. 73). Next, inquiry regarding the family's economic status and primary breadwinner is followed by questions asking the client to describe "what sort of person" both his mother and father are/were, as well as the status of their marriage over time, Sullivan then inquires about each job the client has held as well as level of education.[2] Finally, he asks about the current marital status of the (adult) client, focusing on current satisfaction with the marriage and the client's reasons for getting married in the first place. Regarding a rationale for obtaining the above data, Sullivan states:

Of the labels which the patient's neighbors and casual acquaintances attach to him, I've tried to pick out those that have some measure of probable significance for understanding what he does. He feels that I know a great deal about him—in part because a good deal of these data are ordinarily not discussed in his relations with strangers. In a vague way, I do know a good deal, because from now on I just watch which of the customary indices prove to be correct in his case, and wherein he is an exception to the probabilities which are implied in the semi-statistical data of the past, his family position, and so on [p. 77].

While many BCAs, especially those who hold a behavioral orientation, would probably question the utility of collecting extensive and comprehensive historical information across all clients and presenting problems, there is no doubt that the case history holds an important place in behavioral assessment (Goldfried and Davison, 1976; Kanfer and Saslow, 1969; Lazarus, 1976; Rimm and Masters, 1974; Wolpe, 1973). For example, Wolpe (1973) recommends obtaining a "background history" regarding the client's early family life, his education, his employment, and his ability to perform and maintain social relationships. He emphasizes the importance of asking questions regarding the client's sexual life leading up to his current sexual and marital status. Wolpe explains that historical information sets the stage and provides a perspective from which the BCA may construct a program of treatment. In addition, a thorough case history may provide "important clues to the stimulus-response relationships that are currently relevant" (p. 23). Supporting this idea, Rimm and Masters (1974) suggest that case history information may be helpful in generating and supporting hypotheses about the client's current behavior. They point out that the collection of such information may provide an excellent vehicle for initiating rapport. While Goldfried and Davison (1976) state that the ehavior therapist's focus "is on current situations" (p. 43), they emphasize the important role of past historical information when the client's presenting problem is complex. An exploration of the client's past experiences with the problem event may provide important clues as to the current conditions maintaining the behavior. These authors tend to de-emphasize the role of the case history when the client presents "thoroughly delineated problems, such as phobias [where] knowledge of the historical antecedents will probably provide little help on how to proceed therapeutically" (p. 43).

While agreeing that the case history may provide useful information for some clients and in certain therapeutic situations, virtually every investigator has raised questions about its place in the assessment. Both Brammer and Shostrum (1968) and Hansen, Stevic, and Warner (1972) suggest that the case history may shift responsibility from the client to the therapist when it consumes large amounts of time within the interview process. Hansen et al. (1972) state:

It may ... be argued that asking the client to give a schematic account of himself may increase his resistance in concealing some significant facts about himself. The client may also assume that once he has made the report of his history he can sit back and expect the counselor to solve his problems [p. 197].

In addition, Brammer and Shostrum (1968) argue that extensive history taking may detract from the job of "building the relationship solidly" (p. 143), and give the assessor the false illusion that the mere collection of an orderly set of facts provides data necessary for treatment planning. Rimm and Masters (1974) emphasize that the interview must proceed rapidly from history taking to the "here and now" and an understanding of the client's problem in the contemporary situation. They state:

Clients, especially those who have been exposed to more traditional forms of psychotherapy, frequently have a set to engage in a seemingly endless discussion of their past life (traditional approaches tend to reinforce such behavior). From the point of view of the behavioral therapist, this can be very counterproductive since it is antithetical to his "here and now" orientation, which stresses problem-solving rather than passive reflection. It is recommended that clients be gently dissuaded from undue dwelling on such past experiences. At the same time, however, care should be taken not to communicate to the client that he is forbidden to bring up relevant background material that, perhaps through embarrassment, he avoided during the initial interview [pp. 41–42].

It is quite beyond the scope of this chapter to present a comprehensive compendium of the many case history formats offered in the literature. Instead, a series of commonly employed *categories of case history information* will be presented that might be included depending on the characteristics of the presenting problem, the amount of time available in the intake process, and the BCA's orientation regarding the importance of historical information. The format to be presented proceeds in a somewhat orderly way from the client's birth through those categories of information most relevant to adult functioning; however, it should be emphasized that the order of categories presented here reflects only my own biases. Interviewers should feel free to explore these categories in a variety of different ways.

Categories of Historical-Developmental Information

For each of the categories to follow, the interviewee could be asked about aspects of his own life history or report this information as it relates to someone else. In the latter case, the interviewee is an "informant" providing information to augment the "targeted" client's self-report (e.g., a spouse or parent provides auxiliary case history information about the client). Other informants include parents reporting for a young child or relatives or other close associates reporting for an adolescent or adult client who lacks the verbal and/or cognitive skills necessary to handle the interview. Following a presentation of information categories and a rationale for their use, a discussion of methods and issues suggested by the history will be offered.

Description of Birth

This category includes information about the *pregnancy* of the client's mother, as well as any complications in birth.

Rationale and Comment. Most adult clients will remember little of what their parents told them about their birth, and this information would usually not be assessed for the adult client unless some specific reason was suggested by the presenting problem. In contrast, this category is often usefully explored when the BCA collects information from a parent (informant) regarding a young client. For example, birth-related problems might be implicated in neurological deficits or other physical disabilities or deficits which may define as well as delimit possibilities for intervention.

Developmental History

Information is obtained about the *onset of important developmental epochs* as well as any resulting problems or complications. Categories typically include: age of sitting, standing, walking, first use of functional language, control of bladder and bowel, onset of puberty, and other developmental data of interest to the BCA.

Rationale and Comment. Again, most adult clients will not recall with certainty the times and conditions of their early development, unless they varied considerably from the norm (and heard about this from their parents). When a young child or adolescent is the client, the parent-informant should be able to provide details regarding current developmental status and any problems or concerns. Such information permits the BCA (and parent) to evaluate the child or adolescent's current behavior and possibilities for behavior change in the context of current abilities, repertoire skills, and developmental status. The BCA should explore *how* the parent handled important events such as walking, talking, and toilet training to obtain some notion of the parent's expectations for the child (are they realistic? within the norm?) as well as the parent's repertoire of child-management skills (what procedure did the parent employ to toilet train the child?). An exploration of pubertal development (e.g., growth spurt, secondary and primary sexual characteristics) and parent and adolescent response to it provides a useful frame of reference for understanding current life behavior of adolescent clients. (A thorough reading or re-reading of a developmental textbook can assist the assessor in determining whether or not the targeted child is within normal limits and provides a useful perspective from which to evaluate this information.)

Medical History

The BCA inquires into the *nature and dates of injuries, accidents, notable operations, and illnesses* other than the ordinary "childhood" diseases, as well as physical handicaps. In addition, many investigators explore *medications and regimens of treatment* prescribed from the past through the present, health restrictions (e.g., from physical activity), and obtain a listing of any physicians consulted, particularly if the client's medical problem seems to be related to a current concern.

Rationale and Comment. As might be imagined, physical disease, bodily insult, or physical handicap can have an important impact on the client's development and response to his environment. For some clients, episodes of hospitalization, painful and traumatic injuries, and the like evoke considerable anxiety and discomfort that may be related to a client's current behavior (e.g., a fear of becoming ill, obsessional cleanliness, etc.). Or, a client's present problem may include physical components that can best be understood from the vantage point of a thorough medical history. In addition, the impact of such medical problems on the client's early opportunities to develop social skills and perform academically, or even as delimiters of occupational possibilities, may provide information useful in understanding the client's current behavioral deficits. Finally, in obtaining such information, the BCA achieves an understanding of how the client views his own physical health (Thorne, 1955), as well as current nutritional or health habits. It cannot be overemphasized that all clients should undergo a thorough physical examination prior to approaching the nonmedically trained BCA. This is particularly important when the client's presenting problem is characterized by physical discomfort or other neurological and/or physical signs.

While the nonmedically trained BCA is not competent to evaluate the client's current medical status, the medical history provides an understanding of how this history may have affected the client's behavior and perhaps limited certain behavioral possibilities for him during his development. It may be particularly important for the BCA to obtain the names as well as the locations of any physicians consulted, particularly in the recent past, as this information is collected. A release of information from or direct collaboration with a physician may be most useful and ethically responsible when the client's medical status limits treatment possibilities or suggests a combined medical and psychotherapeutic approach.

Characteristics of Family and Family History

Following a categorization of all family members in terms of age, ordinal position, sex, and current status, the BCA may wish to obtain a more detailed account of *significant family members* (e.g., those present during the client's early development), focusing on how the client interacted with each. Writers have varied considerably regarding the detail with which a client should be asked to describe each family member. Regarding the parents, for example, Wolpe (1973) suggests inquiring: "What kind of person did [the client's] father seem to him to be? Did he show personal interest, did he punish, and if so did it seem just or not? As well as details of parent's death (if relevant) as well as the client's response to it. The same questions would be asked regarding the client's mother" (pp. 26–27). Thorne (1955) suggests obtaining information regarding occupation, education, health, temperament, and personal peculiarities as well as such disabilities as alcoholism, nervous or mental disorders, diseases, or criminal or antisocial tendencies.

Rationale and Comment. Given the important role of parents and siblings in defining and limiting the client's early learning environment, as well as in modeling social and parenting skills, this information may provide clues as to why the client holds certain beliefs (perhaps "irrational") or behaves in a particular fashion. In addition, frequent family moves, separation or divorce of parents, and other family events can have important implications for a client's opportunities to try out and to learn both appropriate and inappropriate strategies for coping with his environment. As a subcategory of the family history, the BCA may wish to inquire about the economic status of the family, as well as any financial limitations which may have restricted the client's opportunities.

Interpersonal Skills

This category defines the client's *ability to instigate and maintain relationships with persons outside the immediate family*, focusing on described excesses or deficits in social-skills behavior, anxiety or discomfort in social situations, or other problems of an interpersonal nature. It is important to evaluate the interpersonal situations in which the client has experienced maximally satisfying social relationships as well as social situations in which the client has had difficulty. Careful evaluation of the client's social relationships within and across periods of his development permits the BCA to determine consistent patterns of interpersonal behavior. In some cases, the client will refer to a previous social situation that provoked considerable anxiety or discomfort and seems to be causal in terms of the client's current social difficulties. The BCA should obtain information about the specific characteristics of that event to determine its possible relation to the client's current social-skills deficits and/or avoidance of social situations.

As a subcategory, the BCA may wish to focus on the client's relationships with members of the opposite sex in the early dating situation, as well as relationships resulting in sexual intimacy. *Alternatively, this information may be handled in a separate category defining dating, sexual behavior, and the client's past and current marital status.*

Rationale and Comment. It is obvious that many problems in living limit the client's opportunities to instigate and maintain interpersonal relationships. While a detailed interpersonal history is maximally important when the problem presented is of a social-interpersonal nature, such information may also be useful across other problem categories in defining persons who may serve as resources and in providing a more complete picture of the client's behavior. The client's reported "problem" may be secondary to problems in interpersonal functioning (e.g., the client who reports that he is "depressed" may also lack the social support of others).

Educational History

This category is often approached from two perspectives. First, the BCA is interested in *schools attended,* academic *grades* achieved, and the client's own characterization of his *performance* within and across academic years. The BCA might usefully explore how the client responded to success and failure as well as how he appraises his performance in the structured academic setting and his general view of his achievement. Significant discrepancies between the client's capability and academic achievement should be followed up with careful questioning.

A second area involves the client's response to the *social environment of school,* in terms of his relationship with both teachers and peers. Problems in adjustment to the school setting are focused on with specific questioning. This category obviously overlaps with that of interpersonal history; the BCA may wish to combine the two categories and focus on academic as well as social functioning during *each* period of school life in the client's development.

Rationale and Comment. All individuals traverse the education process, and it may be important to learn how the client responded to the structure of the academic setting, dealt with success as well as failure experiences, and generally interacted both with persons in authority and peers. Often there is a significant relation between the client's functioning in the school and home environments. In many cases behavior problems, fears, and other poor life adjustments are first detected by teachers and staff in the academic system. In addition, the teacher and/or school counselor are among the persons most likely to be sought out as problems in living emerge, prior to the parents' or child's seeking out more formal psychological or psychiatric services.

The demands placed on the developing child forced to cope with changing school environments (e.g., single versus multiple-teacher situations), the manner in which he deals with social relationships and pubertal change vis-à-vis his peers, as well as his responses to situations calling for achievement, are among influences that have shaped the adult client's current behavior and response to his environment. More specifically the skill behaviors learned during this period may well predict the adult's responses to social and vocational demands. Finally, for the child or adolescent client, adjustment to the academic setting may itself become a focus for intervention.

Sexual Development

Sexual development may be defined broadly as a *description of the client's sexual behavior* with opposite or same sex persons extending from the client's earliest sexual arousal and masturbatory experiences to his present sexual experiences.

Rationale and Comment. While it is obvious that this category would be explored in detail when the client presents a problem having to do with current sexual relationships or functioning, many writers have suggested that the sexual area be explored as an ordinary part of the case history. Houck and Hansen (1972) make the point: "One most important area which is far too often ignored is the history of sexual development. Because sexuality is such a pervasive and integral part of life, it demands detailed exploration" (p. 156). They suggest that sexual information provides useful insights into the client's development of a social role, and may be related to the client's present view of himself. While a sexual history is particularly important for some psychodynamic orientations, many other BCAs find that marital problems as well as problems in interpersonal functioning can often be related to the client's expectations for his own sexual behavior, as well as his current sexual functioning. Unfortunately, interviewers as well as clients often experience discomfort in discussing sexual behavior, so that most writers recommend that this topic area be handled in a matter-of-fact fashion and "without evidence of morbid curiosity" (Hauck and Hansen, 1972, p. 156). Chapter 3 presents some questioning strategies (e.g., the use of a progression of questions) that may be useful.

Occupational History

Virtually every case history format includes a gathering of information regarding *characteristics and dates of employment*, the client's *attitude toward his work*, his *occupational goals*, and the *plans* he has to meet those goals. An important focus is on the client's explanation of difficulties in the job situation or reasons for termination of employment, and his ability to get along with authority figures and peers. Occupational preferences or experiences that are not congruent with the client's abilities and current skills should be explored carefully, as well as any specific problems the client experiences in his work. This information is particularly relevant when the BCA is providing the client with vocational counseling. In this case a more comprehensive occupational history may be necessary.

Rationale and Comment. Just as the child or adolescent spends much of his waking time in the academic setting, the adult must prepare for a particular vocation, seek out employment, maintain a pattern of work behavior, and perhaps advance himself in his occupation. In addition, the employee must respond to work related traditions and regulations and to persons in authority while adjusting to the interpersonal demands of working with others in an often competitive situation. The client's response to these demands is a rich source of information. Writing from a psychiatric perspective, Thorne (1955) states: "The work record is one of the most important indicies of mental health. Mentally unhealthy persons are the last to be hired and first to be fired. A history of frequent job changes, discontent or inability to get adjusted should be regarded as a danger signal indicating personality problems" (p. 126). Behavioral excesses, deficits, or other categories of inappropriate behavior may well be reflected in the client's adjustment to the job situation. In addition, many clients find it easier to discuss life information (e.g., finances, interpersonal problems) within a vocational history than in isolation.

Methodological Issues

The BCA must choose from the foregoing categories those that provide information useful in understanding the client's current behavior and in planning intervention. In doing so, it is obvious that certain categories may not apply to particular clients. Thus, for the child or adolescent, the parent may serve as informant, providing detailed history across birth, developmental, medical, family, interpersonal, and educational categories. Other categories may or may not apply depending on the age and experience of the young client. In contrast, the BCA may wish to collect case history information *directly* from the adolescent client, perhaps comparing these data with similar information obtained from the parent or relevant others. Depending on the adolescent's age and experience, a sexual as well as occupational history might be included. For the adult, all categories are potentially relevant, and it is up the the BCA to explore in detail the categories that will most probably provide information useful in understanding the client's present behavior. Given the selection of particular categories to be explored in the history, the BCA is confronted with the task of deciding on methods for obtaining this information.

Organization of the History

The BCA must decide the order in which the various categories will be entertained.

Within-Category Approach. One approach is to investigate a given category from the client's earliest recollections to the present time *prior* to proceeding to another category. Taking education as an example, the BCA might explore each educational experience encountered by the client (e.g., dates and academic and social adjustment for each school attended) up to the client's present situation. This might include a detailed account extending from preschool or "nursery" experiences through high school or undergraduate college training. A major advantage of this approach is that the client is encouraged to maintain a consistent "set" for discussing his educational experiences, and this focus is not altered until all relevant information in this area is reported. In addition, the interviewer is in a better position to discriminate consistent patterns characterizing a client's response to this life area and can ensure comprehensive and detailed coverage. A drawback to this approach is that the client is continually forced to shift his attention and memory to different life periods within each category assessed.

Developmental-Unit Approach. An alternative approach that eliminates this drawback is to compartmentalize the client's life into a series of developmental units (e.g., preschool, grammar school, high school, college, post-college, present) and explore all relevant information categories *within each developmental unit* prior to proceeding to the next developmental period. Thus, within the "grammar school" unit, the client would be asked to provide information across categories such as medical history, family history, and interpersonal adjustment, as well as his educational experiences. While requiring numerous shifts of focus as questions explore various categories of life history, this approach permits the client to offer comprehensive recollections about a particular period of his life prior to moving to a later period that may be easier to recall. Also the interviewer may be in a better position to determine the interrelationships of the various aspects of the client's life *within* temporal periods (e.g., how did a family move affect educational or interpersonal adjustment?).

Open-Ended Approach. A final approach uses an open-ended format to instigate the client to talk about his past history. For example: "I would like to learn something of your past history as this will help me to understand some of your present concerns and also give me an opportunity to know you a bit better. What aspect of your past life stands out for you? . . . Perhaps that's a place where we could begin."

The interviewer elicits comprehensive information within the category the *client* offers, then encourages the client to move on to other self-stated categories of interest. While this approach places responsibility on the client to take an active role in the interview and reveals aspects of the life history that the client finds particularly meaningful, it is possible that certain information may not be revealed by the client. To avoid the discomfort attendant on discussing personal information that violates certain taboos or other social norms (e.g., in a sexual history) or is unpleasant for other reasons (e.g., provokes anxiety because of previous aversive experiences), the client may avoid discussing categories that might be useful in understanding his present behavior. While the interviewer obviously cannot force a client to reveal any information beyond his free choice, a more structured interview format requiring the client to address all major areas of his life may elicit a response that would otherwise not be offered. The fact that the interviewer asks questions about these "difficult" areas may communicate to the client that it is "okay" to discuss them, that the interviewer will not be offended or think less of the client.

While each of these three formats address the same historical categories, it is clear that they differ significantly in the organization and order with which categories are addressed.

In the first interviews, the BCA should evaluate how the client seems to respond differentially to questions varying in structure provided for a response (e.g., open-ended versus focused questions), and the client's ability to organize his account of current problems or concerns. Clients able to handle the open-ended, less structured format in an organized, comprehensible fashion (and who seem to prefer this approach) might be offered the "open-ended" case history format, while those who cannot do it easily should probably not be assessed in this way. Once this discrimination is made, choosing between the "within-category" or "developmental-unit" approaches depends most on the interviewer's style and preferred manner of organizing case materials.

Questioning Strategies

Within each category, the BCA should ensure that approximate dates of occurrence and characteristics of reported phenomena are obtained (e.g., "What was the first position you held? Could you tell me exactly what job you performed? Roughly what were the dates of your employment and how long did you hold that position? Why did you leave that job?"), as well as the client's own response to reported phenomena, (e.g., "When your mom and dad used to fight, what would you do? How did you handle that?"; "You mentioned that you had a hard time adjusting to junior high school. *Can you tell me how* you handled that?"; "When toilet training Billy, *how* did you and your husband approach that? What did you do?"). I tend to emphasize the open questions described previously, letting the client provide a behavioral description of his adjustment to responses in the situations described. This provides the BCA with detailed information regarding the manner in which the client approached a variety of persons and situations in his past. This behavior, as it unfolds and changes over time, may provide a useful background for understanding the client's current responses to phenomena in his environment.

Often it is useful to inquire about the attractiveness of particular phenomena (e.g., "In your classes in junior high school, which subjects did you like best ... which least?"; "You mentioned that there were certain kids that you didn't get along with very well in high school. Could you describe them for me?"; "Of the jobs that you've had, which did you find most satisfying ... least satisfying?"). This information provides some notion of the characteristics of those persons, situations, or objects that the client seeks out or avoids. Such information may be useful in defining positive and negative consequences to be capitalized upon in changing his current behavior. Finally, many writers find it useful to explore the problems and concerns experienced by the client in describing certain life history phenomena, as well as unusual behaviors or feelings experienced (e.g., "You mentioned you had a hard time in making dates during high school. *What were your concerns in that situation?* What was hard for you?"; "*What were the problems*, if any, you experienced in getting along with the guys [in high school, in a job described]?"; "*Could you describe any problems* you and your wife experienced during the first year of marriage?"). The reader should note that each of the questions in the examples above leads the respondent to provide a verbal description of the designated behavior, rather than a mere "yes" or "no" response. In a case history, it is desirable to emphasize open questions (see Chapter 3), so that the client describes events in his own words. This provides a much better opportunity for the BCA to observe the client's behavior as such information is described. Also, if the BCA's questions are too structured, it is easy for the client to avoid certain anxiety-provoking or embarrassing categories (e.g., Interviewer: "Any sexual problems in your marriage?"; Interviewee: "No").

The Autobiographical Approach

Another way of collecting case history information or augmenting the case history interview is to ask the client to write an account of his life in a systematic or open-ended way. In the systematic approach (called the "time graph" by Brammer and Shostrum, 1968), the client is asked to provide written information regarding specific aspects of his past history that are prelisted in a written inventory and often organized in time-sequential fashion. In the open-ended autobiographical approach, no specific topics are outlined, and the client is free to develop his own style in presenting the content that he wishes to share with the BCA. A major advantage of the autobiographical approach is that the BCA obtains information regarding aspects of the past history that the client wishes to present. The manner in which the client describes himself (e.g., in a socially desirable fashion) may be illustrative of the client's current view of himself and surroundings and/or the way he wishes others to view him. A major problem, of course, is that the BCA may be faced with a disorganized, perhaps sketchy account of the client's life, without the advantage of being able to probe verbally certain significant areas or to observe the client's behavior as his life history is recounted. Perhaps the autobiography could usefully precede a case history interview, serving to provide suggestions to the BCA regarding aspects of the client's history that might be emphasized and perhaps probed more deeply in the interview format.

Footnotes

[1] A thorough reading of Sullivan's classic, *The Psychiatric Interview*, provides a nice foundation and in some cases counterpoint for the material that follows.

[2] Sullivan rather interestingly de-emphasizes the often-employed educational history, believing that educational progress is frequently determined by a combination of "foresight and blind ambition on the part of the parents, wealthy relatives, as well as the patient" (p. 75).

UNIT II-B Written Methods

WRITTEN SELF-REPORT METHODS

Paper-and-pencil self-reports of the client's overt or covert behavior continue to hold a prominent place when BCAs are asked to list assessment instruments they frequently employ. This approach requires the client to self-generate the data for assessment by responding to typically structured written stimuli. Responses are then scored and in some cases "interpreted" to reveal some presumably important aspects of the client's behavior; however, the means by which conclusions are drawn vary considerably across theoretical orientations of BCAs. Perhaps paper-and-pencil instruments have remained in vogue for so long because they are economical to administer and frequently provide the BCA with a "place to start" in outlining an assessment strategy.

This chapter will focus on the use of paper-and-pencil instruments to assess the client's phenomenological view of his behavior and life situation. In line with the goals of this text paper-and-pencil approaches to the assessment of personality traits, intellectual functioning, abilities, or interests will be omitted. Two excellent textbooks are recommended to the interested reader (Cronbach, 1970; Wiggins, 1973).

One means of categorizing a written self-report instrument is to define the degree of structure provided for the written responses to items. While a highly structured instrument might require a simple "yes" or "no" to indicate agreement or disagreement with a series of statements, a less structured approach might permit open-ended or free responses (e.g., in the respondent's "own words"). A client, for example, might be asked to describe one or more of the problems that caused him to come to the clinical setting, to write an autobiography, or to answer an open-ended question that explores some content area of interest (e.g., "Would you please describe your view of marriage?"; "What is your philosophy of child rearing?...Please use as many pages as you feel are necessary"). Obviously the instructions would vary as a function of particular assessment goals and the client's ability to express himself in writing.

Compared to other methods for obtaining the self-report, written methods seem to offer the following advantages. First, as with more structured forms of interviews, the client's responses can be directed to a standard theme or content area of relevance (e.g., social skills, child rearing, vocational goals) and recorded in a format that facilitates scoring. Second, in contrast to the interview, the client *directly* translates his responses into a written record, thus reducing ambiguity in encoding the response. As with any self-report approach, ambiguity of response is increased as the instructions permit a less-structured response. In contrast, more structured written formats may provoke highly discrete, unambiguous data (e.g., numerical ratings, yes-or-no responses), and this information may be sufficiently reduced to permit direct scanning of response sheets for computer analysis, thus dramatically reducing the BCA's coding/summarization activities. Third, many of these instruments have been standardized (e.g., norms have been established), and the results of assessments of reliability and validity studies are frequently reported.

Following a presentation of methods, a discussion of criteria by which the BCA may evaluate the usefulness of a written self-report instrument will be discussed along with certain issues that should be considered in employing such data for decision making.

Assessment Methods

Free Response Measures

While the written stimulus may vary from an open-ended question to an incomplete sentence, this approach permits the client to make relatively unrestricted written responses. Free response measures are often employed to obtain the client's initial description of the referral problem or other life events as a prelude to more formal assessment procedures. One of the advantages of this format is that it provides the BCA with an inexpensively gathered account of the topic area *as the client perceives it,* devoid of the structure and demand characteristics present in the ongoing interview. Regardless of the accuracy of the client's self-report in terms of independent criteria (e.g., convergence with the reports of other persons, observational data, or interview findings), a written self-statement may yield useful information regarding the client's style of communication, his general vocabulary level (often a useful predictor of intelligence), the organization of his cognitive processes, and other items that may be capitalized on as the clinical assessment becomes more focused. In addition, the written format may provoke much different responses than those made to similar verbal probes in the interview, given that the client has time to consider and reflect upon each response without the pressure of having to reply at once. In fact, written responses may provide "leads" that can be followed up or "probed" more extensively in succeeding interviews.

A more structured example of the open-ended approach is the *paper-and-pencil analogue* (Nay, 1977), which requires the respondent to describe how he would behave in response to certain situations that might ordinarily occur in his environment. For example, an analogue aimed at assessing a client's assertive skills might present the following scene and instructions.

Situation: You are standing in line in a supermarket when a rather loud and aggressive man pushes in ahead of you without saying a word. Please write down what you would do and/or say in response to this situation.

The client could be given a variety of instructional sets to guide his responses (e.g., "respond as you actually would if this were to happen to you today," "respond as you would *ideally* like to respond") depending on assessment goals.

Most free response instruments are devised around the specific needs of a particular setting, and few are published for general use. Perhaps the most widespread exception is the sentence-completion format, which provides the respondent with a sentence stem (partial sentence) and asks him to complete the sentence as he sees fit. Frequently employed as a projective test for personality assessment, sentence-completion measures can be subjectively or empirically scored. The Michigan Sentence Completion Test (in Kelly and Fisher, 1951), for example, consists of 100 incomplete sentences relating to numerous areas of one's life situation, such as self, parental figures, likes, dislikes, authority, and aspirations. The test is frequently used with parents of problem children. Sample items include: "The thing about my home———"; "Because of Mom, I ———"; "I despise ———". Kelly and Fisher (1951) administered the sentence completions to both parents in order to determine the degree of discrepancy between their perceptions and attitudes of the problem child.

While numerous sentence-completion tests are available, few offer standard scoring criteria for responses. This points to a major problem of free response measures: How are free form, idiosyncratic responses to be scored or summarized to yield information useful to assessment goals? One approach is to administer the instrument to large, highly defined client populations to determine normative responses. Another approach is to submit responses to a panel of "expert" judges who then sort responses into particular categories of relevance (e.g., high vs. low aggression, high vs. low parental control). Based on the judges' categorization of particular responses (consistent placement across multiple judges), a scoring manual can be developed that prelists potential responses by category. The BCA may then tabulate the frequency with which each client's responses fall into particular categories or the proportion of each category response to total responses made (e.g., "35 percent of responses are categorized as high parental control"). A more limited approach would be to score protocols using a purely face-validity approach—in what category does it appear this response should be placed, based on what I know about child rearing?

While useful as a preliminary screening device to direct the BCA's efforts to particular problem areas, the free response format leaves much to be desired when employed as the sole assessment method.

Checklists

Perhaps best typified by the problem checklist, this approach asks the respondent to indicate presence, absence, or agreement (via a check mark, a yes or no) in response to a fixed set of stimulus items. Although checklists have long been employed in the medical sphere (Davie, Butler, and Goldstein, 1972), they have only recently become prominent in clinical assessment. Using the parent-child relationship as an example, parents might be presented with an array of problematic behaviors and asked to endorse whether or not these behaviors are a problem for their offspring. The Louisville Behavior Checklist (Miller, Hampe, Barrett, and Noble, 1971), for instance, requires the parent to respond in a yes-or-no fashion to such items as: "cries easily over little things," "shockingly cruel with animals or people," "has habits such as picking or hitting her (his) fingernails, twisting her (his) hands, rubbing her (his) eyes, pulling her (his) hair," and "frequently complains of headaches." The instrument is self-administered and comes in two forms, one for girls and one for boys. In this particular case, reliability and factor analysis data have been reported by the authors.

Obviously, such data might be evaluated in terms of face validity or more formally scored, and would be most amenable to any kind of statistical analysis. Major advantages include: checklists are self-administered and can be readily scored using computer scanning formats or response keys for hand scoring; they provide discrete, readily interpretable information to a standard set of stimuli within and across clients; and normative, validity, and reliability data are often reported. In addition, a checklist is relatively easy to construct and can be adapted to virtually any assessment question where the BCA has determined the domain of potential responses in advance.

Rating Approaches

In contrast to the checklist, the rating approach requires more than a mere yes-no or presence-absence response. Instead, the client is asked to rate the stimulus item along some dimension of interest (e.g., degree of agreement, intensity, "relevance to me"). Thus, in response to the stimulus "my son (daughter) engages in temper tantrums," the respondent might be required to rate the degree of intensity of the tantrum behavior, given its occurrence. Such ratings permit the respondent to make fine discriminations within the dimension of interest, which a checklist does not permit. Such discriminations may be most useful in assessing therapeutic change. For example, prior to as well as following treatment, a parent might feel compelled to respond "yes" to a statement regarding temper tantrums ("Are temper tantrums a problem?"), because the child still engages in the behavior at some level of frequency. In contrast, the rating approach permits the parent to denote whether or not the intensity of the tantrum, its frequency, or some other dimension of interest has in fact changed, given its continued occurrence, and this information might be useful in evaluating therapeutic efficacy (e.g., direction of change, differential degree of change across problem behavior targets).

As might be imagined, many variants of the rating scale exist. For example, the Likert scaling method presents the respondent with a statement (e.g., "I prefer indoor activities to outdoor activities"), and asks him to indicate the degree to which he agrees with the item by responding on a scale ranging from definite disagreement to definite agreement. Within the original Likert format, the respondent might be provided with seven possible categories, each reflecting some degree of agreement with the statement (strongly agree, agree, slightly agree, uncertain, slightly disagree, disagree, strongly disagree), and asked to circle the response that most accurately reflects his view. Each of the potential responses is then assigned a number for scoring purposes (e.g., strongly disagree = 1, strongly agree = 7), so that a total agreement score for each category of statements can be determined by adding numerical acores across items in that category. Pfeiffer and Heslin (1973) point out that investigators have moved away from employing the middle category ("uncertain" or "unsure") because it permits the respondent to avoid committing himself. They propose an alternative set of four responses (disagree; unsure, probably disagree; unsure, probably agree; agree) to increase the interpretability of findings. The authors state: "Even though his uncertainty is acknowledged, the respondent is asked to indicate which way he tips slightly. On the other hand, if he is sure of his reaction he can indicate that his conviction is sure" (p. 34). Other variants of the Likert approach include seven, five, or three items, with the extremes as well as the midpoint of the scale anchored by defining statements, so that the respondent is aware of the range within which he makes his reponses.

While degree of agreement is frequently employed, almost any dimension of interest could be presented to the respondent, with ratings made and scored by preassigning numbers to each of the potential points along the scale. For example, the Symptom Check List (SCL) developed by Patterson, Cobb, and Ray (1973) is employed with children ranging in age from six to fourteen years who are classified as "aggressive" or "out of control." The parent respondent is required not only to endorse whether or not a particular problem category is of concern in typical checklist fashion, but also to rate the degree of desirability of the child's behavior on a seven-point scale ranging from "extremely undesirable" to "extremely desirable." The behavior categories include: "anxiety," "destructive," "defiant," bizarre behavior," and "delusions or hallucinations." In addition the parent is asked to estimate the current frequency of occurrence for each category following the rating. This rating scheme supplements information gathered using behavior observation methods within the home proper.

As another example, the Marriage-Adjustment Schedule (Burgess, Locke and Thomes, 1971) requires both husband and wife to rate a series of predefined characteristics of a well-adjusted marriage. The respondent's agreement with questions in each category is assessed. An example item, with the weighted score for that item in parenthesis, is shown below.

To what extent were you in love with your spouse before marriage?
"Head over heels" (8)
Very much   (7)
Somewhat   (6)
A little   (5)
Not at all   (4)

As might be imagined, this schedule, employed as a diagnostic instrument, may help the BCA to identify areas where difficulties exist within a distressed marriage.

Using the Likert (category) approach, it is important that each potential response be defined operationally in precise, behavioral language. While each numerical point may not be described or "anchored," it is most important to anchor the ends and midpoint of such a scale, so that the respondent is clearly apprised of the meaning of the numbers. For example, if a client were rating the degree of anxiety he experiences in standing before an audience on the following scale, he might be confused as to what each of the numbers means.

       1   2   3   4   5
      Low   High
    Anxiety   Anxiety

The words used to define the numbers in this scale are obviously very imprecise and poorly define the experience to be rated. Given a similar grouping of "anxious" clients, there would probably be much variability across raters since each could conceivably view the "low" versus "high" anxiety designation in a different way. As the anchors become more operationally defined, the BCA can be more assured that the scale's numbers (ratings) have a similar meaning for all respondents. Then differences in clients' scores can be attributed to real individual differences across clients, rather than to the scale's ambiguity (method variance). The following scale defines anxiety in terms of muscle tension.

1	2	3	4	5
Little Anxiety		Moderate Anxiety		High Anxiety
(muscles loose)		(muscles somewhat tight)		(muscles very tight)

As an alternative to the Likert-style rating scale, the Graphic Rating Scale (Guilford, 1954; Wiggins, 1973) presents the respondent with a geometric representation of the dimensions to be rated. Several descriptions that serve to anchor various points along the dimension are placed beneath a straight line and the respondent is asked to make a rating by placing a mark on the line.

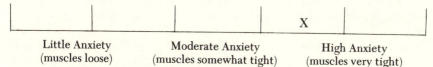

Little Anxiety	Moderate Anxiety	High Anxiety
(muscles loose)	(muscles somewhat tight)	(muscles very tight)

Rather than limiting the respondent to a finite number of possible ratings along the dimension, the continuous scale, a variant of the Graphic Rating Scale, provides the respondent with an unbroken line and asks him to make a check or mark on the line at *any point* to indicate his rating. An example of this scale appears below.

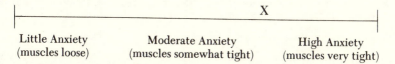

Little Anxiety	Moderate Anxiety	High Anxiety
(muscles loose)	(muscles somewhat tight)	(muscles very tight)

With this last approach the respondent's potential rating is limited only by the length of the line (representing the dimension of interest). As the reader might imagine, the BCA determines the client's rating by measuring the distance from one end of the dimension (usually the low extreme) to the point at which the respondent makes his endorsement, and this distance is then translated into a numerical rating. For example, given a line of five inches which is arbitrarily divided into 100 units, an endorsement made exactly two inches from the left (low) end of the scale translates into a rating of 40 units. The major advantage of this approach is that it provides the respondent with increased flexibility for indicating his rating and detects rather subtle discrepancies from the end and middle points so often endorsed when a Likert scale is employed. Thus, a respondent who might avoid taking a stand by checking off the midscore (3) on a five-point Likert rating scale, is forced to respond unequivocally to a less structured situation, and even a small degree of discrepancy from the middle point may reflect a directionality of the opinion, attitude, or description of some phenomenon of interest to him. (Obviously, slight discrepancies from the midpoint may also indicate a client's sloppiness in making his rating or certain perceptual-motor biases on the respondent's part.)

One of the Likert-style rating scales most commonly employed in behavioral assessment is the Fear Survey Schedule or FSS (Wolpe and Lang, 1969; see Tasto, 1977), which is designed to assess client or subject responses to various items that have been found to provoke avoidant responses. The FSS describes objects and/or situations (ranging in number from 50 to 122) and asks the respondent to rate the degree of fear aroused by each item on a scale ranging from 1 to 5 or 1 to 7 (5 or 7 indicating highest level of fear). A total "fear" score is obtained by summing numerical ratings across items; however, perusal of respondent ratings of individual categories is most useful for clinical assessment. Normative studies evaluating the responses of large samples of subjects across divergent settings have consistently shown higher fear scores for women than men (Lawlis, 1971; Tasto and Hickson, 1970). Factor analysis of a 122-item version of the FSS (Rubin, Lawlis, Tasto, and Namenek, 1969) identified five conceptually pure factors, including: (1) fears related to small animals, (2) fears of the precipitators and manifestations of hostility, (3) primitive moralistic and sexual fears, (4) fears of isolation and loneliness, and (5) fears of anatomical destruction and physical pain. The authors found that only 40 items were necessary to tap each of these five factors optimally; thus they modified the original FSS considerably. In addition, several investigators have assessed reliability and concurrent and construct validity by correlating FSS scores with data obtained using other measures of emotionality and fear (see Tasto, 1977).

The Semantic Differential

In order to evaluate the affective meaning that persons ascribe to various objects in their environment (e.g., groups, organizations, people, practices), Osgood, Suci, and Tannenbaum (1957) had large numbers of subjects employ bipolar adjective scales (e.g., good/bad, fast/slow, hard/soft) to rate a wide variety of concepts. In a substantial number of studies three factors—*evaluation* (clean/dirty, valuable/worthless, good/bad), *potency* (large/small, strong/weak, heavy/light), and *activity* (active/passive, fast/slow, noisy/quiet)—emerged as the major categories of affective meaning across a wide variety of raters, scales, concepts, and even across divergent cultures. In most Semantic Differential (SD) scales used for clinical assessment purposes, some or all of the bipolar adjectives within the evaulation dimension are employed to rate an object or concept (sweet/sour, beautiful/ugly, tasteful/distasteful, kind/cruel, pleasant/unpleasant, bitter/sweet, happy/sad, sacred/profane, nice/awful, good/bad, clean/dirty, valuable/worthless, fragrant/foul, honest/dishonest, fair/unfair). The scale between the adjective pairs may be numbered from 1 to 7, or is sometimes numbered –3 to +3. In any case, for scoring purposes ratings are often given a positive number designation (e.g., –3 = 1; +3 = 7) since minus numbers are more difficult to deal with statistically.

Below is a sample SD item used to assess student trainees' views of institutions to which they were assigned.

1. *A mental health institution is:*
Good: ____:____:____:____:____:____:____: Bad
Ugly: ____:____:____:____:____:____:____: Beautiful
Clean: ____:____:____:____:____:____:____: Dirty
Belligerent: ____:____:____:____:____:____:____: Peaceful

Note that adjective pairs are systematically reversed in terms of direction (positive versus negative evaluation score) to ensure that the respondent is accurately reading and rating each dimension rather than responding haphazardly by marking all ratings at one end of the scale without regard to direction. For scoring purposes, the numbers beneath each point on the scale would yield the respondent's scale score, with all scores across the bipolar scales added to yield the total evaluative score. An example is given below.

Good: ____:____:____:____:____:____:____: Bad
    (7) (6) (5) (4) (3) (2) (1)

Ugly: ____:____:____:____:____:____:____: Beautiful
    (1) (2) (3) (4) (5) (6) (7)

Clean: ____:____:____:____:____:____:____: Dirty
    (7) (6) (5) (4) (3) (2) (1)

Belligerent: ____:____:____:____:____:____:____: Peaceful
    (1) (2) (3) (4) (5) (6) (7)

The concepts or objects rated using the Semantic Differential have ranged from parent assessments of their children's behavior (Patterson, Cobb, and Ray, 1973) to ratings of snakes made by "snake-phobic" persons (Bandura, Blanchard, and Ritter, 1969; Lira, Nay, McCullough, & Etkin, 1975). Persons, objects, statements, or other phenomena that could potentially be rated using the Semantic Differential format are limited only by the BCA's creativity and the specific assessment question.

Idiosyncratic Rating Schemes

In some cases a highly idiosyncratic rating system is constructed by the BCA and client to assess some dimension of relevance to the client's treatment goals. For example, the client could systematically rate the intensity of a targeted behavior prior to, during, and following treatment as well as at follow-up periods. The subjective degree of discomfort or SUDS approach developed by Wolpe (1973) is an excellent example. The client subjectively rates his fear of some object (snakes, social situations, etc.) on a scale from 0 to 100 SUDS units. Points along the dimension are anchored using behavioral referents of the target following a discussion between client and BCA. Such behavioral anchors are highly specific, very discrete, and explicit. The continuous scale that follows might be employed to assess a client's anxiety as carefully defined by behavioral referents consistently present when the client reports "anxiety."

00	50	100
Muscles loose; heartrate not noticeable; breathing unrestricted; palms dry	Muscles moderately tight, particularly the back; heartrate slightly noticeable; respiration rate somewhat elevated; palms moist	Muscles very tight, particularly back and neck; heart pounding; respiration very shallow; palms very wet

This scale, derived prior to treatment by requiring the client to focus carefully on his body when anxiety-arousing stimuli are presented (*in vivo* or imaginally), can now be employed as a measure of behavior change and permits the BCA to evaluate quantitatively the course of self-reported anxiety within treatment. Any one of the previously described rating formats could form the basis of idiosyncratic ratings.

A more formal approach to idiosyncratic ratings is Goal Attainment Scaling (GAS), devised by Kiresuk and Sherman (1968). The GAS provides the BCA with five scales on which each of five separate behaviors "targeted" for change can be listed. For each target scale, the BCA (and optionally the client) defines at least three behavioral anchors that describe possible outcomes of intervention ranging from "most unfavorable" to "best anticipated." Each point on the target scale is assigned a letter (A–E) so that behavior change can be defined by attainment of specific outcomes (as defined by the assigned letter) as treatment progresses. An example of a completed GAS scale, designed for a drug-addicted client, is shown in Figure 5-1.

	1/14/78 Difficulty making social contact with nonaddicts	1/14/78 Heroin	1/14/78 Unable to identify problems	1/16/78 Employment	1/16/78 Group Participation
Most Unfavorable Treatment Outcome Thought Likely (A)	His only friends are heroin users.	Continues to use heroin—next 4 urinalyses all show heroin use.	Says, "I have no problems; there is nothing specific wrong in my life," or equivalent.	Makes no effort to get a job.	Will not speak in group sessions for next month.
Less Than Expected Success With Treatment (B)	Tries to renew or establish contact with nonaddicts once or twice, but does not follow through.		Says within 4 sessions, "I feel like things have improved," but can't identify what or why.	Meets once with prospective employer, but does not follow through.	Will not volunteer anything in groups but will answer direct questions.
Expected Level Of Treatment Success (C)	Although most friends are still addicts, he spends about an hour a week with a "straight friend."	Will have 2 of the next 4 urines clean of heroin.	Is able to identify at least 1 problem area within 4 counseling sessions.	Gets a job and keeps it for 3–4 weeks.	Will volunteer at least one comment per group.
More Than Expected Success With Treatment (D)			Can identify 1 or 2 problems and states general intention to change them.		
Best Anticipated Success With Treatment (E)	Sees at least 2 straight friends regularly for 4 or more hours per week.	All of the next 4 urines will be clean of heroin.	Can identify 2 or more problems and suggest specific ways to work on changing them.	Stays on the job for 8 weeks, reports that he does work well and enjoys it.	Speaks freely in groups, makes several comments each session.
	Ⓐ B C D E	A B C D E (circled A)	A B Ⓑ C D E	Ⓐ B C D E	A B Ⓑ C D E

Figure 5-1

GAS scale for drug-addicted client.

This scale was completed during initial assessment as client and BCA were able to define goals. A first priority goal agreed on by client and BCA has to do with "heroin" usage. Using behaviorally specific language, three levels of potential outcomes are carefully described. The circled "A" at the bottom of the "heroin" target scale shows that at the time of assessment this client was experiencing the most unfavorable outcome ("continues to use heroin"). At preagreed-upon times during the course of intervention, client and therapist evaluate whether or not desirable behavior change has occurred (movement up the scale from A = most unfavorable to B, C, D, or E as defined by the client's behavior). The following guidelines for writing behavioral objectives (McCullough, 1973) are based on a previous GAS manual constructed by Putnam, Kiesler, Bent, and Stewart (1972) for use by student therapists in a mental health agency.

The basic rule of GAS construction is that the therapist write in goal levels for each scale in language that is concise, clear, and behavioral. So often goals are talked about in abstract terms which imply different meanings to different people. For example, to say that at the end of treatment a client should have a "better marriage" is not a clear behavioral description. "Better" can mean many different things depending on the user. If you want to know more clearly what is meant by "better marriage," you have to determine what specific things the individual will be doing in regard to his spouse, and these can be many. Thus, a more behavioral description of this same goal might be any one or all of the following: (1) "mutually satisfactory sexual relations at least three times a week," (2) "spends at least a half-hour each day conversing with each other alone," (3) helps the wife with some chore at least three times a week," and so on.

You will notice that the more specific and detailed the description of a particular goal—that is, the less abstract, more concrete it becomes—the easier it is for the reader to *visualize* the client actually doing something. This is the first principle of valid GAS descriptions—*they must be written in such a way that their meaning is clear and unambiguous to any reader*, so they point to actions by the client which the reader can visualize. The second principle of GAS descriptions is that they *include some count, frequency, or amount of time within which client behaviors occur.* A client, then, must "do something" so many times, "not do something" for some period of time, "do something so many times in a certain period, etc. If counselors adhere to these two basic rules of GAS descriptions the resulting GAS forms can function as objective and reliable measuring devices. As a consequence, at any moment in time several judges can observe (directly or through analysis of factual records) what the client has accomplished in regard to each goal, and these several judges can independently arrive at the identical rating (A, B, C, D, or E) of progress [pp. 9–10].

Finally, Putnam et al. (1972) offer a quick summary of the guidelines for GAS scaling offered by Kiresuk and Sherman (1968).

1. Never fill in less than *three* scales (columns) on the GAS form.
2. For any given scale, you must fill in descriptions of at least three levels.

3. You must have more than one problem or goal on each scale. Each scale must limit itself to a single problem.
4. Don't use abbreviations or catch phrases which another later scorer will not understand. Don't scribble.
5. Don't list goals that are too general to be useful. Goals should be behaviorally specific.
6. Avoid vague goals like "get my head together" or "learn to relate to people."
7. Don't list goals that cannot be told apart, one level from another.
8. Keep follow-up scores in mind. List goals based on data you are sure can be located.
9. There should be no "expected" levels which are so high that there is no possible "better than expected" level. Nor should there be "expected" goals which are so low there is no possible "less than expected" level.
10. You cannot list scales which go lower than "most unfavorable outcome thought likely" nor higher than "most favorable outcome thought likely."

Important Considerations in Selecting a Written Self-Report Instrument

Norms

In many cases it is important to be able to compare the endorsed problems, ratings, or other categories of self-report of a client or population of clients to some larger reference population. It may be diagnostically useful to know how a given client's total score or pattern of responding on an instrument like the Fear Survey Schedule compares with the responses of a population of demographically similar clients. Similarly, when a client completes a problem behavior or symptom checklist as an initial means of "screening" his problems and concerns, the BCA may wish to know if the scores within and across categories are within or beyond "normal" limits. Of course, it is difficult to define what "normal" is and many writers have ignored normality in favor of describing certain characteristics of abnormal behavior (e.g., Buss, 1966). While an individual with a shoe size of 12 is obviously abnormal from a purely statistical point of view, this bit of information would be useless to the BCA interested in evaluating that individual's ability to function effectively and with minimal discomfort in his environment. Obviously, then, the BCA can evaluate a client's responses using his personal judgment (clinical prediction) or base decisions exclusively on information collected using valid and reliable assessment instruments (statistical prediction). This controversy is not new (see Meehl, 1954; Holt, 1958; Wiggins, 1973). While statistical criteria have been found to be generally superior to clinical judgments in aiding the BCA to make successful predictions regarding a client's behavior, the controversy has by no means abated.

In summary, a norm provides a context or frame of reference from which the BCA may evaluate a client's responses. A given individual's responses to some instrument may be classified as statistically abnormal when norms are used, but this may hold little significance in terms of clinical considerations and must be evaluated in the light of other information obtained.

When a paper-and-pencil instrument is "normed," we mean that the instrument has been administered to a sufficiently large and well-defined population of persons for certain descriptive, statistical statements to be made regarding the distribution of responses. The degree of confidence we have in those statements depends on the size of the population to which the instrument was administered. For example, comparing our client's responses to norms established across a small sample of 25 persons might lead to erroneous conclusions. The average or mean responses of such a small group might be strongly influenced by the extreme scores of a very few respondents. Also, the scores could show high or low variability because of the criteria employed to select the sample, and this variability might bear little relation to the degree of variability in responses shown by the reference population at large. Variability in responding is usually expressed in terms of standard deviations (e.g., +2, -1) above or below the mean for the population, so that the BCA can know the degree to which a given response approximates the mean.

As the size of the normative sample is increased, the BCA can feel more secure in generalizing from that population's norms to his client's responses. In addition, the BCA should evaluate the extent to which the demographic characteristics of the targeted client (e.g., age, sex, socioeconomic level, number of years of education) compare with those same characteristics displayed by the reference population. The norm becomes less meaningful the more the client differs from the reference group. One measure of the utility of a set of norms is the number of different, well-defined, and sufficiently sampled reference populations for which normative information is provided.

Reliability

Paper-and-pencil self-report measures can be subjected to the same kinds of reliability assessments that might be employed to evaluate a personality test, interest inventory, or aptitude scale. Reliability may be assessed within three major categories: *internal consistency, stability,* and *generalizability,* as in the formulation of Cronbach, Glesser, Nanda, and Rajaratnam (1972), which views reliability as multiply determined across a number of dimensions the BCA may wish to generalize his findings to. These dimensions might include *occasions* (specific occasions within which the client completes the instrument), *persons* (persons to whom the instrument is administered), or *settings* (specific locations within which the client is asked to self-report some aspect of his behavior). A related and more thorough presentation of the rationale and methods of generalizability theory appears in Chapter 10 which focuses on the reliability assessment of observation instruments.

With regard to internal consistency, our goal is to assess the degree to which individual questions, statements to be rated, or other item dimensions within an instrument measure the same behavior or characteristic. Internal consistency is often assessed by correlating odd and even items or items in the first half with second-half items. Pfeiffer and Heslin (1975) describe internal consistency in terms of homogeneity of items.

If two statements are measuring the same thing, then as scores go up on one, they go up on the other; as they go down on one, they go down on the other. They vary together, or they are said to "co-vary." Homogeneity (all the same) is a characteristic of a good measure; if an instrument is purporting to measure a certain trait. . . . Scores of the various statements on the scale should vary together, although they should not vary together perfectly, as then we would have duplicate measures of exactly the same thing, and that would add no new information [p. 30].

A criterion of internal consistency does not necessarily apply to many instruments, particularly those of the checklist variety. Statements relating to a wide variety of problems and/or potential concerns would not be expected to show internal consistency unless all of the statements were related to some specific problem dimension (e.g., difficulty in social situations, child management problems). Even when the items present different aspects of the same core problem area, internal consistency might realistically remain quite low. For example, a problem checklist describing various categories of child problem behavior (a core theme) might include such items as "difficulty in getting them to go to bed" or "difficulty in getting him to clean his room." If the problems a client describes are quite specifically focused and there is little generalization across problem categories, we would expect little correlation in scores between the checklist items. In contrast, the rating scale or checklist purporting to measure some trait or dimension of personality is often refined using factor-analytic procedures (the items that tend to cluster together when correlational methods are employed) to produce scales for which each item contributes to measurement. In this case items would be expected to show internal consistency. In summary, then, the degree of internal consistency expected for a self-report instrument depends on the degree to which items within the instrument are selected to measure some core dimension or theme, as opposed to surveying a wide variety of discrete and perhaps mutually exclusive categories of life events.

With regard to stability, a self-report instrument is administered on several occasions to the same population of subjects. If scores vary considerably (given the presumption that the behavior or other phenomenon assessed should show stability over time), then the BCA may conclude that the respondent's endorsements are due more to guessing, chance or momentary factors, ambiguous wording of items, or other deficiencies of the instrument proper (method variance) than to characteristics of the client's life situation. The correlation coefficient is employed to measure the degree to which endorsements agree or converge across administrations. Particularly when instrument administrations occur in close temporal proximity, low or nonsignificant "test-retest" correlations indicate *either that* the instrument is unreliable for some of the reasons mentioned above, or that repondents *in fact* displayed considerable variability across time in the problems/concerns tapped by the instrument, perhaps due to situational events in their life environments. Pfeiffer and Heslin (1975) note that correlation coefficients of $r = .85$ or higher are generally reported to be acceptable in the literature.

Validity

By validity we mean simply: Does an assessment instrument measure what it purports to measure? While internal consistency and test-retest reliability checks are frequently performed for self-report instruments, perhaps due to the ease with which such assessments can be made, it is unfortunate that validity data are rarely reported. Before discussing validity, it should be understood that validity and reliability are in fact related, in that a measure must show some moderate, acceptable degree of reliability to be useful for measuring a behavior category. Thus, validity is limited by reliability. In fact, the correlation between an instrument and an independent measure of the criterion (what the instrument is to measure) can never be higher than the square root of the correlation between two forms of the instrument (Cronbach, 1960). Thus, if reliability is .81, validity cannot exceed .90.

Each of the categories of validity will be discussed, with pertinent examples from the literature employed for illustration purposes.

Content Validity. By content or "face validity," we mean that the items chosen for inclusion within a self-report instrument seem to be related to the behavior category or dimension of interest because of their obvious content characteristics. Thus, "on the face of it," items such as "bedtime problems," "disobedience," "destructive behavior," "verbal and physical aggressiveness" are categories of behavior that might reasonably be included in a checklist or rating scale that attempts to assess parents' concerns about their "problem children." Obviously, the extent to which these categories validly represent the problems that parents actually experience in the natural environment depends on the BCA's knowledge of that environment. A popular self-report instrument employed in clinical assessment is the Reinforcement Survey

Schedule (Cautela and Kastenbaum, 1967), which employs a rating scale to assess respondents' preferences of various objects and activities potentially useful as incentives for client effort. Goldfried and Sprafkin (1976) criticize the content validity approach Cautela and Kastenbaum employed in selecting items for their "survey."

> The items within the survey were apparently generated on an *a priori* basis, reflecting what the authors believed would be reinforcing to various individuals. Had Cautela and Kastenbaum used an empirical approach in the construction of their measure, they would have undoubtedly discovered a number of items not included in the present survey, among which might have been such situations as pleasing a loved one, walking barefoot through the grass, or having one's back scratched [p. 307].

By an empirical approach, Goldfried and Sprafkin are suggesting that Cautela and Kastenbaum might have begun their item selection procedures by systematically sampling (perhaps via interviews) some large population of adults to determine the objects, activities, or thoughts most frequently reported as pleasurable. Or a large number of items could have been generated with the help of "experts" who have some knowledge of the behavior dimension of interest, and these items could then have been submitted to the subject sample of interest for initial preference ratings. As an adjunctive or alternative method, the subjects could have been systematically observed as a means of generating an item pool. Observing directly or via videotapes of subject behavior-in-setting, observer-judges could have defined the activities or objects that subjects most often selected.

Regardless of the method, the resulting pool of items frequently shown to be of positive value to this initial population (based on some *a priori* criteria, e.g., at least 50 percent endorse as very pleasurable) would then be included in the final instrument, perhaps after additional refinement (excluding very similar items, resubmitting the items to another population for ratings). These procedures for a "situational analysis" (Goldfried and Kent, 1972) are described in more detail in Chapter 7 as a means of selecting categories for an observation instrument.

Concurrent Validity. Another method of assessing validity is to *compare subjects' responses on the proposed instrument with their responses elicited by other assessment methods that presumably tap the same behavior dimension.* This method has frequently been employed in the validation of personality instruments, and the "goodness" of this approach obviously depends on the choice of "criterion" measures used for comparison. If the criterion measures are questionably valid, high intercorrelations between the proposed and criterion instruments may produce misleading or ambiguous results. The criteria employed within concurrent validation might be another self-report measure, direct observations, physiological responses, a score or product, or some other indicant of the behavior dimension of interest. Blunden, Spring, and Greenberg (1974), for example, assessed the concurrent validity of the Classroom Behavior Inventory (CBI), an instrument that purports to measure behaviors associated with children's hyperactivity in class. The authors correlated scores from each of seven factors derived from teachers' completion of the CBI with students' actual classroom behavior in each of the seven categories. The authors asked: If a child is rated by a teacher as being high on the CBI scale of "restlessness," will that child also show behavioral indicants of restlessness defined by independent observations? While the approach of these authors is laudable, unfortunately only one of the scales of the CBI was significantly correlated with classroom behavior, thus showing very limited concurrent validity for this instrument. A similar approach was employed by Johnson, Bolstad, and Lobitz (1976) for a home problem behavior rating scale endorsed by parents (Becker, 1960) and a school problem checklist completed by teachers (Walker, 1970). The authors found very low and nonsignificant correlations between the school behavior checklist and the percent of deviant behavior actually displayed by children in the school situation and between the home rating scale and deviant behavior displayed in the home proper. In explaining the low current validity for these two self-report instruments,[1] the authors pointed to the potential for significant error when a variety of different raters employ the same instrument:

The correlations should be examined with a full recognition of the considerable error variance that can be introduced by the use of different raters responding to the rating scale forms. It is known that the trained observers operate under highly similar response sets examining children's behavior, but it is to be expected that different parents and teachers approach rating scales with different reponse sets. This factor introduces considerable error variance in the scores obtained and would at least partially account for the low correlation obtained in other research where different raters were used [p. 170].

The authors are suggesting that the poor reliability with which parents and teachers employed the self-report measures may have limited the possibility for acceptable levels of concurrent validity. In validating an instrument, the BCA must be sure that variability in reponding attributable to unreliable use of that instrument (e.g., poor training of raters, lack of standard instructions) is held to a minimum so that the correlations obtained are relatively unconfounded by method variance and the results are interpretable.

The term "convergent validity" is often employed to describe concurrent validation: to the extent that these different measures of the same behavior dimension converge or correlate, the instrument would be said to display convergent validity. The term "discriminant validity" might be thought of as the opposite side of the coin. Here, measures that purport to assess behavior dimensions unrelated to the criterion behavior are correlated with the targeted instrument. The targeted instrument is said to exhibit discriminant validity if it fails to correlate significantly with the unrelated measure. It is obvious that an instrument that converges with similar instruments but *also* with instruments that measure other, unrelated behavior dimensions (failure to achieve discriminant validity), would be of questionable utility in predicting a client's behavior or placing him in a problem category.

The rationale behind assessing both convergent and discriminant validity is provided by the multitrait-multimethod validation procedure suggested by Campbell and Fiske (1959). Originally designed to assess the validity of certain measures of personality traits, this procedure sets up a matrix within which two or more different traits or behavior dimensions are assessed by two or more measures. The intercorrelation matrix clearly shows whether or not multiple measures that are supposed to measure the same trait converge while also showing little correlation with measures of some other trait (discriminant validity). A more thoroughgoing presentation of multimethod validation, as it relates to independent observational methods appears in Chapter 7. It should be noted that the procedures of convergent-discriminant validation are frequently employed as one means of defining the construct validity of an instrument.

Construct Validity. In some cases, items are selected for inclusion in an instrument because they are consonant with a theory or hypothesis about human behavior held by the constructor. Thus, in devising a self-report instrument that attempts to measure incidences as well as degree of fearful behavior displayed by some population of adults, a pool of initial items may be chosen purely for their content or face validity, but also inevitably reflect the constructor's assumptions of what constitutes "fearful" behavior. This is true even though the BCA has no formal theory of fearfulness and does not view fearfulness as a trait that shows generality across situations within which a person functions. While many BCAs are interested only in the empirical (statistically significant) and/or functional relationships of behavior to events within the environment, obviously the manner in which such data are collected, combined, and interpreted (e.g., when a child's behavior is labeled "disruptive," "aggressive," or "deviant") presupposes certain theoretical assumptions regarding *what* behavior does and does not characterize each of these designations. Without belaboring this issue further, I shall present some of the methods employed in construct validation.

One way of assessing the validity of a *construct* is to determine whether or not it enables the BCA to make certain predictions. Thus, a rating scale for parents that purports to measure child behavior problems should reasonably be able to discriminate between parents whose children display problematic behavior (e.g., at a rate and frequency sufficient to call them to the attention of the parents, teachers, or other persons in a supervisory role) and parents of children who do not behave in this way. Clearly, in selecting a "problematic" and a "normal" population of children the BCA has already made numerous assumptions regarding the nature of "problem" and "normal" behavior. This *group comparison* approach has frequently been employed as a measure of construct validity. For example, to assess the validity of Becker's (1960) Bipolar Adjective Checklist (a rating schedule consisting of 72 bipolar, seven-point ratings scales with pairs of adjectives defining the extremes, i.e., social/unsocial, happy/depressed, likes school/dislikes school), Lobitz and Johnson (1975) administered the instrument to 28 referred and 28 nonreferred control families. The referred or problem group consisted of families who had themselves instigated contact with a university psychology clinic for treatment of a child between the ages of four and eight years. The nonreferred families, each having a child within the age range of four to eight years, were carefully screened to ensure that the child had not been previously referred for behavior problems and had not at any time sought psychological or psychiatric treatment. The control families were carefully matched to the referred sample for age and sex of the targeted child, socioeconomic status of the parent, father absence or presence, number of siblings, and, for 20 of the cases, position of the targeted child in the family. The authors report that it was possible to achieve a close match between the two groups. Both parent groups completed the checklist and also permitted independent observers to view the family in the home as well as in a structured laboratory observation setting. Analyses of parents' checklist responses showed that the referred children were perceived as significantly less relaxed, more withdrawn-hostile, more aggressive, less intellectually sufficient, and more prone to conduct problems (the five scales of the Becker checklist) than the nonreferred children, attesting to the validity of this self-report instrument. Also, the referred children displayed a significantly greater proportion of deviant and high-intensity problematic behaviors than did the nonreferred children. Differences were also noted in the parents' responses to their children in the standardized laboratory situation. Thus, the authors' assumptions about the construct of "child deviance," as defined by the self-report and behavior measures described, was in fact validated for this population of subjects.

A similar approach was employed by Borkevec, Fleischmann, and Caputo (1973) in validating various measures of social anxiety within an analog laboratory situation. The authors found that 17 socially anxious and 17 socially nonanxious males, defined by a self-report instrument that measures anxiety and distress within the social situation (the Social Avoidance and Distress Scale, Watson and Friend, 1969), responded in a significantly different fashion when exposed to a stressful situation. In support of the authors' hypotheses, the high-anxious subjects reported greater anxiety and showed more physiological activity during the stress-evoking situation than did the low-anxious subjects. In addition, two of three behavior measures of social anxiety assessed each minute (number of words, number of overt anxiety signs, and number of speech disturbances) showed a strong trend toward differentiating the two groups in the predicted direction, although the differences were not statistically significant. The results thus provide some evidence attesting to the validity of this self-report measure.

Another means of assessing construct validity is to employ the multitrait (behavior)-multimethod approach already discussed. If an instrument in fact taps a behavioral construct of interest then it should show acceptable levels of convergent and discriminant validity.

Response Sets

One problem that has plagued the constructors of paper-and-pencil instruments is the possibility that self-reports may be colored by an expectancy or demand suggested by the situation of instrument administration or by other response biases the client brings with him. Among possible response sets that could bias one's responses, *social desirability* has perhaps been most frequently addressed in the literature (Crowne and Marlowe, 1964). This is the idea that certain individuals tend to respond in a socially desirable manner—in a sense, they "fake good." A number of instruments have been developed that attempt to assess a client's proclivity for responding in this way (Crowne and Marlowe, 1964; Gough, 1952; Edwards, 1957). In some cases, subject responses to a social desirability scale (which often presumes social desirability as a trait construct) are employed to correct a subject's responses for bias. The Minnesota Multiphasic Personality Inventory (Hathaway and McKinley, 1967), a popular personality test, employs this kind of correction when subject responses are scored. Another method forces the respondent to select, between items matched for social desirability, the statement or behavior description which best represents his choice or response. An example of this approach is given below.

Of the pairs of activities to be presented, choose the activity you prefer most by placing an X in front of it. Check only one activity for each pair.
1. Playing a contact sport like football.
   Listening to a favorite stereo album.

Obviously this approach might also force the respondent to choose between two rather socially undesirable alternatives. Among other problems in using this approach are the costs of performing a preliminary analysis to match items for social desirability, the impossibility of employing this approach for many self-report instruments, and the fact that this approach frequently irritates respondents by requiring them to choose between two equally attractive or unattractive alternatives (Pfeiffer and Heslin, 1975).

Another response style, *acquiesence,* is the tendency of certain respondents to agree that a statement or behavior description is self-descriptive, independent of its content. According to Wiggins (1973), "to qualify as a response style, such a tendency should refer to an organized disposition within individuals to respond in a consistent manner (true, agree, yes), across a variety of substantive domains" (p. 423). Wiggins points out that the tendency to agree with items can to some extent be predicted by their content. One common method for reducing acquiescence is to balance the way that true versus false, agreement versus disagreement items are keyed or scored. In the example below, items from a scale attempting to measure a respondent's anxiety in a social situation are shown, along with the direction that they would be scored (number of points attributable to each item).

1. Sometimes I become uncomfortable when a stranger is introduced to me.

   1   2   3   4   5   6   7
   agree   disagree

2. I rarely experience discomfort when I meet new people.

   1   2   3   4   5   6   7
   agree   disagree

Agreement with item one is scored in the direction of a respondent's experiencing social anxiety whereas agreement with item two would indicate a relative lack of social anxiety. The respondent must carefully read each item, given that items vary in terms of their directionality, rather than merely endorsing one end of the rating scale (agreement) across items. A respondent who consistently responds "strongly agree" to each of the items will produce an uninterpretable protocol and will easily be identified. While such balancing does not ensure that items are completely unconfounded with acquiescence, it certainly seems to be an inexpensive step in the right direction.

Footnote

[1]Obviously this study was also examining the validity of the observational procedures if the self-report instruments are thought of as a "criterion."

UNIT II-C Observation Methods

6

SELF-OBSERVATION:
Methods and Issues

Many events of interest to the BCA do not occur in the clinical setting where they might be observed, nor do they occur with sufficient frequency in the natural environment for trained, independent observers to record their characteristics and incidences. In fact, many potential targets may not be observable to any person other than the client himself. Private or covert phenomena include thoughts, feelings, sensations, and the like, and such events (e.g., negativistic depressed thoughts, sensations of tension in a muscle group) may themselves be targets for change or function as a prelude to some target of importance (e.g., an "urge" preceding the smoking of a cigarette). It is difficult for a client to report reliably on such events unless they are recorded on an ongoing basis in the natural setting so that their immediate characteristics can be described. The reader, for instance, might find it difficult to describe carefully and systematically the anxiety experienced two days before when speaking to a group. Thus, it may be important to train the client to self-observe carefully certain aspects of his behavior, since he is always present when such events occur. In fact, clients and research subjects have been asked to self-record an extensive array of target events within numerous formats which will be discussed in this chapter. Such diverse categories as weight, caloric intake, and exercise (Stuart, 1971; Mahoney, Moura, and Wade, 1973); urges and incidents of smoking (McFall, 1970; McFall and Hammen, 1971; Chapman, Smith, and Layden, 1971; Lipinski, Black, Nelson, and Ciminero,

1975); obsessive thoughts and feelings of depression (Mahoney, 1971; Jackson, 1972); alcohol consumption (Sobell and Sobell, 1972); interactional and sexual behavior of married couples; certain academic behaviors appropriate to the classroom setting (Johnson and White, 1971; Gottman and McFall, 1972); hair pulling (McLaughlin and Nay, 1975); and even nail biting (McNamara, 1972) have been the focus for self-observations. In addition, students in a variety of classroom settings have been required to self-monitor the frequency of disruptive, problematic behaviors and often earn rewards based on their self-rated performance (Fixsen, Phillips, and Wolf, 1972; Santogrossi, O'Leary, Romanczyk, and Kaufman, 1973).

While initial interest in self-observation was directed toward defining behaviors for change and assessing the results of treatment (Kazdin, 1974a), it was soon found that the frequency of the targeted behavior often changed merely as a function of the monitoring procedures. Whenever assessment methods themselves alter a behavior in some fashion, we say that the behavior is reacting to the assessment process and term this "reactivity." In clinical practice and research we are typically interested in assessing the untreated, unbiased frequency of some event *before* we manipulate the behavior in any fashion. If an observational procedure is reactive, then this criterion has obviously not been met. However, while such reactive effects may reduce the usefulness of self-observation as an assessment procedure, the behavioral change induced by self-observation is interesting in its own right and may have practical clinical value. McFall (1970), for example, found that student smokers asked to self-monitor the times that they wanted to smoke *but did not* during a class period significantly reduced their smoking, presumably as a result of self-observation. Their smoking was observed by nonsmoking students in the classroom before self-observation as well as during treatment. Interestingly, another group of students asked to self-monitor incidents of smoking (and not the urge) paradoxically increased the number of cigarettes they consumed within the class period. While this study shows the reactive effects of self-monitoring, it also clearly demonstrates that such effects may depend on the category of targeted behavior observed. In fact, more recent investigations have shown reactivity to be influenced by a variety of factors some of which have become the focus for research efforts. A later section will discuss these research issues in more detail.

While the rationale for self-observation has often been based on assessment or therapeutic considerations, some investigators have incorporated self-monitoring in theoretical speculations as to how persons come to self-control their own behavior (Kanfer, 1970, 1975; Mahoney, 1975; Mahoney and Thoreson, 1974). We know from earlier findings that a person's performance is enhanced when he receives feedback or knowledge of results regarding his responses (Locke, Cartledge, and Koeppel, 1968). In fact, immediate feedback has become a major part of the programmed learning approach to education, largely based on earlier findings by B. F. Skinner and his colleagues (e.g., Skinner, 1953). The student is asked a question, makes a response, and then, by merely glancing to the right (or left) of the page, is provided with immediate feedback as to the correctness of his response. If the response is incorrect, the student is referred to preceding portions of the text for a quick review before answering the question again. Thus responding and feedback are an ongoing process which ultimately results in mastery of the task. This feedback model may also be applied to nonacademic aspects of an individual's everyday behavior; for example, social behavior. Through the social transactions we have with others (positive and negative feedback), as well as the instructions we receive from significant persons or entities (parents, the church, societal rules and regulations, each of us adopts self-standards to evaluate our own behavior. In certain therapeutic practices the definition of such standards is a major goal of intervention, and presumably when the client adopts values or standards he is comfortable with, therapy is complete.

The process of setting standards and monitoring one's behavior in terms of these standards are two important aspects of "self-regulation." Self-regulation depends on intrinsic, internal mechanisms by which an individual directs his own behavior in the absence of positive and negative feedback from others (extrinsic agents). For example, if a child fails to take a cookie from a cookie jar prior to dinner time when his mother is present, one might imagine that this is because of his fear of (desire to avoid) immediate negative feedback. If he fails to take the cookie under similar conditions (presuming that he is hungry and motivated) when his mother is *not* present, we might say that this is because of internal mechanisms: he is exerting *self*-control in the absence of external controls. In Kanfer's model of self-control (see Kanfer 1975), the individual must first learn to monitor his behavior systematically so that it may be assessed in terms of self-standards. This process of assessment has been termed *self-evaluation* by Kanfer and is presumed to occur whenever an individual behaves in a pro- or contra-standard fashion. Following this self-evaluation, the individual may provide positive or negative feedback to himself either through the medium of self-statements (e.g., "I'm really getting better at that"; "Terrible job, I've got to improve") or perhaps by self-initiated, overt activities (e.g., rewarding himself by watching television or eating a desired food). While this is a very simplified presentation of Kanfer's theoretical rationale for self-control, it should be noted that self-monitoring seems to be an essential first step in the self-control programs proposed by several investigators (e.g., Kanfer, 1970, 1975; Mahoney, 1975; Mahoney and Thoreson, 1974).

In summary, self-monitoring may be employed variously as an assessment tool, to promote certain therapeutically desirable behaviors (reactivity effects), or as an initial step in training a client to gain control of specific behaviors in the "self-regulation" framework. Following a presentation of procedures for gathering self-observed data, important issues suggested by self-observation will be discussed, with recommendations offered to assist the BCA in training the client to be a reliable observer.

Definition of the Problem

Once it is decided that some domain of the client's behavior is to be observed, the BCA must define *precisely* what the client is to observe and record. Let us imagine that the focus of self-observation is to be "anxiety." The following case example illustrates the definition process.

A 24-year-old female is referred to an inpatient psychiatric setting because of frequently occurring episodes of "anxiety" and "restlessness." These episodes began about two years prior to her admittance and have gradually become more frequent and intense. No specific life history events account for the anxiety attacks, according to both client and spouse reports. These attacks currently interfere with the client's ability to perform her management job, as she is often so overwhelmed by feelings of anxiety that she cannot concentrate on her work. While tranquilizing medication somewhat reduces the anxiety, only continuous sedation has proven to be completely effective.

Since she has been in the institutional setting (two weeks), two nurses as well as one aide who have interacted with her report that she often trembles to the point of not being able to hold a cup in her hand. She has been observed to cry on a few occasions. These staff members report that her "attacks" seem to occur "about equally across all settings," although no systematic observations by staff have been carried out.

After reading the case history (which in this case offers little useful information about specific referents of the client's behavior), then evaluating the brief reports of the three staff members, the BCA decides to ask the client to self-observe her anxiety episodes. The goal is fourfold:

1. To establish the *frequency* of these attacks over time prior to formal treatment. Because client and referral reports use such terms as "frequent," "always," "continuous" in an imprecise way, the BCA wishes to establish exactly how often these episodes occur.

2. To obtain information about possible *controlling conditions*. Information regarding the times, locations, and other specific conditions of each occurrence might reveal certain events controlling the onset and/or maintenance of the client's behavior.

3. To obtain further information about *what* the client labels "anxiety" and "restlessness." A term such as "anxiety" (or "depression," "nausea," "uneasiness," "aroused," for that matter), may mean markedly different things to different people. Other than to say that she feels a "great numbness in my chest," the client is virtually unable to describe specifically what she thinks about and feels physically during an anxiety attack. By asking the client to carefully observe such experiences, the BCA obtains additional information about the targeted behavior's characteristics.

4. Based on information that the client collects, the BCA hopes to ultimately *train* the client to observe carefully her own behavior on a permanent

basis. If self-observation enables the client to detect the beginning of the various sensations which culminate in a full-blown "attack," she can be trained to use some course of intervention (e.g., self-relaxation or interrupting her anxiety-producing thoughts by engaging in some activity incompatible with anxiety). Careful self-observation is a skill many clients must learn prior to being trained in specific treatment procedures. Treatments obviously cannot be competently applied unless the client can identify precisely when a problem behavior is about to occur or has occurred. Furthermore, as previously mentioned, self-observation often leads to self-directed behavior change, thus should be thought of as exhibiting potential therapeutic properties.

Because "numbness in my chest" is the only referent that the client reports occurs reliably (each time) she experiences an anxiety attack, the BCA defines anxiety as: "a numb feeling which typically begins in my upper chest." It is incumbent upon the BCA to now define carefully for the client precisely *what* she is to observe. One or two events that consistently occur as part of the targeted behavior (referents) may be used to define its occurrence. It may be that many separate covert and/or overt events occur together and are labeled as the problem; however, to ensure accurate observations, the BCA may limit client observations to one or two referents.

In order to accomplish the observation goals already mentioned, the BCA asks the client to record more information than a mere frequency count. To ensure that the client understands exactly what she is to record, the BCA writes the following in the front of a small notebook:

Definition of anxiety: a numb feeling (a tingling sensation) which typically begins in my upper chest. When "anxiety" occurs, I am to record:
1. The *date* and *time* (e.g., 2/5, 9:15 A.M.).
2. *Where* I am located (e.g., my room, dining room, occupational therapy).
3. *Who* I am with, if anyone.
4. The *activity* (e.g., eating lunch, watching TV, participating in group therapy).
5. What I am *thinking about* (specific thoughts, images).
6. What it *physically feels like* other than the numbness (e.g., a tightness in my upper arms, cold sensation in my feet).

Note that the BCA not only describes the information that the client should record, but also *provides examples* for each category.

Recording Procedures

The client must now be given instructions about the method of recording self-observational data. The client exhibiting "anxiety attacks" was asked to make a written record of a number of pieces of information outlined above. Although *written recording* of client self-observations is a popular technique (Stuart, 1971; McFall and Hammen, 1971), a number of other recording methods are available to the BCA.

Mechanical Devices

Many BCAs supply the client with a mechanical or electronic device for indicating that a behavior has occurred. For example, Chapman, Smith, and Layden (1971) required smokers interested in decreasing their consumption of cigarettes to depress a counter (worn on the wrist) each time a cigarette was smoked.

Various timing devices may be used in obtaining duration measures. The client may be provided with a stopwatch that provides a cumulative record of duration (Ciminero, Nelson, and Lipinski, 1977), a stove timer, or wristwatch with built-in timer (readily available in many department stores; see Katz, 1973). Mahoney and Thoreson (1974) employed a simple switch to control onset-offset of a common electric clock to measure elapsed time spent studying. The client was asked to switch the clock on at the beginning of each study period and off at the end. More sophisticated electronic counting-timing devices, usually employed by independent observers rather than the client himself, are described in Chapter 7.

For simple counting, a client may be asked to move poker chips or coins from one pocket to another at each instance of an event (Alban and Nay, 1976), which allows an end-of-the-day tally of the behavior by merely counting objects per pocket. Any means by which the client *manipulates some material object to count defined behaviors* is considered a *mechanical* procedure. Of course the possible counting mechanisms are limited only by the creativity of the BCA (and client!). Advantages of *mechanical* procedures include the following:

1. Procedures such as depressing a counter are usually easy to perform, and do not require much of the client's time.

2. Mechanical recording procedures can be carried out in any setting and in various situations where other procedures, such as writing down information, may not be feasible. For example, a teacher may have time to deflect a wrist counter while presenting class material, but may be unable or unwilling to pause to write something. An executive in a board meeting, a mechanic engaged in his work, or a client in a group therapy meeting, present possible examples where mechanical recording may be the only way to gather data.

3. The discrete data produced by a simple frequency count may display the information, thus providing behavioral feedback to the client. With a wrist counter, for example, the client receives an immediate summary of his behavior merely by looking at the tally on his wrist. The provision of *immediate feedback* of self-recorded data may be particularly advantageous when the BCA wishes to maximize reactive behavioral change (Kazdin, 1974a, 1974b).

Notable *disadvantages* of mechanical recording procedures include:

1. Mechanical procedures limit self-observational data to simple frequency counts or duration measures. The BCA may desire to obtain much more information, particularly when self-observation is used for pretreatment

assessment. The "anxious" client described earlier was asked to record information as to the time, location, conditions, and cognitive and physical referents of her "anxiety attacks." Such information would be lost if a mechanical approach was chosen.

2. The equipment required for mechanical data collection may not be available to the BCA (e.g., wrist counters, although these are quite inexpensive) or the client may refuse or be unable to use such devices for cosmetic or other reasons.

Product-Related Methods

Webb, Campbell, Schwartz, and Sechrest (1966) suggest that many behaviors produce some product or debris which may be evaluated as an indicant of behavioral frequency. Here we will interpret *product* rather broadly to include *any observable material effect on the setting elicited by client behavior*. Clients have been asked to record such products as weight displayed on a scale as a measure of food eaten (Stuart, 1971) or number of hairs collected as a measure of hair pulling (McLaughlin and Nay, 1975).

A client may find it difficult to record each time he eats a snack, but an evaluation of snack foods remaining at the end of the day (e.g., in his refrigerator) may be a useful indicant of snack consumption (providing others are not partaking also). Similarly, an accumulation of cigarette butts may provide an easily gathered measure of smoking frequency. In the academic realm, tests, papers, or even usage of task materials (e.g., number of sheets of paper, amount of single-use typewriter ribbon, etc.) may serve as accurate indicants of task-related efforts.

The kinds of behaviors that produce some product are numerous, and many such behaviors become the focus of intervention efforts. More will be said about product methods in Chapter 7. Meanwhile, a number of *advantages* of product-related client monitoring are worth noting.

1. The product is readily available for precise and accurate evaluation—a certain number of cigarette butts, pounds of weight, sheets of paper typed, parts of a room cleaned and ordered, automobiles washed, and so forth.

2. Product-related measures often require little effort on the client's part, and may involve only a once-a-day product evaluation. Thus the client is able to carry out daily activities in a more or less normal, uninterrupted fashion, counting or evaluating the product only at certain limited times each day (e.g., first thing in the morning, each evening before bed, only after mealtime, etc.). Observation methods do not interrupt, disturb, or exert controls on the client's ongoing behavior, thus reducing potential reactivity. In fact, product-related measures are probably the least reactive among observational methods, because assessment takes place outside the sequence of behavior at infrequent intervals.

Disadvantages of product-related measures include:

1. As with mechanical methods, the data obtained are limited to "how many," "how much," and/or "quality ratings," and do not provide information regarding possible controlling conditions.

2. The client does not *directly* observe the targeted behavior, but some product of it. The immediate feedback gained from observing specific occasions of a behavior may provide useful information to the client.

3. Many behaviors, most notably covert events (thoughts, physical sensations, etc.), do not produce an overt product, and thus are not amenable to product-related observation. As a product is often easier for a client to monitor than an imprecise covert event, the BCA should evaluate possible overt events linked to covert behaviors (Nelson and McReynolds, 1971). Nail biting, for example, might be a reliable referent of anxiety for a particular client (occurs whenever s/he is anxious), and is easy to monitor via length of nails (McNamara, 1972). Or a client may be able to monitor the degree of wetness of his shirt (perspiration) as an indicant of anxiety.

4. The product must be carefully evaluated to ensure that it is a direct reflection of the targeted behavior of interest and not due to other client behaviors, the actions of others, or environmental factors beyond the client's control, such as aging or climatic conditions.

5. Lastly, and probably most important, product measures may not be sensitive to slight frequency changes in the targeted behavior which often serve as indicants of improvement to the BCA and client. Such indicants often reinforce the client (Kanfer, 1970; Kazdin, 1974a) and enable the BCA to monitor progress more precisely.

Written Records

Written recording includes *any occasion when the client is asked to make a written response about his behavior.* There are a variety of ways that a client may translate behavior into a written record. Two major variants are *nonspecific* and *specific* record keeping. For example, the BCA might ask the client to make a complete record of his behavior for some particular time each day (e.g., everything he does from the time he arrives home from work until bedtime). Such a diary is a nonspecific record in that the client's observations are not directed to any specific class or category of behavior, but toward all behavior occurring within this time frame. In contrast, specific recording procedures exclude all events other than one or more targeted behaviors (e.g., "each time you feel anxious, as defined by a tightness in your chest," or "each cigarette you smoke"). The client may also be asked to record information as to time, location, physical and cognitive events, and other conditions that describe the behavior; however, such information is recorded only on the incidence of the target. Sometimes, a client may usefully be asked to use some combination of nonspecific and specific records.

Nonspecific records. Because collecting a complete record is a difficult task for the client, and may interfere with ordinary activities, its use is usually limited to certain time blocks or situations of particular interest. This approach may provide useful information to the BCA when the client cannot define his problem or has difficulty describing his life situation. Nonspecific recording may thus help the BCA to "target" certain behaviors as a focus for later *specific* recordings or for treatment. In addition, a nonspecific record of activities allows the BCA to define certain frequently selected behaviors or events that may be used as incentives for behavioral change.

Finally, a nonspecific record may be useful in providing the client with a means of describing feelings of anger, depression, or other events he cannot verbalize. Such records, collected on an ongoing basis, may be valuable when brought to the therapy situation as a means of focusing on important covert events.

Specific records. This more structured written approach often provides the client with a coding sheet, checklist, or rating form to complete as the targeted behavior occurs. One example of a structured coding sheet is provided by Stuart and Davis (1972) for clients completing a weight-control program. On "daily eating record forms," clients record information about possible variables controlling thier eating: "time," "food consumed," "how much?" "where," "who is with you?" and "how do you feel?" Lewinsohn and Atwood (1969) required a depressed female client to "keep track of her moods" using an adjective checklist that provided a daily score of mood state (Lubin, 1965).

Watson and Tharp (1972) suggest a simple recording format which offers much flexibility. The client is given an abbreviation or *coding symbol* for each behavior to be reported. As an example, the authors describe a self-observational approach to smoking:

An older woman wanted to stop smoking. She began by counting the number of cigarettes she smoked daily. She also noted the *situation* in which smoking occurred. She had already established categories for these situations and codes for the four major categories:

Category	Code
After or during eating or drinking	E, for eating
While nervous in a social situation	S, for social
While driving the car	D, for driving
Other times	O, for other

Each letter is the code for one category. Using an abbreviation makes recording less tedious. Her daily 3 x 5 card looked like this for the first Monday:

Smoking Record		Monday, the 7th
Morning	*Afternoon*	*Evening*
EEDOSSSE	OSSDSEEE	EO

She was surprised to see her pattern of smoking so clearly revealed [pp. 83–84].

Thus, on a single 3 x 5 card, which the client could readily carry with her, information as to time of day (mostly morning and afternoon), specific events during which smoking occurred (mostly during eating and social events, rarely at other times), and frequency (18 cigarettes) was obtained. The use of a coding symbol cuts down on the amount of writing the client must do, thus perhaps decreasing potential aversion to the recording task. Obviously this format could be adapted to a variety of targets.

Because it is important that the client be able to observe progress over time, a recording system should allow the client to readily see the pattern of his behavior over hours, days, or weeks. A client might be asked to graph or chart the frequency of a target as a part of the recording task. For example, a 32-year-old "depressed" male was asked to record each occurrence of a self-critical thought. He was asked to carry a 4 x 6 printed recording sheet in his shirt pocket and merely darken a small box on the chart each time he experienced the targeted event within each hour of the day. His chart for one day is shown in Figure 6-1.

Behavior to be observed: "Whenever I experience any negative thought about myself."

Examples: "I'm not doing as well as X is." "This won't work." "He (my boss) probably won't like it," etc.

Date: Tuesday, October 10

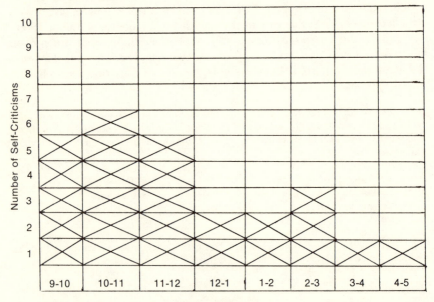

Hours of the day

Figure 6-1
Record of targeted behavior on a 4 × 6 recording sheet.

By sequentially darkening a box for each incidence of the targeted behavior within hours, the client could readily discriminate patterns of behavior over various times of day. He was not only counting, but displaying his behavior. It soon became obvious to him that he was experiencing more depressive thoughts in the morning than in the afternoon, which provoked him to examine this period of the day (he had a different work supervisor in the morning).

Of course, this format could also be used to record events over whole days, thus providing the client with a weekly display. Then one column on the chart would represent the number of behaviors each day instead of each hour. Such a format can be easily adapted to fit the goals of observation and specific characteristics of many behavioral events.

Among the *advantages* of written record keeping are:

1. The written approach allows the client to collect information other than a frequency count. Such information is often useful in defining controlling variables.

2. A number of formats are available for recording information such as diary description, use of symbol systems, checklists, and self-ratings. In addition, many formats allow the client to obtain immediate visual feedback as to the frequency of a targeted behavior over time.

3. Written recording allows the client to use greater precision in describing what he is experiencing. He can place a behavior within the context of other events and describe its subtle characteristics, which a mechanical or product-related measure does not allow.

4. Written recording is often more "reinforcing" to the client than other more mechanistic procedures, as the client has more of an investment in a written account. Some clients are "put off" by procedures that seem to be mechanistic or artificial. For such clients a written approach may make more sense.

Among the *disadvantages* of written recording are:

1. It may be difficult or impossible for a client to make a written response in some settings (e.g., while swimming, driving, playing tennis, sailing).

2. Written recording tends to interrupt a behavioral sequence such as a verbal interaction, and thus may produce more reactive measurements.

3. Depending on how much information the client is asked to record and the client's view of the recording task, written record keeping may have aversive properties for certain individuals, and in fact has been used as a response-cost procedure by some investigators (McLaughlin and Nay, 1975). *The BCA must be certain that the written demands made on the client are not viewed as unpleasant,* as the client may not accurately perform the task.

In choosing a recording approach, the BCA must consider several important factors, such as the kind of information required, the setting or activity within which data are to be gathered, and the client's expectations and interests. Careless or mechanical assignment of methods to clients may confound a primary goal of self-observation: to collect accurate and reliable information regarding a client's behavior.

Setting

The setting in which a client is asked to self-observe may be determined by a number of factors. Usually, the BCA sifts through the client's case history, verbal self-report, staff reports, and other preliminary information to obtain some initial "locus" for the behavior. In some cases a behavior may be known to occur across all settings, in which case self-observations must be directed at as many settings as can feasibly be self-monitored. In other cases it is apparent that the behavior is limited to some specific setting, and this then becomes the focus for data collection. For example, marital problems, child-management problems, and self-care problems might occur exclusively in the home setting, thus immediately limiting the focus of self-observation. Because of the poor quality of many client verbal reports and existing records, initial self-observation across all settings might be desirable (say for one week) to ensure that the settings chosen for treatment are inclusive of those settings in which the targeted behavior occurs. Obviously, the BCA must carefully evaluate as many avenues of preliminary information as possible before focusing self-observation exclusively on one or more settings. Even if treatment is only directed at one high-rate setting (say the home), it may still be useful to have the client collect data for the targeted behavior in other settings to determine whether treatment effects generalize to those settings (if such generalization is desirable).

Sampling

There are two major approaches to the question of "how often" the client should record a targeted event. In *event sampling* the client is asked to record each specific instance (event) of the targeted behavior. If the behavior does not occur, nothing is recorded. This is by far the most commonly used approach. In *time sampling* the client is asked to self-record during certain predetermined intervals during the day or at randomly selected times. This approach can drastically reduce the amount of time the client systematically observes a target behavior while maintaining a representative sample of that behavior across time. Time sampling may also prompt the "poor observer" to become more systematic in examining some aspect of his behavior. The time prompt, in a sense, forces the client to self-observe on a regular basis which he might not do otherwise. The primary problem with a time-sampling approach is that the client must be able and willing to monitor times. As the frequency of sampling increases, it may become more difficult for the client to accurately self-monitor the more abbreviated time sequences. In this case the BCA should provide an external cue for observations. A wristwatch alarm, stove timer, or other readily available timing device can serve to cue the client if reset (e.g., for one-half hour each time) immediately following its signal. More complicated portable electronic devices may be devised which signal the client via a soft tone or vibration on a preset schedule and permit very elaborate observation schedules. Chapter 9 will provide a more extensive presentation of sampling methods and issues, particularly as they relate to independent observational approaches.

Another important question is how many "samples" or specific observations of some behavior constitute an overall sample that accurately reflects the behavior's incidence. Before intervention, we must have an accurate account of baseline frequency; however, suggestions as to the number of observations necessary to ensure an accurate baseline are inconsistent in the literature. Published case studies often report baselines that include many observations, but over only a few days; or a few observation sessions over a longer period of time (e.g., three weeks). Although there are no hard and fast rules, the following recommendations would seem to be minimally acceptable guidelines for baseline sampling:

1. With *low-rate* behaviors such as acts of aggression, fire setting, or stealing, the number of days of baseline data collection must be increased to ensure an accurate assessment. You may sample every day for a week and find only one occurrence of the behavior. Three to four weeks of monitoring might be necessary to obtain a more accurate occurrence per day baseline for the behavior.[1] The increased sample of behavior that a *high-rate* behavior provides (e.g., smoking, many verbal behaviors) permits the observer to obtain an accurate assessment (e.g., rate per day, rate per hour) over a more abbreviated time span.

2. Sampling should typically be performed as *frequently as possible* both *within days* and *across days*.

Within days: When a client self-observes within restricted, predetermined times or conditions, an extraneous variable exclusively present during those periods could be responsible for the incidence or characteristics of the target. Thus, computing an hourly or daily rate from such a limited sample may yield inaccurate results. To take a simple example, let us assume that Mrs. Jones self-records her smoking behavior in the morning from 10:00 A.M. to 12:00 A.M. each day. Her data reveal an average of 20 cigarettes smoked or 10 per hour (suggesting 80 per eight-hour day). However, a particularly "nerve-wracking" business meeting that consistently occurs between 10:00 A.M. and 11:00 A.M. each day provokes a high rate of smoking, thus elevating her frequency of smoking during the two-hour self-observation period. When asked to extend her self-recording over the entire eight-hour work day, she is found to smoke an average of 50 cigarettes or about six per hour. Thus, by extending the observation times *within* the day, a more accurate account of hourly frequency is obtained, and the BCA is more certain that some unknown variable is not unduly influencing the results.

Across days: In addition to sampling extensively within days, the BCA must also sample frequently enough across days to obtain an accurate accounting of daily and weekly frequency. Taking the same example, Mrs. Jones may be found to smoke 48, 45, and 40 cigarettes on each of three consecutive baseline days, suggesting a mean daily rate of about 44 per day. Collecting daily data over a full two weeks however, yields the following outcome:

Week 1		Week 2	
48		42	
45		50	
40		41	
42		38	
39		37	
37		35	
37		32	
287/7	= 41.14 per day	275/7	= 39.29 per day

The data for each full week show a somewhat reduced mean number of cigarettes smoked per day over each seven-day period (41.14 and 39.29)— lower than the three days of observation would imply. In addition, it may be noted that more cigarettes per day are smoked at the beginning than at the end of the week. Thus, by extending observations across days, we are ensured of a more representative sample, and daily and weekly trends are revealed more precisely. It makes sense that more extended *within* and *across* day sampling increases the representativeness of baseline, process, or outcome data.

The *variability* of the targeted behavior across days should also be considered. Many authors suggest that baseline data collection should proceed until a stable baseline is achieved (little variation in frequency across days). Sidman (1960), for example, suggests that stability should be defined as no more than five percent variation in the range of frequencies across some period. Unfortunately it is often difficult to achieve this criterion, and practical and ethical demands often force the BCA to initiate intervention before some predetermined criterion of stability has been reached. It is safe to say, however, that the BCA can be more assured of the stability of baseline frequency by extending observation across days. Chapter 13 will discuss important issues suggested by the "baseline" in more detail and relate the baseline to various research designs which may permit the interested BCA to evaluate more systematically the effects of intervention.

Important Issues

Each of the issues to be discussed represents a major area of research interest defined by the recent literature. Rather than provide a complete review (for reviews of the literature, see Kanfer, 1970; Kazdin, 1974a; Ciminero, Nelson, and Lipinski, 1977), this chapter will summarize the findings so as to assist the BCA in designing self-observational strategies.

Reactivity

It has already been mentioned that behavior change occurring as a function of client self-observation is called "reactivity." It was also noted that the usefulness of self-monitoring as an assessment device is concomitantly limited as reactivity effects are enhanced and that the manner in which reactivity is viewed depends on the goals of self-observation. In fact, many BCAs employ self-observation primarily as a means of altering a behavior of interest and may thus wish to maximize reactivity effects. The present discussion will explore the variables that seem to enhance reactivity.

First, it is important to note that while some studies have shown dramatic therapeutic effects following self-monitoring for such classes of behavior as cigarette smoking (McFall, 1970; McFall and Hammen, 1971), studying or class participation (Johnson and White, 1971; Gottman and McFall, 1972), and time spent on academic tasks (Mahoney, 1973), few investigators have employed follow-up measurement to assess the maintenance and durability of self-monitoring effects. When such follow-up has been done, the effects of self-monitoring have been shown to "attenuate with time" (Kazdin, 1974a). Stuart (1971) and Mahoney, et al. (1973) for example, found mild weight loss when clients were required to self-monitor eating behaviors and weight, but these effects dissipated over a period of weeks. Mahoney, Moura, and Wade (1973) found no difference between self-monitoring and no-treatment control groups when these conditions were compared to self-reward and self-punishment procedures for weight reduction. In general, self-observation has not been effective in altering the weight of obese persons when it has been the sole treatment.

Other negative findings include those of McNamara (1972), who attempted to dismantle self-monitoring into component parts. With the goal of reducing nail biting in an undergraduate population, McNamara divided his 42 subjects among the following conditions: self-monitoring of an incompatible response, engaging in an incompatible response with no self-monitoring of nail biting, self-monitoring of a resistance response, self-monitoring of nail biting only, and a no-treatment control condition. While subjects in all treatment conditions improved in comparison to the no-treatment group, no one condition showed superiority, suggesting that certain nonspecific effects (e.g., perhaps expectancies set by the "therapist") may have operated to produce the observed therapeutic gains.

Fixsen, Phillips, and Wolf (1972) found that six institutionalized "delinquent" boys were very poor self-observers of their room-cleaning behavior (poor reliability) and that mere self-observation did not change the frequency of room cleaning. Numerous other studies could be discussed, but it is obvious that the reactivity effects of self-monitoring have proven quite inconsistent as reported in the literature. In an excellent review, Kazdin (1974a) summarized the reactive nature of self-monitoring:

> At the present time, one would have to conclude that the effect of SM (self-monitoring) in altering behavior has not been consistently found. Several studies reviewed here failed to find any behavior change when subjects recorded their own behavior. In many studies in which SM was effective, a variety of other procedures already known to influence behavior (for example, contingent praise, desensitization, therapist contact, and suggestion to alter the behavior) co-varied with SM. Few studies have attempted to dismantle therapeutic treatments of which SM is a part [p. 230].

With the above statement in mind, it is still important to attempt to define conditions where the BCA has the greatest probability of obtaining reactivity effects, and the literature does provide sufficient information to make some educated guesses.

The nature of the *specific target* chosen for self-monitoring may have an important bearing on the results obtained. On the face of it, it makes sense that there are differences between recording an "urge" to do something and recording the behavior once it has occurred. Particularly if the behavior holds reinforcing consequences to the self-observer (e.g., eating, smoking), "occurrence" recording permits the behavior to occur, thus reinforcing the client again. Each additional trial that reinforces the client would tend to further establish the strength of the response. On the other hand, the self-recording of an urge prior to the occurrence of a targeted behavior permits the client to immediately predict and perhaps control the onset of that behavior. If the behavior has not yet occurred, its reinforcing properties have not yet been directly experienced, thus it may be easier for the individual to exert self-controlling responses (e.g., engaging in an incompatible response; physically removing the source of temptation, such as e.g., a cigarette). While many findings in the animal literature support this speculation, there is only limited support in the self-monitoring literature. McFall (1970), for example, found that students actually increased their smoking when asked to monitor incidences of smoking, whereas students asked to monitor "resistances" to temptation decreased the frequency of smoking. Although both groups showed a mean decrease in the time spent smoking per cigarette, notable differences were found when self-recording was discontinued. While the group that monitored smoking continued to smoke at a higher rate than was observed prior to treatment, there were no within-phase differences (baseline-treatment-baseline) for the group that monitored resistance to temptation. These results were, however, clouded by the obvious demand characteristics imposed by the experimental situation (Orne, 1970). Along similar lines, Gottman and McFall (1972) found that high school students who monitored their verbal participation in class correspondingly increased such participation, but decreased participation when asked to monitor their nonparticipation (not talking when they wanted to talk, for whatever reason).

Romanczyk (1974) assigned 70 overweight subjects to one of five groups: no-treatment control; self-recording daily weight; self-recording daily weight and daily caloric intake; behavior management and stimulus control instruction; and behavior management, stimulus control, and self-recording of daily weight. Self-recording of daily weight produced no significant change in subjects' weight following four weeks of treatment. However, subjects who recorded daily caloric intake as well as weight showed behavioral changes as extensive as the subjects exposed to the more extensive treatment conditions. The author concludes: "One possible explanation for the previous inconsistent findings of the reactive nature of self-monitoring lies in the particular parameters of the self-monitoring process. Care must be taken in choosing the particular behavior to be monitored in relation to the presenting problem. Thus, in the case of obesity, monitoring of daily weight does not appear to interact with the variables that maintain over-eating, whereas monitoring caloric intake does have a significant effect" (p. 38).

These findings suggest that the BCA should carefully consider choice of target. If the goal of intervention is to directly alter a covert event (e.g., an urge) that reliably precedes an overt target, or if the goal is to disrupt the chain of behavior that begins with an urge and ultimately leads to the problematic response, then it is compelling to reason that the target should be the covert event *and not* the overt behavior itself. Conversely, if an overt event is of primary interest, then it makes sense to have the client monitor that behavior. For example, if the goal of treatment is to increase a client's speaking out in public, it would make more sense to have the client self-monitor that specific class of overt events. Unfortunately, these suggestions are clouded by another aspect of the targeted behavior which has recently received attention: the *valence* of the behavior for the client.

Regardless of the characteristics of the targeted behavior and the precision with which it is defined, a behavior negatively valued by the client (negative valence) may not increase in frequency no matter how often the client self-monitors that event. Here the role of cognitive events comes into play; the client is not simply a passive participant in the therapeutic regimen. Kanfer (1970) was among the first to speculate that negatively valenced behaviors would be more likely to decrease in frequency, while positively valenced targets increase, as a result of self-monitoring. Tied in with valence is the idea of *motivation,* which we will define here as the degree of effort the client is willing to exert in altering the behavior of interest. A client will likely be poorly motivated to change a behavior that is neutrally valenced and increasingly motivated to alter a behavior that is valenced positively or negatively. In fact, in reviewing the literature on self-observations, Kazdin (1974b) has stated that "most self-monitoring investigations show behavior change in the direction predicted from the value of the behavior" (p. 705).

Kazdin (1974b) performed a well-controlled evaluation of the role of valence in determining the effects of self-observation on behavior. Rather than employing clients who would definitely be motivated to alter problem targets, Kazdin had undergraduate subjects monitor the number of "I" or "we" pronouns they used in constructing sentences from stimulus words—a neutral task. Three groups of self-monitoring subjects were provided with instructions that placed a positive valence, a negative valence, or no valence on the sentence-structuring task. Positive valence was developed by informing subjects that self-referencing statements such as "I" or "we" were made more frequently by intelligent, creative, sensitive, and secure persons. Negative valence subjects were given the identical rationale, except that the frequent use of self-referencing statements was associated with "*less* intelligence, less creativity, less sensitivity, insecurity, a failure to accept oneself or others" (p. 706). No-valence subjects were not told anything about the personality characteristics associated with self-referencing statements. Three additional groups performed the sentence-structuring task, but were not required to self-monitor; each of these was given one of the valence instructions just described. There were thus six experimental conditions. All subjects were required to complete 40 sentences after being given the valence instructions. Their scores were the combined number of "I" or "we" sentences constructed. Results showed that regardless of valence instruction, subjects who self-monitored evidenced greater behavioral change from baseline condition than did subjects who did not monitor their sentence constructions. Among self-monitoring subjects, valence did seem to have a pronounced effect. Subjects provided with a positive valence significantly increased their use of personal pronouns, while those provided with a negative valence siginficantly decreased their use of personal pronouns. Further, monitoring subjects who were not provided with any valence showed no significant change. Thus, valence appeared to be an important ingredient in influencing the direction and magnitude of behavior change.

More recent research has supported Kazdin's findings with different targeted behaviors. Nelson, Lipinski, and Black (1976) found an increase in the frequency of a socially desirable behavior (conversation), no change in a neutral behavior (object touching), and a decrease in an undesirable behavior (face touching) when groups of retarded persons were asked to self-monitor these targets. While none of the findings were statistically significant, they provide suggestive evidence to support Kanfer's original speculation. Cavior and Marabotto (1976) also found the same relation between valence and direction of behavior change for verbal behaviors self-selected as positive or negative by subjects.

Another factor that might reasonably affect reactive behavioral change is the provision of a standard by which the monitoring client can evaluate performance. It has already been mentioned that such standard setting is a prerequisite for behavioral change in the self-regulation models suggested by many writers. Using the same sentence-construction task described above, Kazdin (1974b) evaluated the role of a performance standard for subjects who self-monitored, subjects who were monitored by others, and subjects whose performance was not monitored at all. Subjects provided with a performance standard were informed that a total of 35 out of 40 "I" and "we" statements was the cutoff for a really good performance. Results indicated that subjects who received the performance standard used the targeted pronouns more frequently than subjects who did not receive the standard. Of subjects who were provided with the standard, about 31 percent achieved the specified goal (35 out of 40 "I" and "we" statements), while only 8.3 percent of no-standard subjects achieved this goal. In addition, the self- and other-monitoring groups used the targeted pronouns significantly more frequently than the no-monitoring subjects.Finding no significant difference between the two monitoring conditions suggested that monitoring oneself or being monitored by another are equally reactive.

In a final study, Kazdin (1974b) found that subjects provided with a digital display of their self-recorded frequency of personal pronouns (performance feedback) used significantly more targeted pronouns than those who did not receive such feedback, and that this feedback seemed to enhance the effects of employing a performance standard. Further, performance feedback significantly increased the use of personal pronouns even for subjects who did not receive the performance standard.

Among other findings related to the nature of the target, Hayes and Cavior (1977) found that monitoring of two or three behaviors (face touching, nonfluencies, or value judgments) provoked significantly less reactivity than self-recording a single target.

To summarize, self-monitoring has been inconsistently shown to promote reactivity effects for the neutral, laboratory manipulations described and for the largely undergraduate student population employed, and when evident, these reactivity effects seem to be enhanced by a number of factors. First, reactive behavior change occurs in the direction suggested by the valence, positive or negative, of the behavior. Second, the setting of clear, predetermined standards for the client's performance seems to enhance the reactivity effects of self-monitoring, and lends support to Kanfer's speculations regarding the role of self-monitoring and standard setting in self-regulation. Third, while not necessary, performance feedback also seems to enhance the reactivity effects of self-monitoring. Regarding this last observation, several investigators have provided ways of giving subjects feedback; however, this feedback is often a summary of previously collected data, and is not provided on an ongoing basis as the client self-monitors. Rutner and Bugle (1969), for example, posted the self-recorded hallucinations of a psychotic patient on a graph placed on a wall visible to the client in his ordinary interactions. Both Kanfer (1975) and Kazdin (1974a) feel that graphing client behavior change for the client and others to see increases the client's social reinforcement for his efforts, and they maintain that this social reinforcement is most important in maintaining self-instigated behavior. In a previous section, the recording of self-observations in a graphic format and the use of wrist counters to provide an immediate display of frequency were both illustrated. It would seem to be most important that such feedback be provided on a regular basis if it is not ongoing.

Reliability of Self-Collected Information

Because self-monitoring has frequently been employed as a means of assessing the frequency and other characteristics of client targets prior to, during, and following treatment, it is critical that the client become a reliable self-observer. By reliability we mean that a client's self-recording of the target should consistently coincide with recordings made by an independent, unobtrusive observer (if he were present in the situation). However, many client targets make it difficult or impossible for an unobtrusive observer to assess reliability. For example, certain very low frequency behaviors may occur so rarely (yet still be of clinical importance) that it would not be feasible to have another observer continuously present. Similarly, it is often impractical for the BCA to traverse the natural setting, and if independent observers must be employed, the costs of assessment increase. Also, some targeted behaviors are private and occur at a covert level. For these behaviors it may be impossible to assess occurrence independently (Simkins, 1971).

Given the limitations, a first question is: Can clients learn to self-record targets at acceptable levels of reliability? The answer here is a clear yes. Azrin and Powell (1969), for example, found 98 percent agreement between psychiatric residents' self-reports of pill-taking and the reports of independent observers, and Ober (1968) noted a high correlation ($r = .94$) between self- and peer-reports of cigarette smoking. Similarly, Drabman, Spitalnik, and O'Leary (1973) found that children were accurate observers in assessing on-task classroom behavior when their self-reports were compared to those of adults, while Santogrossi et al. (1973) showed that adolescents' self-recording of disruptive classroom behavior correlated highly with data collected by independent observers. While reliability averaged an acceptable $r = .95$ across the phases of implementing a behavior modifcation program, the students' determination of their own rewards (tokens) based on such self-ratings was ineffective in altering problem behaviors. This is clearly a case where reliable self-monitoring did not automatically provoke reactive behavior change, thus suggesting that *reliability and reactivity may not be related*. In support of this, Herbert and Baer (1972) found that while the accuracy of mothers' observations of their children's appropriate behavior was poor (approximately 45 percent agreement with an independent observer), self-recording did lead to desirable behavior change for their children. In further support of previous findings, Hayes and Cavior (1977) found low correlations between accuracy and reactive behavior change across three targets self-monitored by undergraduate student subjects. For one behavior, "nonfluencies," independent observers and the subjects showed no correlation in their endorsements; yet this target displayed a high degree of reactive behavior change.

As for reactivity, it is hard to draw any firm conclusions from the literature since methodology and targets vary considerably. Given that clients *can* become reliable in their self-endorsements (the literature is clear on *this*), the BCA must ensure that the client is trained in observation methodology and that accuracy is assessed *prior to* formal data collection. The following recommendations should be considered.

1. When the target is clearly defined and the methods of monitoring and time demands are commensurate with the client's capabilities and apparent level of motivation, the BCA should *verbally review* the observation task with the client, *demonstrating* (modeling) how the target is to be recorded. The BCA and client might consider together events that would interfere with monitoring and review possible solutions in advance.

2. The client should be given an opportunity to *practice* self-monitoring the targeted behavior. If it ordinarily occurs when the BCA is present, the client can be asked to practice self-monitoring during the remainder of the clinical "session." If the target does not occur during regularly scheduled meeting times, the BCA might attempt to elicit it by having the client imagine himself in situations that ordinarily provoke its occurrence or by physically role playing such situations with the client (see Nay, 1976).

3. If the target is overt, the BCA can simultaneously record with the client as a means of *checking reliability*. If the client fails to detect the target or records improperly, the BCA can provide immediate verbal feedback. The BCA might even go into the client's natural environment to independently observe the target when the client is self-monitoring. Chapter 10 suggests a number of methodological options and issues to be considered when reliability is assessed. One issue concerns the impact of checking reliability upon the observer's accuracy. It is well-established that the reliability of independent observers tends to be significantly higher when they are aware that reliability is being assessed, and such reliability drops when assessment is unobtrusive (Reid, 1970; Romanczyk, Kent, Diament, & O'Leary, 1973). Only one investigation has systematically evaluated the role of obtrusive versus unobtrusive measurement with self-observers (Lipinski and Nelson, 1974). Given a neutral target (face touching) in a classroom situation, subjects were required to self-

record each time they touched their hands to their faces with an observer present (obtrusive) and under conditions when they were not informed that reliability was being assessed (unobtrusive). For obtrusive reliability assessment a correlation of .86 was obtained over a total of 48 observations. This correlation dropped to .52 over the same number of observations during unobtrusive assessment, suggesting that subjects were more accurate when they were aware that reliability was being assessed. Another interesting finding was that a decrease in face touching (presumably a negatively valenced behavior) which occurred during phases of self-observation was not maintained when subjects were no longer required to self-monitor, thus suggesting the temporary effects of self-monitoring as a therapeutic agent.

A number of BCAs have reported client failure to carry out monitoring procedures and that the frequency of monitoring seems to dissipate with time (Boren and Jagodzinski, 1975), so that it may be important to provide incentives for accurate data recording. For example, a number of investigators have found that children and adolescents can be trained to be accurate self-observers when specific positive or negative incentives (e.g., tokens, response costs) are provided for their efforts (Risley and Hart, 1968; Fixsen, Phillips, and Wolf, 1972; Lyman, Rickard, and Elder, 1975). Similarly, adult clients may need the structure of a formal therapeutic contract (e.g., I *[name]* agree to monitor [behavior specified]; *methods* specified; *times* client agrees to monitor; *contingencies* for monitoring or failure to monitor, i.e., access to desired activity; *signature*) to enhance motivation. Nelson et al. (1976), for example, found that adult retardates could accurately self-monitor behaviors such as face touching, with reliability significantly enhanced when positive incentives (McDonald's Gift Certificates) were made contingent on subjects' matching with independent observers.

4. If a goal of training is that clients will *continue* to self-monitor once the therapeutic relationship is terminated, it is important that the BCA program such *maintenance* by ensuring continued availability of incentives for monitoring in the client's natural environment or by instituting a self-control program (see Kanfer, 1975; Nay, 1976) that provides intrinsic motivation for the client's monitoring efforts.

While there are often problems in assessing reliability of self-monitored overt behaviors, this category of target at least permits such assessments. With private, covert events such as thoughts, imagery, and urges, it is obviously impossible for an extrinsic agent to observe the target directly. In fact, some writers have suggested that assessment and treatment procedures focusing on covert phenomena are inherently of such questionable reliability that we should consider not employing them (Simkins, 1971a, 1971b). Simkins feels that the data collected within covert paradigms may be intentionally or unintentionally falsified (if the client's criteria for response differs from the therapist's), and interobserver checks (*not* possible for covert phenomena) are the only means of assessing reliability.

In reply, Nelson and McReynolds (1971) agree with Simkins that the reliability of such covert self-recordings cannot be directly ascertained. They suggest that overt behaviors linked to covert targets might be independently assessed as indirect measures of the covert target. For example, while it may be impossible to observe an "urge" to smoke a cigarette directly, an extrinsic observer may observe the overt act of smoking. This assumes that an "urge" reliably precedes the smoking and that one needs to observe only the overt act itself to determine the covert phenomena that precedes it. Obviously there are a number of problems with this suggestion. For one thing, there is no way of knowing for sure that the covert and overt behaviors reliably occur together (e.g., in some cases the client may smoke without any awareness of an urge, or the client may control an urge, and not smoke a cigarette). Second, it may be very hard to establish a covert-overt chain for many covert events. For example, what overt events are reliably associated with fantasizing, daydreaming, or other kinds of imagery that do not usually lead to overt behavior? On the other hand, if therapists and clients tend to find reliable relations between a covert event and overt behavior across occasions as well as situations (e.g., client blushes or perspires in response to anxiety), and this overt response can be assessed by an independent observer, the recommendations of Nelson and McReynolds are justified and perhaps provide the only means of assessing reliability within the covert paradigm.

In addition, Nelson and McReynolds point out that one can assess the reliability of the *effects* of self-monitoring (reactivity) when those effects are overt in some fashion. It is important to note, however, that a reduction in the target may have been due to a host of factors other than self-observation. For example, the client may have been responding to certain expectancies that his behavior would change (Orne, 1969), may desire to please the examiner, or may even be responding to certain contingencies in his environment (e.g., his spouse or friends will not permit the target any longer). Any one of these events may produce change in the overt referent. Because the therapist has only the client's word that self-monitoring has even taken place, cause-effect statements regarding the effects of monitoring must be made even more cautiously when covert targets are assessed.

Clearly, the development of more reliable methods for assessing covert phenomena would be a welcome addition to the literature (Mahoney, 1977). Mahoney summarizes the current state of the art with regard to cognitive events:

There are promising signs of progress in the assessment of cognition. In the past, our psychometric instruments were primarily trait dependent and psychodynamic. The current trend seems to be toward more direct and situational methods of assessment. In addition to self-report questionnaires, researchers have begun to use such methods as self-monitoring and electrophysiological recording. Likewise, some of the old prohibitions seem to be weakening. It used to be unheard of for a behaviorist to inquire about dreams, but this is less so today. With a few of our theoretical prejudices aside, it may turn out that even some projective techniques may offer valuable information on perceptual biases and other cognitive tendencies. Moreover, we can learn much from the cognitive psychologist regarding methods of perceptual and conceptual assessment [p. 11].

Footnote

[1]Obviously, the BCA would be ethically bound to restrict baseline assessment and provide suitable intervention when the client's welfare is compromised by extending self-monitoring or any assessment strategy.

7

INDEPENDENT OBSERVATIONS: Description, Development, and Validation of Methods

While the BCA may well decide to train the client to self-observe along the lines suggested in Chapter 6, self-collected data may be limited by the client's ability and willingness to record his own behavior as well as the feasibility of carrying out such observations in certain settings (e.g., while engaged in a particular task). The reliability of self-recorded observations may thus be questionable, and the extent of the behavioral sample may be limited by these and other factors. In addition, although a given child's ability to systematically self-observe probably varies with cognitive and attentional variables (e.g., intelligence, ability to maintain a set), no one would question that age is a limiting factor. In general, the child of 10 years or less could probably carry out only the simplest observation procedures in a reliable fashion. The mentally retarded, psychotic, and infirm also may not be able to employ observation methods.

As an alternative to self-observation, the BCA may train persons other than the client to observe and encode client behavior in some prearranged fashion. Such "independent" observers are often trained to develop and/or employ quite sophisticated observational procedures. Among the major advantages of independent observation methods are:

1. Information detected and recorded by well-trained, reliable observers may provide the BCA with a more systematically gathered sample of a client's behavior than self-observation can provide. Independent[1] observers are free from the ordinary demands of the setting and may attend exclusively to the observation task.

2. Self-observation procedures cause the client to interrupt ongoing behavior so that a recording can be made. While independent observations do not usually interrupt the client, they may promote some measure of reactivity. The issue of reactivity as it relates to the independent observer (e.g., effects of observer's presence on client behavior) will be discussed in detail in Chapter 8.

3. Given self-observations may accurately reveal the frequency of the recorder's behavior, only independently gathered data directed at the setting as a whole (e.g., observations of entire classroom, cottage, or ward settings) can provide accurate information as to the behavior of others who interact with the client.

Following a review of those *methods* that might be employed to independedently assess client behavior-in-setting, the methods and issues suggested by *selecting, defining, and validating* those event classes chosen for systematic observation will be explored. This material should assist the reader in developing and evaluating an observation instrument that could be employed across intervention settings for clinical or research purposes.

Method Options

Selection of particular methods will depend on the nature of information to be obtained as well as certain resources available to the BCA (e.g., persons to serve as observers, access to certain equipment). To assist the reader in selecting a method that best suits an assessment question and can be practically implemented, certain advantages and disadvantages of each method category will be elaborated. In line with the general emphasis on employing multiple measures of the same event when feasible, it should be underscored that more than one of the observation methods described below might be simultaneously employed.

Mechanical Approaches

Like the self-observer who employs mechanical methods (see Chapter 6), the independent observer can employ a simple golf (wrist) counter (Lindsley, 1968), grocery counter (Kipp, 1971), or some physical means of noting the occurrence of a targeted event, such as transferring coins from pocket to pocket (Alban and Nay, 1976) or marking a piece of Scotch tape placed around the wrist (Hawkins, Axelrod, and Hall, 1976). While limiting data to simple frequency counts of events, these mechanical methods are particularly suited to the participant observer who must collect observational data as a part of other responsibilities.

At a somewhat more sophisticated level, portable electronic counters ensure accuracy of recording, given reliable detection of an event by the observer. Wolach and his colleagues report a simple procedure for converting a variety of popular (and increasingly available) low-cost electronic calculators into frequency counters (Wolach, Roccaforte, and Breuning, 1975) as well as the use of stopwatches to measure the duration of some event of interest (Wolach, Roccaforte, and VanBerschot, 1975). Unfortunately, the observer can encode only one behavior at a time with these methods; often it is desirable to observe and record multiple behavioral events simultaneously. One alternative is to employ a multichannel recorder permitting the recording of up to 20 separate behaviors on a continuous basis. For example, Lovaas, Freitag, Gold and Kassorla (1965) used an Esterline-Angus 20-pen recorder (cumulative paper record) to encode nine behaviors displayed by autistic children in a classroom setting. Five pairs of observers learned to depress one of 12 buttons (activating a microswitch) on a hand-held panel, which in turn activated a pen on the recorder. The buttons were arranged on the 7 x 14-inch panel in the configuration of the fingertips of an outstretched hand to enhance ease of recording. Once the position of particular buttons (behaviors) was learned, the observers were able to record the children's behaviors while maintaining continuous visual contact. In addition, the continuous paper record made it possible to recognize certain time-behavior and behavior-behavior (functional) relations that simple frequency recording does not permit. The paper record of frequency also made it easy to assess the level of agreement between observers.

Because the presence of an observer may provoke reactivity effects within a setting (Patterson and Harris, 1968; White, 1972) audio-video taping devices have been employed as an alternative means of data collection (Johnson and Bolstad, 1975; Johnson, Christensen, and Bellamy, 1976; Johnson and Lobitz, 1974). When verbal behaviors are of interest, clients may be audiotaped quite inexpensively. Johnson and Bolstad (1975), for example, employed a simple cassette tape recorder in sampling the behavior of family members during a standard 45-minute period each evening. While the authors speculated that this procedure would be less obtrusive (hence less reactive) than employing an observer, the fact that a family member was responsible for activating the recorder at a standard time makes such a speculation questionable. In fact, merely having a microphone or tape recorder obviously present may provoke behavior different from that with concealed, unobtrusive recording methods (Roberts and Renzaglia, 1965), thus suggesting the potential reactivity of even these less obtrusive mechanical approaches. Questions of reactivity aside, a tape recorder can be programmed to time-sample the clients' verbal behavior in a setting by having onset controlled by a timer which turns the recorder on and off at fixed or varied time periods over the course of a day (Bernal, Gibson, William and Pesses, 1971). For example, verbal behavior might be recorded for five minutes every half hour so that a one-hour audiotape would include data from 12 samples made throughout the day at fixed times. Or a variable time sample might turn the recorder on for five minutes of recording at random times each hour to provide 12 randomly selected samples of client verbal behavior. These approaches ensure a more representative sample of behavior over time.

As an alternative, the client/subject might be outfitted with a transmitter capable of transmitting verbalizations to a receiver-recorder within or outside of the setting proper. In using such a device, Soskin and John (1963) and Purcell and Brady (1965) found that references to being observed or about the equipment declined to zero level during the first few hours of recording. However, even though subjects talked less about the transmitter (suggesting some adaptation to its presence), one cannot conclude that their behavior was uneffected.

Videotape records (camera and microphone concealed) may be made similarly to audiotape recordings when both *verbal* and *nonverbal* client behaviors are of interest under continuous or time-sampling conditions. These tapes may then be viewed by observers at a convenient time so that a written record of client performance may be compiled. Recordings also provide the BCA with the option of using such tapes for training purposes. For example, audio or audiovisual recordings of client behavior may be played for the client to provide "feedback" (Bailey and Sowder, 1970) regarding important targeted behaviors. Clients may be asked to self-record certain behaviors from such tapes to provide them with "focused feedback" (Hersen and Eisler, 1973) and/or to train them to self-observe their own behavior systematically, as discussed in Chapter 6.

It seems reasonable to assume that potential reactivity will be greatly reduced or eliminated to the extent that the persons to be observed are unaware of the schedule of observations and cannot detect the onset of recording equipment. Johnson, Christensen, and Bellamy (1976) used this approach to "bug" the verbal behavior of five children believed to display active behavior problems (e.g., aggressiveness, destructiveness, temper tantrums). Employing a transmitter, a receiver, a 24-hour timer, two 15-minute time switches, and two reel-to-reel tape recorders, the parents activated the transmitter and fastened it to their child's belt for morning, afternoon, and evening time blocks totaling approximately five hours each day. Stored in a trunk placed in the home (to eliminate parent detection of recorder onset), the receiver was wired to the two tape recorders. One recorder was activated for 15 minutes at three predetermined "random" times each day without parent awareness. The second recorder could be activated by the parents during a time "picked" by them to record a problematic occasion. As might be expected, data collected during the "picked" times were significantly more sensitive to child behavior change resulting from an ongoing 12-week treatment program (see Eyberg and Johnson, 1974) that all parents completed. In fact, the "random" data collection substantially failed to detect the incidence of problem targets prior to and following intervention. Obviously data collected during the "picked" times are open to questions of reactivity (and demand for "improvement"). The authors recommend high-density "random" taping to meet this objection. Among the problems encountered with their methodology, the authors reported difficulty in obtaining compliance with instructions with particular families (e.g., getting the child to wear the transmitter, recharging the transmitter).

When audiovisual recordings of client behavior are made, the BCA should be certain to obtain the *prior permission* of each client (or a legal guardian). The specific nature, frequency, and potential uses of such recordings should be made clear and should be so stated verbally or in a written release. In fact *any* observations of a client should be dealt with in a similar manner. Most settings use a standard release form which includes a description of the nature of observational data to be obtained. Failure to inform a client that such observations are being made presents ethical and possibly legal problems (see Martin, 1975). Also clients should be permitted to turn off the device at their choosing and perhaps even "censor" records before they are employed by the BCA (Johnson and Lobitz, 1974; Johnson et al., 1976).

Other mechanical devices may be directed at recording the frequency of a *specific* targeted behavior—for instance, if a *complete* record is not desired. One investigator known to the author constructed a playroom in which microswitches beneath individual floor tiles were connected to recording equipment. Data as to the frequency and extent of mobility around the room were gathered for a group of young children with this approach. Ultrasonic devices which detect the movement of air molecules caused by the client could be used with a group of over- or underactive clients to record treatment progress. Level of noise (as in a disruptive classroom, cottage, or ward situation) could be detected and recorded using audiometric equipment. Hoats (1975) describes a variety of electronic filters that can be used to detect certain audio and ultrasonic frequencies. Unfortunately, many of these procedures are impractical because they physically limit client interactions or are too expensive. The possibilities for mechanical measurement, while certainly limited by the characteristics of the behavior to be detected, are a function of the investigator's creativity. For example, because of the impracticality and expense of many mechanical measures of "hyperactivity" in child subjects (e.g., chair stabilimiters), Bell (1968) constructed a simple and inexpensive device consisting of a packet containing two small, hand-wound wristwatches without balance wheels. These were worn by subjects, whose movements provoked mechanism movements and were thus translated into time recorded on the watch. This measure was found to correlate significantly with other measures of activity.

One final note, the telephone can be employed economically to collect self-reported information from clients (Jones, 1974), or a telephone record can itself be scored for certain targeted events (e.g., signs of anxiety, "depressive" verbalizations).

The *advantages* of mechanical recording procedures include:

1. Recordings may be made without an observer's being physically present within a setting, thus reducing or eliminating reactivity effects.

2. Mechanical procedures produce data that are reliably obtained in a standard and systematic fashion, while observers may not maintain saisfactory levels of reliability (O'Leary and Kent, 1973).

3. Mechanical devices reduce the costs of assessment. Although initial and maintenance costs vary with the type of equipment used, even videotape equipment is becoming increasingly accessible to most clinical settings. In addition, the data generated by mechanical equipment may be summarized (e.g., coded from the recording) and evaluated by staff members at convenient times.

Significant *disadvantages* of mechanical recording procedures include:

1. If recording equipment cannot be concealed in the setting, its presence, like that of an observer, may affect client behavior (Roberts and Renzaglia, 1965). Also, many natural settings (e.g., homes, wards, outdoors) do not permit the concealment of recording equipment.

2. The data obtained by certain mechanical methods (e.g., floor tiles, sound detectors) may be limited to simple frequency counts, and no data regarding possible controlling variables are obtained.

3. In most cases data recorded on audio and videotape media must be observed and written recordings of targeted behaviors made so that systematic records of progress can be assessed. Of course, staff can make such records at their convenience. However, this advantage may be offset by the limitations of *any* mechanical recording of human behavior: it is often difficult to discriminate certain words, sounds, or nonverbal behaviors even on the best of audio or videotape recordings. Noise level in a setting, for instance, may make detection of a specific individual's verbalizations difficult or impossible.

As to videotaping, a camera typically maintains a fixed position and some clients may be blocked from view by objects or persons so that facial expressions and body language, often important referents of a behavior, may be lost as a client moves around (Lytton, 1971). In contrast, the observer who is physically present in the setting can move about as necessary and is better able to discriminate sounds and subtle behaviors than is possible with recording equipment. Of course, many disadvantages of mechanical recording can be overcome by using multiple cameras and microphones, using a "camerman" (e.g., through one-way glass) who can differentially focus on certain clients, and in general, by increasing the sophistication of recording procedures. To a great extent, the characteristics of the targeted behavior predict the usefulness of mechanical methods. If the behavior is discrete and discriminable enough for accurate detection (e.g., a physical interaction, standing vs. sitting), then some of the disadvantages of audiovisual recording may be overcome.

Product-Related Measures

The product-related measures described for self-observation may also be assessed by the independent observer as a noninterfering measure of some targeted behavior. Such product-related measures are often described as being "unobtrusive" (Webb, Campbell, Schwartz, and Sechrest, 1966) because they do not require that an independent agent be placed in the setting as client behavior occurs. Unobtrusive measurement would thus be one means of reducing the potential effects of an observer on targeted behaviors. Webb et al. (1966) have suggested three sources of unobtrusive data which have been relatively "untapped" by researchers: *erosion measures*, *trace measures*, and *archive measurement*.

By *erosion measures*, the authors mean that wear and tear, damage, or other physical change in a setting occurring as a result of a behavior may be evaluated as an independent assessment of that behavior. Using a standardized means of assessment, the extent of erosion of floor varnish in a children's setting might indicate the degree of overall physical activity of the youngsters. In addition, marks on the walls, the degree of wear and tear on the furniture, the frequency with which the setting requires cleaning, and various other "erosions" all might be related to physical activity in the setting.

As with any product-related measure, one must be careful that some extraneous variable does not contaminate the relation between the product measure and the targeted behavior. For example, the degree of erosion of a floor might be influenced as much by a new system of floor cleaning, or even by the hiring of a new janitor who cleans the floors more frequently, as by the clients' foot movements. Product assessment ideally includes data from several physical locations in the setting, each perhaps representing a different modality of the targeted behavior (e.g., floor erosions as a measure of foot movements, marks on the walls as indicants of hand activity or play). When a cluster of such "erosions" occur together the BCA can be more satisfied that no unknown variable is responsible for setting change.

Decay and breakage measures might also be included in the erosion category. For example, the frequency with which a vacuum cleaner requires repair or replacement can probably be related to the frequency of its use and is thus an indirect measure of the soiling of carpeting in a setting. Often, such decay measures may prove to be valuable indices of targeted events. For example, in a setting where children are encouraged to make use of certain objects as part of treatment (e.g., mathematics games, books, magazines, toys), the frequency of required replacement of such objects might indicate frequency of usage. In addition, the breakage or destruction of objects in a setting may be a direct indicant of active physical behaviors. In implementing a token economy in a training school for adolescent females (Nay, 1974), the author noted a remarkable drop in the number of windows broken each month following the establishment of the treatment program. While the relation between windows broken and the reduction of certain targets (e.g., physically aggressive behavior) can only be hypothesized, these data, in combination with direct observational data showing a reduction of aggressive acts, led the author to believe that the program was accomplishing its goals.

It should be noted that measures of erosion, decay, and damage must be evaluated in the context of ordinary wear and tear that might be expected even if targeted events did not occur. Once norms for ordinary wear and tear are established, any excessive erosion, decay, or breakage may be related to client targeted behaviors with more assurance.

Webb et al. (1966) have defined *trace measures* as those objects deposited by clients in a setting or the ordinary debris left by client interaction with or consumption of material. Examples given by the authors include: the number of cigarette butts in airport ashtrays before and after a major crash as an indicant of anxiety, the variety of fingerprints on a book or display case, or the frequencies at which push-button radios are tuned as a clue to where a car has been. Regarding client behaviors, the placement of movable furniture in a day room might indicate the manner in which clients interact with one another while seated (e.g., chairs clustered together, rather than placed in isolation). The following are additional examples of trace measures: the quantity of food containers and other food-packaging material as an indicant of snack foods consumed; the movement of magazines and books to other locations within the setting as an indicant of reading behavior; movement or rearrangement of task materials (e.g., sewing, handicrafts, art supplies, etc.) about a setting or to client rooms as an indicant of use; the amount of food left on a plate, or the amount of food remaining of the total amount delivered, as an indicant of "appetite." Trace measurement must use a standard methodology for assessing the number, "degree," or other relevant characteristic of trace materials in some setting. Lyman, Rickard, and Elder (1975), for example, developed a formal checklist to assess "cabin cleaning" (e.g., clothing stored properly, floor clean) with a group of campers trained in cleaning skills. Literally any object that the client moves about some setting that remains following the client's departure might be employed as a trace measure of the behavior that presumably deposited it, and the creative BCA may employ such measures very economically (e.g., measure once a day or once a week).

The third category postulated by Webb et al. (1966) is *archive measurement*, which includes such records as tombstones in a cemetery, information in the Congressional Record, voting records, and records of accidents. Often, record keeping at the global level of a city or county indicates changes in certain behaviors (e.g., frequency of marriages, divorces, deaths) with certain seasons of the year, certain times of the day, and certain important external events.

While the kinds of records just described are not directly relevant to clients, most treatment settings do maintain a compendium of records which may be useful. The time between intake and discharge, the frequency of readmission to a clinical setting, the length of time following discharge during which behavioral gains are maintained, the length of time that a client maintains a given job, client level of income following discharge, and a host of other statistics might be valid indices of client progress. Martin and Lindsey (1976) discuss the problems in employing one such measure, irregular discharge, as an unobtrusive measure of discontent within hospital programs. They point out that discharge can be determined by so many variables that it becomes difficult to relate it to any one phenomenon. This may be true of many archival evaluation systems.

Another product category that does not fall as obviously into the schema of Webb et al. (1966) might be termed "task" measures. In the academic realm, for example, the number of completed papers or other assignments, accuracy of printing, erasures in math problems, and projects completed (Hawkins, Axelrod, and Hall, 1976) are among the task products that could be unobtrusively measured and may reflect some target of interest (see Hawkins et al., 1976, for a more extensive discussion).

Table 7-1 shows a variety of *trace* and *archive* measurements of the behavior of adults in a psychiatric inpatient setting, evaluated in a research program by Palmer and McGuire (1973). The authors show the correlation between each measure and a number of criterion variables: rate of readmission; rate of discharge; median days of hospitalization; and clinical judgment of independent assessors. The "starred" correlation coefficients indicate that a significant relation exists beyond that which might occur by chance alone. While a number of the measures listed did not correlate well for this population of psychiatric clients, they suggest categories of unobtrusive measures that the reader might employ and evaluate.

Baseline assessment of the erosion, trace, or archival product should be

Table 7-1
Correlations between Various Measures and Criteria of Ward Performance

Measure	Rate of readmission	Rate of discharge	Median days of hospitalization	Judges' ranking
MILIEU				
1. Bedside furniture (tables, dressers, etc.)	39	26	-23	00
2. Attractive bedspreads (nonissued)	-18	33	-23	-10
3. Current bulletin board	23	39	-06	-12
4. Curtains in day hall (yes or no)	02	28	16	25
5. Rugs in day hall (yes or no)	-12	09	-10	43*
6. Current magazines in day hall	24	13	14	08
7. Pictures on wall of day hall	-13	-28	11	05
8. Games visible (pool table, bingo)	19	34	02	-36
9. Clean clothes issued daily	38	33	20	00
10. Showers available daily	59†	31	23	42
11. Private lockers (patient has key)	-04	-18	-29	00
12. Dining room decorated	-26	-26	33	-05
13. Ward radio in day hall	-37	08	-27	-34
14. Washer, functioning	-15	14	-34	-19
15. Dryer, functioning	-14	14	-34	-19
16. No. chair groups	02	45*	-08	12
Total subscale	10	31	-08	00
PATIENT PROGRAMS				
17. Ward patient government	27	00	18	20
18. Privilege panel (patients decide penalties for asocial behavior)	49*	-18	-11	-12
19. Ward canteen	40	18	-21	09
20. No. regular social events per month (birthday parties)	08	-01	-22	32
Total subscale	40	00	-11	16

Measure	Rate of readmission	Rate of discharge	Median days of hospitalization	Judges' ranking
COMMUNITY INVOLVEMENT				
21. No. visitors	-13	27	00	35
22. Pieces of patient mail (incoming)	-32	06	-04	57†
23. No. patients on home visit	40	10	26	77‡
24. No. man hours spent by family in group therapy	19	52†	-16	48*
25. No. man hours—volunteers	23	38	-13	-33
26. No. man hours—community representatives (probation)	01	35	-08	28
Total subscale	10	44*	-14	54†
TREATMENT				
27. No. referrals to vocational rehabilitation	31	43*	-14	44*
28. No. patient—individual therapy	-20	34	-24	34
29. No. occupational, recreational sessions (cooking, bowling)	00	16	19	26
30. No. small therapy groups	-14	24	05	34
31. No. all-ward meetings	33	06	-13	58†
Total subscale	21	32	07	60†
PATIENT MORALE				
32. No. AWOLs	-20	-20	-13	38
33. No. special incidents (fights)	-50*	-27	-22	05
34. No. patients "pacing"	-43*	-02	-11	-08
35. No. patients sleeping	-18	24	-14	-32
36. No. patients sitting alone	-25	15	-26	-41
37. No. patients "talking to self"	-43*	-06	-02	-46*
38. No. patient groups (need not be talking)	-13	38	-21	17
39. No. patient groups talking	03	46*	-11	28
40. No. patients wearing own clothes (of first 10 observed)	62†	46*	23	09
Total subscale	47*	23	11	40

(continued)

(Table 7-1 continued)

Measure	Rate of readmission	Rate of discharge	Median days of hospitalization	Judges' ranking
STAFF MORALE				
41. Nursing station door open	34	39	25	19
42. No. disciplines in ward meetings	25	04	-18	27
43. No. disciplines leading group therapy	04	-05	52*	48*
44. No. staff seen with patients	06	-11	63†	55†
45. No. staff out of station	18	30	15	48*
46. No. staff in street dress	35	-11	15	-20
Total subscale	27	-22	44*	49*
47. Amount of drugs used	-38	61†	-38*	-34
48. Sex of ward (male = 1, female = 2, 10 segregated wards)	-56*	22	-29	17
49. Sex of ward (male = 1, female = 2 vs. integrated wards)	60†	20	30	—
50. Segregated = 1; vs. integrated = 2 wards	52†	10	-09	39
Total score (six subscales)	37	21	13	52†

Note: Decimals omitted in body of table
*p ∨ .10
†p ∨ .05
‡p ∨ .01

made prior to the implementation of treatment, with assessments made throughout intervention as well as following termination. In addition, product measures should ideally be employed in conjunction with assessment methods that require the client or independent observer to be present in the setting to record behavior of interest. This permits an assessment of the convergence between multiple and divergent measures and permits a comprehensive view of behavior-in-setting.

Perhaps the greatest value of product measures is that behavior is assessed without being potentially contaminated by measurement (e.g., the presence of an observer). Product-related measurement is also an ideal alternative when measurement by an observer is impractical or impossible. In an excellent review of the current status of unobtrusive measurement, Sechrest (1976) reports:

> Unobtrusive, nonreactive measurement is an approach offering many advantages but serving only as supplementary or complementary to surveys. There are sufficient problems with unobtrusive measures that they should not be regarded as substitutes for other measures; rather, they are most useful and most justified when thought of as providing additional and often confirmatory data. Since the idea of unobtrusive measurement was first proposed there has been disappointingly little additional systematic work on types and properties of unobtrusive measures, and there clearly are potential psychometric problems with such measures. More work on unobtrusive measures is called for and can be justified by their potential [p. 106].

Written Methods

The most frequently employed means of encoding behavior is to make a written report. Written record-keeping usually falls into two major categories: (a) records encompasssing all behaviors in a setting and thus *nonspecific* regarding particular targets to be observed, and (b) approaches that predefine *specific* categories of behavior as the exclusive focus of recording. The *nonspecific* approach implies that the observer is interested in the total picture of behavior over some fixed period of time, while the *specific* approach implies that targeted behaviors have already been chosen. Both approaches have advantages and disadvantages which will be presented and evaluated.

Nonspecific Records. Perhaps the best example of a nonspecific approach is the specimen record-keeping procedure originally proposed by Barker and Wright (1949). More recently, Wright (1960) has defined a specimen record as *an unselected sequential, narrative description of behavior and the condi-*

tions within which it occurs. Using this approach, an observer employs a narrative form to record *all* behaviors occurring over some time period. According to Wright (1960), the observer is in no way selective about what he records, but is deliberately unselective in recording everything that occurs. The idea is to obtain a complete picture which includes specific behaviors emitted, the effects of those behaviors, and cause and effect relations between persons and objects as behavior occurs. Wright has summarized the various instructions investigators have provided to "specimen" observers of child behavior:

1. Begin reporting each observed sequence with a description of the scene, the actors, and the ongoing action. Report throughout in everyday language. Describe the situation as fully as the behavior. Thus include "everything the child says and does"; but also "everything said and done to him."
Describe the larger "adaptive actions" of the child, but weave in as well the "hows" of these actions as much as possible. "Non-adaptive aspects of behavior" (Stone, 1941) are important on this account. These include hunchings, turnings, twistings, and the like, which often illuminate such properties of behavior as intensity, effect, and efficiency.
2. Do not substitute interpretations that generalize about behavior for descriptions of behavior, but add such interpretations when they point to possibilities of fact that might otherwise be missed. Segregate every interpretation by some such device as indentation or bracketing. Strict reporting must be left to stand out.
3. Notes on the scene of observation, which obviously are needed for sufficiently detailed and accurate description, can be kept in improvised shorthand. These field notes can be enlarged in writing immediately after each observation, or they can serve then as a base for dictated narration of the observed behavior sequence. Also, a co-worker can hear this account through and at once question the observer where it is thin and unclear. The original dictation plus the interrogation and the observers' responses can be sound recorded. All of the recorded material can be copied and revised in an improvised running account.
4. Observations can be timed to permit various measures of duration. Timing of the field notes at intervals of approximately one minute or even 30 seconds (Fite, 1940; Jersild & Fite, 1939; McFarland, 1938) has been found practicable. When long records are made, observers can work in rotation; and the time of each observing period can be regulated to minimize effects of fatigue upon ability to see and remember an always fast train of events [1960, 84–85].

These recommendations go far toward ensuring that the observer constructs an unbiased account of behavior. In addition, employing several observers who each observe during particular time periods reduces the possibility that fatigue or boredom will interfere with observations. Simultaneous audio or video recordings would allow written data to be compared to the taped recording as an indicant of reliability, thus ensuring a comprehensive record. What follows is an example of a specimen record made in an adult psychiatric ward by an observer who attempted not to interfere with ongoing behavior.

Setting: Room 245
Present: Mrs. L., Mr. M., Mrs. W.
Time: 8:45–9:00 A.M.
Observer: W. S.

Mrs. L. walked very slowly over to the south window, looked out of the window for about one minute, and said to Mr. M., who was sitting approximately five feet away in a soft chair, "What a lovely day. I sure wish I could go home. Don't you?" Mr. M. looked over at Mrs. L., shook his head [looked very disgusted with her comment], turned back to a book that he was reading, and made no further response. Mrs. L. then turned toward Mr. M., and with her arms outstretched, asked, "Why didn't you answer me? What's the matter with you? Why don't you ever talk to anybody?," She then then moved two steps toward Mr. M. Mr. M. made no response. Mrs. L. then turned away from Mr. M., and looked across the room at Mrs. W., who was sitting rigidly upright in a hard chair and staring straight ahead. Mrs. L. said to Mrs. W., "What's the matter with him? Don't you know?," Then she sighed and turned back to again look out of the window. Mrs. W. made no observable response to Mrs. L., and continued to look, with fixed expression, straight ahead. Mr. M. looked over at Mrs. L. for about 30 seconds, then looked at Mrs. W. for about 10 seconds, shook his head, and resumed reading his magazine.

This specimen record indicates the time of observation, the specific behaviors observed, aspects of the setting, and information regarding the relation between the behavior of Mrs. L., Mr. M., and Mrs. W. An observer interpretation of these events is separated from the record proper using brackets.

There are a number of *advantages* of the nonspecific approach:

1. Specimen records can register literally everything that observers can see of ongoing behavior, using the array of words available in the English language (there are 17,953 words defined by Allport and Odbert, 1936) to describe the characteristics and subtleties of setting events.

2. Specimen records describe behavior in the context of the situation in which it occurs. As Wright (1960) has said, "Everyone knows, at least intuitively, that the meaning and significance of an action and even its occurrence depends directly upon the coexisting situation. So, without checklists, rating scales, or precoded categories to confine him, an observer who makes a specimen record naturally works the situation into his running account, moment by moment and action by action" (p. 87). Such records provide extensive detail regarding the specific characteristics of the behavior, and there is a direct, written relation between behavior and environmental events. Thus, while knowing that the children in a classroom called out eight times in one hour may be useful information, a specimen record might provide the additional information that all of those calls were related to events in the playground outside the classroom window, not to ongoing class routine.

3. Nonspecific record keeping may be useful in defining behavior categories to be used as a measure of behavior change with treatment (e.g., the "situational analysis" to be discussed in the next section). Until the BCA has a

complete picture of behavior in a setting, it is very difficult to select the specific categories that should be observed to the exclusion of others.

Significant *disadvantages* of the nonspecific approach are:

1. Specimen record keeping could be directly limited by the observer's descriptive vocabulary, which is influenced by his previous experience with behaviors and situations similar to those observed. The observer-recorder must be able to express himself in an organized and concise written fashion in response to moment-to-moment events. The creative writing skills, fund of information, and vocabulary required may be beyond many potential observers who could, however, master a limited coding language (e.g., specific symbols).

2. As the number of interactors (clients, staff members, others) in a setting increases, the practicality of the specimen approach diminishes. When the observer is forced to summarize across several persons, information will be lost. Also, the probability that the observer's own biases will color the record is enhanced as he must choose what to write down from many ongoing behaviors (Weick, 1968). An approach that limits the categories of data to be recorded or sequentially time-samples each person in the setting would be better suited to larger populations.

3. It may be difficult to train observers to gather nonspecific data reliably due to the number of symbols (words describing behavior) possible and the inferences that must be made regarding ongoing behavior. The specimen observer is, in general, free to use his own symbols. Obviously the agreement between two independent observers is reduced when such idiosyncratic records are kept. Comparisons between events recorded by two observers over time, or between observer records and taped recordings of those behaviors, could serve as a check on reliability.

While reliability is certainly reduced, the nonspecific record does provide considerable flexibility and a comprehensiveness in data gathering not found in specific approaches. Thus, depending on the BCA's goals in obtaining the record, precision may be traded for detail and flexibility, or vice versa.

Specific Records. Systems using predetermined coding definitions typically require the observer to record the frequency of each scorable behavior on standard coding sheets. One approach is to require the observer to note in some fashion whether or not one or more predetermined behaviors occurs in a particular time period. The observer views the clients in the setting for a fixed observation interval, perhaps once every 30 seconds, minute, five minutes, or hour, then merely notes whether or not one or more of the targeted behaviors occurred ("on") or did not occur ("off"). Implicitly, any behaviors that are not a part of the coding system are ignored by the observer. An excellent example of this approach is the classroom behavior coding system developed by Cobb and Ray, (1970) which lists the symbols for each of 19 child behaviors on a format sheet, and asks the observer simply to circle the behaviors a given child exhibits during a brief coding interval. Figure 7-1 shows an example of this format sheet.

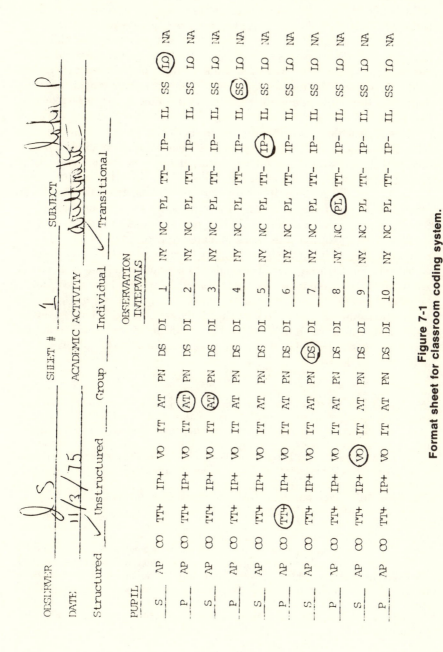

Figure 7-1
Format sheet for classroom coding system.

On the left-hand margin, "S" denotes a particular subject (e.g., targeted child), while "P" indicates other peers in the classroom who are alternatively observed. Thus, the subject is observed for a fixed observation interval (e.g., five seconds, 15 seconds) and the coding symbol that represents the child's behavior during the interval is circled (e.g., LO). Next, a peer observed during the second observation interval is shown to be attending to the teacher's presentation, indicated by the circling of AT. Then, the subject is again observed during the third observation interval, and at this time found to be attending (AT is circled).

This system thus sequentially samples both the subject of interest and other peer-students in the class over time. If behaviors are not circled, this indicates that they were not exhibited during the observation interval ("off"). Listing the coding symbols on the recording sheet saves the observer from having to record them himself; he can merely make a mark on the sheet to indicate occurrence. Other variants of this method list the symbols and require the observer to make a check, slash, box around it, and so forth, but all are similar in that the observer is merely required to note which of the behaviors represented by the listed symbols occurred. Because each observation interval is defined by a fixed number of seconds of observation, all intervals can be added up to define the total observation time, and specific behaviors can thus be related to time.

Another example of the "on-off" approach is provided below. In this instance a staff member in a psychiatric ward was interested in observing the verbal interactive behavior of five clients in a day room. The following symbols were employed:

X (verbal interaction)
Definition: Coded whenever the observed client is in the process of talking to one or more persons, as indicated by speaking in the direction of the recipient; or is engaged in listening to some other person's verbalizations, as indicated by active, full-face attention. In all cases, the client should be facing the interaction partner.

To code, write the first letter of the last name to identify the person interacted with. Writing this letter indicates that the interaction occurred during the 10-second observation interval.
Examples: Mrs. A. says something to Mrs. B. Mrs. B. looks full-face at Mrs. A. Mrs. B. nods her head while watching Mrs. A. speak.

EC (eye contact)
Definition: To be recorded only when X is recorded. EC indicates that the client is looking directly at the face of the interactive partner, whether talking or listening, EC should be determined by the position of the head in relation to the face of the interactive partner, and requires that the observer discriminate the position of the eyes.

Make a check in the EC column only if the client is engaged in EC while interacting.

Examples: While Mrs. A. listens to Mrs. B., Mrs. A. looks full-face at Mrs. B., nodding her head in agreement. Mrs. A. is directly facing Mrs. B., and Mrs. A's eyes are positioned toward Mrs. B's face.

G (hand gestures)
Definition: To be coded only when the client is engaged in X. G indicates any movement of either hand or arm during the 10-second observation interval. Thus, any one movement during the interval would be sufficient to encode G.

If G occurs, place a check in the G column alongside the client's name.
Examples: Mrs. A. and Mrs. B. are interacting, and during the 10-second observation interval, Mrs. A. raises her arm to illustrate a point. Mr. X. and Mr. Y. are interacting, Mr. X.'s hands are in his pockets, but he moves his elbow toward Mr. Y. during interaction to emphasize a point.

Figure 7-2 shows how these symbols could be used in an "on-off" format.

Note that during the first 10-second observation interval, Mrs. A. is observed to be interacting and maintaining eye contact, but does not use physical gestures. Then, during the second 10 seconds, Mrs. J. is observed and is seen to be interacting with Mrs. A., but not employing eye contact or gestures. In the third 10-second interval, Mr. L. is observed and is found not to be interacting with anyone. In the fourth interval, Mr. M. is found to be interacting with Mr. T., and maintaining eye contact while using physical gestures.

The *field format* variant of the "on-off" approach (Weick, 1968) ensures that observers systematically attend to several aspects of a setting when information beyond mere occurrence is desirable. The specific conditions under which a behavior occurred, its physical location in a setting, and specific clients or objects that the behavior seemed to be related to are examples of information that could be obtained using the field format approach. For example, the observer might be asked to supply information for each of the following rating categories in assessing a client interaction: *behavior* (A, OS, OA, P, V, etc.); in what *location* the behavior occurred (day room, hall, bedroom, kitchen, nurses' station, etc.); what *time of day* the behavior occurred (before breakfast, morning, during lunch, afternoon, during dinner, evening); whether a *staff member was present* in the setting (yes, no); under what *conditions* the behavior occurred (free time, task-vocational, recreational, etc.). The observer would be asked to circle, check off, or make some notation for each of these categories for each observational interval. Along these lines, Melbin (1954), listed six categories on a 3 x 5 card, and asked the observer to pull out the card and rate/check/circle each of the six categories at systematic time intervals for a population of adults in a department store. Virtually any category of information can be assessed using the field format approach.

Due to the limited number of discrete behavior categories assessed with the "on-off" approach, several observers using the same coding system in a

DATE: __4/21___

OBSERVER: ___T.___

TIME BEGUN: ___10:05_____TIME STOPPED:_____

Behaviors

	Client	Interaction	Eye Contact	Gestures
10 sec.	Mrs. A.	J	✓	
10 sec.	Mrs. J.	A		
10 sec.	Mr. L.			
10 sec.	Mr. M.	T	✓	✓
10 sec.	Mrs. T.	M	✓	✓
10 sec.	Mrs. A.	J	✓	
10 sec.	Mrs. J.	A		
10 sec.	Mr. L.			
10 sec.	Mr. M.	T	✓	
10 sec.	Mrs. T.	M		
10 sec.	Mrs. A.			
10 sec.	Mrs. J.			
10 sec.	Mr. L.			
10 sec.	Mr. M.			
10 sec.	Mr. M.	T	✓	✓
10 sec.	Mrs. T.	M		✓
	Etc.			

Figure 7-2
**Use of symbols representing particular behaviors in
an "on-off" format.**

setting are often able to achieve high levels of reliability (Barrish, Saunders, and Wolf, 1969; Broden, Hall, Dunlap, and Clark, 1970; Hall, Panyan, Rabon, & Broden, 1968; McArthur and Hawkins, 1974).

As an alternative to "on-off" formats, the observer might be required to make a continuous record of behavior over some period, using a finite number of coding categories as language. To illustrate this approach a sample recording sheet from the Patterson et al. (1969) Behavior Coding System (BCS) is presented (see Figure 7-3).

The symbols for each of the 29 behaviors of the BCS are listed at the top of the recording sheet in addition to identifying information. This serves to remind the observer of the appropriate symbol to employ, which is particularly useful when an observer is learning the coding system. Along the left-hand margin, the numbers 1 through 10 indicate the beginning of each 30-second observation period defined by an electronic timing mechanism. Beginning at 1, the observer makes a continuous record of ongoing behavior using the symbols listed above, ending at the right-hand side of the page approximately at the end of the 30-second period. When the 30-second cue is heard, the observer then begins at 2, and moves from the left- to right-hand side of the page as a 30-second record is again completed. Each recording sheet thus contains a grand total of five minutes of behavioral observations broken down into ten 30-second intervals. The numbers preceding the coding symbols designate particular members of the family, so that behaviors can be related to persons. The authors use 1 to denote the "deviant" targeted child, 2 for the father, 3 for the mother, 4 for the oldest child, 5 for the next oldest child, etc. A 9 is used when three or more family members are engaged in a similar behavior.

In Figure 7-3 the targeted child (1) was the subject of the observer's efforts. For this five-minute period, the child (1) was observed, and his behavior, as well as any behaviors he elicited from other family members, were duly recorded. Behavior was recorded in sequences which first included some designation of the subject's behavior, followed by the behavior of other family members who reacted to or in some fashion interacted with the subject. In the first coding interval, the observer began at the left-hand margin. Subject 1 was playing while the father (2) made no response. The "slash-1,' in the next six-second block indicates that this behavior continued through the second and third (roughly six-second) blocks. In the fourth, 1 was playing while 2 (father) and 3 (mother) did not respond. This continued through the last block within the first interval. After the 30-second cue, the observer moved back to the left-hand margin and resumed. Now 1 played while the oldest sibling (4) talked.

It is thus possible to obtain information not only about the incidence of particular behaviors, but of the behavioral relation between parties in the set-

Family Number ___50___

ID Number ___50 110461___

BEHAVIOR CODING SHEET

Phase ___/___

Subject ___/___   Observer _JC_   Date _4/04/69_ No. ___/___

Behavior Codes

AP Approval	DS Destructiveness	NO Normative	SS Self-Stimulation
AT Attention	HR High Rate	NR No Response	TA Talk
CM Command	HU Humiliate	PL Play	TE Tease
CN Command (negative)	IG Ignore	PN Negative Phy-	TH Touching, Handling
CO Compliance	In Indulge	sical contact	WH Whine
CR Cry	LA Laugh	PP Positive Phy-	WK Work
DI Disapproval	NC Non-compliance	sical contact	YE Yell
DP Dependency	NE Negativism	PC Receive	

#						
1	1PL 2NR	— /	— /	1PL $^{2NR}_{23NR}$	— /	
2	1PL 4TA	1DI 4HU	2CM 1NC	2CN $^{1CO}_{NE}$	1PL 4PL	
3	1PL 4PL	— /	— /	4DS 1PN	2CM 1CO	Ⓐ
4	1NO 9NO	— /	— /	— /	— /	
5	1DP 3CO	1AP 201	4TA 1LA	1TE 4WH	1NO 9NR	
6	1NO 2PP	1TA $^{316}_{24AT}$	1YE $^{2/3}$DI	1SS 9NR	1SS 9NR	
7	3CM 1CO Ⓡ	1CR $^{3/4}$AT	1TA $^{3TA}_{22AT}$	24U 1DI	3TH 1RC	Ⓑ
8	1WK 9NR	— /	— /	3IN 1RC	3IN 1AT	
9	3IN 1AT	1TA 3NR	1HR $^{2/3}$YED	2CN 1CO	1WK 9NR	
10	1CM 4CO	1AP 4TE	1WK 9NR	1AT 9NR	1WK 4AT	

Description: _Playing before DINNER (1-3), DINNER-time (4-5), DOING HOMEWORK AFTER DINNER (8-10)_

Figure 7-3
Sample coding sheet from the Behavior Coding System. From
"A manual for coding of family interactions," 1969 edition;
by G. R. Patterson, R. S. Ray, D. A. Shaw, and J. A. Cobb.
Reprinted by permission.

ting. It is also possible to relate these ongoing behaviors to time when a time-sampling approach is employed. A similar approach is used by Lewinsohn (reported in Mash and Terdal, 1976) to obtain a record of the "actions" (e.g., physical complaints) emitted by depressed persons and the potential "reactions" (e.g., ignoring, changing topic) of others. Using the format: action—reaction; action—reaction; a complete record of behavior is obtained using a series of predetermined behavioral codes.

Advantages of the *specific* category approach to recording include:

1. The well-defined behavior categories and standardization of method often found in multivariate (multiple targets) coding systems ensure that observations are collected under well-controlled and consistent conditions over observation occasions, thus reducing method variance. This is particularly important when data are to be employed for program evaluation purposes.

2. Specific, well-defined behavior categories enhance the probability that multiple observers can learn to employ the observation system at acceptable levels of reliability and reduce the possibility of bias in summarizing or interpreting ongoing behavior in comparison with nonspecific approaches.

3. Particularly when behavior categories are defined in clear language, limiting the amount of inference required by observers, the possibility that they may be employed across several agencies or communicated to others is enhanced. This may be particularly important when observational data are used for research purposes (e.g., establishment of a behavioral construct or theory testing, as in defining the nature of some class of behavior such as aggression or assertiveness).

Significant *limitations* include:

1. The use of predetermined categories obviously determines *in advance* what information can be detected. As persons and settings change, categories may not permit different (and perhaps clinically relevant) behaviors to be detected. In fact, the use of standard observation categories across clients has frequently been found to be insensitive to highly focused, behaviorally specific change resulting from intervention (Eyberg and Johnson, 1974).

Selection, Definition, and Validation

When the goal of assessment is to assess the characteristics and frequency of some class of events (e.g., social-skills, verbal communications between marital partners), the BCA must logically begin by selecting certain behaviors for inclusion in the observation scheme. Once those targets are selected, one or more of the method variants already described can be employed to detect and encode occurrence.

Selection of Targets for Clients

In selecting certain behaviors for observation with clients the procedures of item selection are similar to those for self-observation presented in the previous chapter. The client's self-report, for example, may be employed to focus the observer's preliminary observations on particular categories of behavior in the natural setting. Because of the problems of unreliability of client self-reports previously mentioned (e.g., Walter and Gilmore, 1973), it is important for the observer to also attend to the *entire* sample of observed behavior. Although a parent may report that his child's "problem" is his "fighting with his younger brother," a comprehensive analysis of behavior-in-setting may reveal that this initial target (a particular child's fighting) is but one of several possible targets for change. For instance, one or both parents might provide immediate and extensive attention to the child when he misbehaves, but ignore the child when he behaves appropriately. In addition, a careful appraisal of the setting itself may show that, rather than occurring "all the time," as the parent reports, the behavior seems to occur at high frequency only when the child is in the recreation room watching television with his brother. Many similar examples could be provided to illustrate the need for a comprehensive analysis of behavior-in-setting to augment the client's self-report.

If the BCA wishes to include independent observations in the assessment, the following recommendations for initially "shopping" setting behavior for behavior categories of clinical relevance seem to be in order.

1. The observer should not be limited by a predetermined and fixed set of behavior categories which are to be the exclusive focus of preliminary observations. Even though a particular category is reported to be *the* problem, a more complete record of each relevant person's behavior should be collected so that the "problem" may be viewed in the context of other behaviors. Often, the BCA's previous experience with similar clients provides a framework for exploring behavior categories not self-reported by clients (Jones, Reid and Patterson, 1975).

This strategy ensures that the observer focuses more comprehensively on a client's complete repertoire of behaviors, some of which may be very adaptive and appropriate to the setting. In addition, the observer may note that certain behaviors unreported by the referral source are beyond normal limits or promote behavioral inefficiency on the client's part and thus might also be targeted for intervention.

2. Rather than limiting the scope of observations to any one "problem" person or subgrouping, persons in the setting who interact with the client(s) should also be observed, so that the focal client(s) behavior may be placed within the context of normative behavior in the setting. The child who is reported to be extremely "oppositional" to teacher requests may be found to display behavior typical of numerous other children in the setting, thus suggesting a more comprehensive approach to intervention, perhaps focusing on

teacher skills. Many writers have suggested that members of a setting will "offer up" one or more persons as being deviant or "sick" when in fact the the targeted individual's behavior must be carefully viewed within its interpersonal context. Because the behavior of persons does not occur within a vacuum, and others may be importantly involved in eliciting and maintaining such behavior, a comprehensive survey of all persons in the setting further refines the requirements for intervention and the scope of future observations.

3. The physical characteristics of the setting should be carefully surveyed to determine the possibility of any functional relationships between setting and behavior (e.g., stimulus control, see Chapter 2). For instance, if the behavior of members of a classroom setting is not "disruptive all the time," as a teacher or principal reports, but exclusively or largely present in less structured settings or at certain times, this may provide important clues to the BCA regarding potential controllers of the behavior and suggest ideas for intervention.

If the foregoing procedures are followed, and particularly if a sufficient number of situations and times are sampled, the BCA can be confident that the behaviors chosen for systematic observation are in fact representative of the setting and not merely the result of the referral source's biases or lack of observational skills. It is obvious that no matter how sophisticated the observational methodology, inadequate sampling of behaviors, persons, or the setting itself may produce information with little clinical utility.

Approaching Validity in Instrument Construction

Because of the costliness of thoroughly "shopping" a setting and constructing highly personalized definitions of behaviors for each client, many investigators employ preconstructed, formal coding systems. The formal coding system typically presents operational definitions, examples, and instructions for observation for each of several behaviors of relevance to some population of clients. The Behavior Coding System (Patterson et al., 1969) has already been presented as an example of using "specific," predetermined observation categories. These authors train paraprofessionals to reliably employ the BCS to observe the behavior of families prior to, during, and following intervention. Thus the investigators and observers, as well as the parents, have a common language, as specified in the coding manual. Given that the definitions do not change, this language becomes a point of reference, providing a vocabulary for describing diverse families across time.

Using this approach, the BCA interested in systematically observing the behavior of some particular client population merely has to choose a coding system that seems to represent behaviors of interest, and ensure that observations are made according to the manual's instructions. However, the usefulness of a coding system is limited by the extent to which important subject/client behaviors are depicted, the specificity and clarity of the behavior codes themselves (so that high levels of observer accuracy may be achieved), and the sophistication of instructions provided to observers. The strategies involved in developing a formal coding system will now be addressed.

In traditional psychometric assessment we would say that an instrument is valid if it measures what it is intended to measure. Assessment of validity often involves the correlation of responses elicited by an instrument (e.g., an IQ test) with responses elicited by some other instrument purporting to measure the same construct (e.g., another IQ test, achievement test) or some set of behaviors thought to be related to the construct (e.g., academic performance in school). In fact, many procedures have been suggested for determining whether some hypothetical, inferred construct, such as "intelligence," "dependency," or "achievement motivation," is a valid one that, for example, generates predictions consistently supported across different situations. Because the notion of certain fixed "trait" constructs is central to the development of "personality" tests, the question becomes: What are the "constructs" of behavioral measures and to what extent do traditional methods of validation apply?

In describing behavioral assessment methods, Goldfried and Kent (1972) address this issue: "Rather than hypothesizing certain underlying constructs (e.g., 'instincts,' or 'needs') which are believed to function as motivational determinants of behavior, the basic unit for consideration involves the individual's response to specific aspects of his environment" (p. 412). These authors suggest that the behaviors a client displays are important in their own right and the logical focus for assessment. Jones, Reid, and Patterson (1975), on the other hand, leave the issue of behaviors versus constructs up to the interpreter of data collected. They state:

The targets of naturalistic observations are signs, indicants, or behaviors and these data may or may not be used to make inferences about inferred constructs. For example, if a child is observed in a natural setting to hit another child, this datum can be noted and recorded as a behavioral fact or event. The user of this datum may wish to infer that the hitter is aggressive (a construct), or may simply treat the datum as a simple fact with no further extrapolation to broader characteristics of the observed child [pp. 45–46].

One could argue that any time the instrument constructor attempts to devise a coding system that samples phenomena such as "oppositional behavior," "cooperative behavior," or "bizarre behavior," certain theoretical assumptions are made about what those categories mean and will predict in terms of the respondent's behavior. Thus, as soon as hitting, pushing, shoving, swearing, etc., are classified as falling within the category of "oppositional," the investigator is employing this dimension as a kind of construct. The implicit assumption is that children or adults who hit, push, or shove show more "oppositional" behavior or *are* more "oppositional" than children or adults who do not display behaviors in this category. To the extent that behavioral assessment instruments can be thought of as attempting to predict certain dimensions of behavior (constructs), traditional procedures for construct validation (e.g., Cronbach and Meehl, 1955) may be usefully applied to these instruments. It is hoped this issue will be further defined in the future.

For the present, though, how does the constructor of a behavioral coding system ensure that behavior categories selected for inclusion are representative of behavior in the relevant (criterion) situation? For example, if the BCA wishes to construct a manual of definitions that depicts "appropriate" as well as "inappropriate" parent-child interactive behaviors and ensure that this coding system is representative enough to be employed across diverse home settings, particular behavior categories must be included or excluded for manual definition based on their generalizability across those settings. Goldfried and Kent (1972) have described this process:

> The assumption that behavioral test responses constitute a sample of certain response tendencies is closely tied to the assumption that the test items themselves consist of a representative sample of situations relevant to behaviors of interest. In the assessment of assertiveness toward authority, for example, a sampling interpretation of the individual's test responses would rest on the assumption that the test items represent an adequate sample of interpersonal situations involving authority figures [p. 413].

Emphasizing *content validity,* that is, *the degree to which test items sample relevant content of interest,* Goldfried and Kent (1972) describe a set of "behavior analytic" procedures (Goldfried and D'Zurilla, 1969) which may be employed to ensure that behaviors chosen for observation adequately represent the setting. This "behavior analytic" method will be expanded on and related specifically to the choice of behaviors to be included in a coding system. For example, let us assume that the coding system we wish to construct will adequately represent the various "aggressive" behaviors young children might display in the home.

1. *The "situational analysis"* (Goldfried and D'Zurilla, 1969). The initial step is to *select a pool of items (behavior categories) classified consistently as "aggressive" by some panel of experts.* These "experts" might include professionals who work with parents full time, child-care workers who have occasion to observe children on a regular baisis, researchers who have developed a theoretical model model that defines the nature of aggressive behavior, or even parents of young children. Selection of experts depends on the BCA's goals (e.g., testing a theoretical model, selection of behaviors suitable for clinical intervention). Because of the possibility of lack of agreement of experts regarding classification of items (as "aggressive"), the BCA may wish to establish some predetermined level of agreement across persons for item inclusion. While the experts may all be chosen from the same category (e.g., theorists,

clinicians, or parents), the BCA may engage persons across divergent categories to perform item selection to ensure that more comprehensive selection criteria are employed for inclusion of items. To make this procedure more concrete, examples of procedures the BCA might use to generate an initial pool of items from which experts would select final behavior categories will now be presented.

First, employing one or more of the self-report variants presented in Chapters 3 and 5, a representative and sufficiently large sample of parents might be asked to respond (verbally or in writing) to the following instruction in an open-ended fashion: "Please list each of the problem behaviors that you feel your child displays at home, either in interacting with you or in interacting with others. For each problem behavior, try to give an example from your experiences and please be as detailed as possible."[2] From a pool of items that a sufficient number of parents (e.g., at least 10 percent) report as problem behaviors, the items judged as "aggressive" by the experts would then be placed in the final item pool.

This judging procedure might be similar to that employed in the construction of certain psychometric instruments, such as the attitude scale. We will digress, for a moment, to provide an example from the social-psychological literature that illustrates this procedure. First, a card-sorting procedure might be employed to discriminate the degree to which certain item statements, such as "I believe the government must continuously demonstrate its power to other nations," represent certain attitudes, such as those about pacifism-militarism. Fishbein (1967) recommends that the item pool of statements, in this case about pacifism-militarism, generated by asking a large group of people to write out their opinions on the subject, be submitted to a series of judges. The judges sort out each item statement into one of 11 piles, which here would range from extreme pacifism (Pile 1) through neutral opinions (Piles 5 and 6) to extreme militarism (Pile 11). Each of the items may now be given a numerical value by noting placement on the scale.

When such sorting has been completed by two or three hundred readers [the judges], a diagram . . . is prepared [see Figure 7.4]. We shall discuss it with the scale for pacifism-militarism as an example. On the base line of this diagram are represented the eleven apparently equal steps of the attitude variable. The neutral interval is the interval 5 to 6, the most pacifistic interval from 0 to 1, and the most militaristic interval from 10 to 11. This diagram is fictitious and is drawn to show the principle involved. Curve A is drawn to show the manner in which one of the statements might be classified by the three hundred readers. It is not classified by anyone below the value of 3, half of the readers classify it below the value 6, and all of them classify it below the value 9. The scale value of the statement is that scale value [below] which just one half of the readers place it. In other words, the scale value assigned to the statement is so chosen that one half of the readers consider it more militaristic than the scale value assigned [p. 85].

This set of procedures could be applied in developing our coding system for "aggressiveness." Once the "problem" items are generated by parents, the judges (our "experts") might be asked to sort parent problem descriptions (prewritten on cards) into one of 11 piles ranging from "nonaggressive response" to "aggressive response," with first and last piles (Piles 1, 2, and 10, 11) representing behavioral extremes, and middle piles (Piles 5, 6) representing a "moderate" degree of aggressiveness. The median or mean rating for each item might then be employed as a quantitative expression of the degree to which judges view a particular behavior as "aggressive" and thus worthy of inclusion in our coding system. A cutoff score (e.g., ≥ 9) could now be chosen for inclusion of items in the coding system. Obviously, the validity of this selection procedure (e.g., how accurately aggressive items are chosen for inclusion) depends on the employment of a sufficient and representative sample of judges chosen according to meaningful criteria of competence.

The above approach suggests a stable construct of "aggressiveness" which includes certain behaviors and excludes others. As already stated, many behaviorally oriented BCAs do not adopt a "construct" point of view. For them behaviors are viewed as the primary focus (endpoint) for assessment and not as signs or indicants of inferred traits like "aggressiveness." If this viewpoint is adopted, the suggested sorting procedure might still be quite profitably employed to scale each behavior in the initial item pool along certain dimensions of interest. Judges might sort items into piles along dimensions ranging from "low intensity–high intensity" to "low priority–high priority," which might aid in selection of items according to practical or other criteria. Patterson et al. (1969), for example, have specified certain codes within their BCS as "high order," and these take precedence over other "lower order" codes if both occur at the same time. Using a systematic sorting approach, experi-

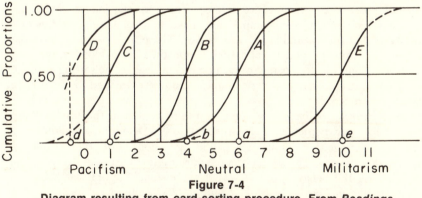

Figure 7-4
Diagram resulting from card-sorting procedure. From *Readings in attitude theory and measurement* by M. Fishbein. New York: Wiley, 1967. Reprinted by permission.

enced coders, parents, or others could provide quantitative information which would aid in making such decisions.

An alternative item selection strategy would employ observational procedures to perform or augment the situational analysis already performed. Using this approach, trained observers might be introduced into a sufficiently large and representative sample of homes of families reporting behavior-management problems and required to make a complete record of ongoing behavior in the setting. Importantly, observers would not employ predefined categories, which might limit the kinds of behavior scanned (and thus defeat the goals of the "shopping" enterprise), but might employ certain nonspecific procedures (e.g., specimen recording, Wright, 1960) to obtain a complete transcript of events that occur. Alternatively, behavior-in-setting of family members might be videotaped to provide the complete record necessary for a situational analysis. Jones et al. (1975) provide this description of early efforts at defining coding categories for the BCS:

> In comparison to contemporary observation procedures, these early excursions were chaotic. Various recording techniques were tried, including extensive note-writing immediately after the observation session, note taking in longhand during the observation session, and even automatic recording during the session with a face-mask device which concealed a microphone and battery-operated recorder. With this apparatus, the observer could unaudibly speak the "stream of behavior" onto permanent tape for later replay. All of these efforts served to sharpen the initial behavior categories and suggest others. A trial set of behavioral categories resulted, with working definitions of the specific behaviors admissable to each category [p. 49].[3]

Thus, observational data are collected via observers or mechanical media, and these complete records of behavior can then be submitted to the judgemental procedures previously described. For example, judges could independently observe the videotapes and make note of specific instances of behavior that they would label "aggressive." Those items seeming to display aggressive content (content validation) would then be included in the resultant item pool. Ideally, scaling or rating procedures like the sorting approach used for written behavioral descriptions would be employed to quantify the selection process.

2. *Definition of behaviors.* Each of the behaviors in the resultant item pool should now be defined as clearly as possible. Definitions should be written in a language that emphasizes specific operations rather than vague, subjective descriptions. The definition or "code" most typically includes: a *name* or label for the behavior (e.g., "verbal aggression," "out-of-seat behavior," "noninteraction," etc.); a *specific definition* of what the label means (e.g., an operational description of the particular elements of the client's behavior that the label encompasses), and *specific examples* of behavioral events that fall within the definition. Often, the use of a symbol for each behavior makes

transcription easier for the observer. Thus, if the aggressive behavior of interest were John's hitting behavior in a classroom, "John-HT" or "J-Ht" would be easier for an observer to write than "John hit another student." Similarly, it would be much easier to write "P" to represent physical aggression, than to write out the words proper.

As an example, the following two codes are part of a coding system developed by O'Leary et al. (1971) which is directed at the classroom behaviors displayed by young children. Note the manner in which the authors defined the purpose, description, critical points, as well as appropriate and inappropriate examples for each behavior.

Vocalization—symbol = V
Purpose: Vocalization is intended to monitor verbal behavior which is usually distracting to both the child and to others.
Description: For the sake of consistency, any *audible* nonpermitted vocalization is to be recorded even though in the opinion of the observer it did not "seem" disruptive. Any nonpermitted "audible" behavior emanating from the *mouth*.
Critical Points: The observer must *actually* hear the vocalization. Inferences are not acceptable except as noted below.
Includes: If vocalization is obvious, but can't be heard (obvious—if another child responds). Answering without being called. Moaning. Yawning. Any noise made with mouth when eating—*unless* child has permission to eat. Any vocalization made in response to the disruptive behavior of another child, e.g., telling another child to return stolen article, crying in response to aggression committed to his person or possessions, etc., if the child has *not* received permission specifically from the teacher to speak. Whispering, belching, crying, shouting, coughs, or sneezes.
Excludes: Vocalization in response to teacher's question. Sneezing. Automatic coughing.
Note: Once a child is recognized by the teacher, vocalization is not scored, regardless of content of the vocalization: crying, yelling, swearing, etc., *until* the teacher specifically instructs the child to stop.

Playing—symbol = P
Purpose: Playing is intended to monitor often subtle manipulative behavior that is distracting to the child and possibly also distracting to others.
Description: Child uses his hands to play with his own or community property, so that such behavior is incompatible (or would be incompatible) with learning.
Critical Points: Child used his *hands* to manipulate his *own* or community property.
Includes: Playing with toy when assignment is spelling. Playing with comb or pocket book. Eating *only* when the hands are being used—chewing gum is not rated as P *unless* child touches or manipulates it with hands. Poking holes in workbook. Cleaning nails with pencil. Drawing on self. Manipulating pencil in such a manner as to make the behavior *incompatible* with learning, e.g., shoving pencil back and forth on desk; waving pencil through air as an airplane. Picking scabs, nails, or nose if the desired "object" is separated from the body and manipulated. Looking into desk and moving arms, but does not come out with a task related object. Working with or reading nontask-related material, e.g., reading page 25 when told to read page 1, doing math when told to do spelling, etc.
Excludes: Touching others' property. Playing with own clothes (Note: Include if ar-

ticle is removed from body, e.g., shoes, tie, buttons, scarf, etc., and is manipulated). Lifting desk or chair with feet (rate N = Noise, if this creates audible noise). Random banging of pencil on desk (rate N = Noise, if audible). Simple twiddling pencil if it is not seen as being incompatible with learning (Note: Include twiddling pencil, banging pencil, or putting pencil in mouth, hair, behind ear, etc., if child attends to such behavior and ceases attending to assigned task). Operational definition of attending: child either looks at manipulated object or begins to manipulate object in nonrandom patterns for more than 5 seconds. Picking scabs, nails, or nose if the desired "object" is *not* separate from the body [pp. 13–15].

Next, three codes from the popular BCS developed by Patterson, Ray, Shaw, and Cobb (1969) are included as further examples of behavioral descriptions. This coding system is directed at the behavior of parents and children interacting in the home.

AP (APPROVAL): Used whenever a person gives clear gestural or verbal approval to another individual. Approval is more than attention, in that approval must include some clear indication of positive interest or involvement. Examples of approval are smiles, head nods, phrases such as, "That's a good boy," "Thank you," and "That's right."

DI (DISAPPROVAL): Use this category whenever the person gives verbal or gestural disapproval of another person's behavior or characteristics. Shaking the head or finger are examples of gestural disapproval. "I do not like that dress," "You didn't pick up your clothes again this morning," "You're eating too fast," are examples of verbal disapproval. In verbal statements, it is essential that the content of the statement *explicitly* states disapproval of the subject's behaviors or attributes, e.g., looks, clothes, possessions, etc. DI can be coded simultaneously with CM = COMMAND. An example of DI and CM being coded together is when father says to the child, "Put on a shirt before you come to the dinner table, I don't like you wearing T-shirts to dinner."

DP (DEPENDENCY): Behavior is coded DP when Person A is requesting assistance in doing a task that he is capable of doing himself. For example, mother is reading the newspaper in the evening and a child who is in junior high school requests her to look up a word in the dictionary; or a child, age 10, asks his mother to tie his shoes. Everyday requests should not be coded as DP; they must meet two criteria: that the person is capable of doing the act himself and it is an imposition on the other person to fulfill the request. For example, asking someone to pass the newspaper which is very close to the individual to whom the request is directed would not be considered DP, since the person would be able to hand the paper to the other individual without an undue amount of effort. If the paper were across the room from where the person is to whom the request has been made, and the person would have to move to get the paper, thus unduly interrupting whatever he was doing, then the request is coded DP [pp. 9–10].

Whenever possible, the simplest wording that accurately describes the behavior should be employed, without excessive use of jargon or words with idiosyncratic meanings. To the extent that the code provides a clear, explicit definition of the behavior, the probability of the observer's being able to employ it at acceptable levels of reliability will be enhanced. Specific procedures regarding how the setting is to be sampled using the final pool of codes should be described in a manual immediately preceding the coding definitions themselves. Procedures for choosing a setting for observation and alternative strategies for sampling will be discussed in Chapters 8 and 9 and will assist the reader in manual construction. Chapter 10 presents a format the assessor might employ in constructing a coding manual.

3. *Evaluation of definition procedures.* To evaluate the manual definitions resulting from steps 1 and 2, an assessment of reliability and validity should be undertaken.

Regarding *reliability*, the BCA must ensure that observers who simultaneously but independently observe a setting agree as to the presence or absence of events as they occur within the stream of behavior. Thus, if an episode of child fighting occurs, two observers must endorse the same code(s) in describing the event (agreement), and must do so each and every time the event occurs to be considered 100 percent reliable, although this level of agreement is typically approached and not achieved. Regarding the observation category itself (excluding the role of observer variables, such as training), agreement seems to depend on the complexity of the behavior observed (e.g., Taplin and Reid, 1973) and, rather obviously, on the clarity and specificity of the coding definition. Issues relating to reliability assessment will be addressed in detail in Chapter 10.

The definition of a behavior category should be refined if observers report difficulties in understanding. When poor levels of observer agreement are found it may be that the definition encompasses too great a range of behavior (overinclusive). For example, "aggressiveness" defined as "any physical interaction between children" would include so many behaviors (e.g., hits, playing "tag," a pat on the back) that it would be questionable as to when not to endorse it, and no information regarding the specific nature of aggressive acts would be obtained. Conversely, definitions so restricted as to exclude important component behaviors (underinclusive) may enhance reliability because of their narrowness, but provide unrepresentative and misleading information. For instance, "physical aggressiveness" defined as "one child kicking another child" excludes many physical interactions of possible interest (e.g., hitting with hands, pinching, shoving with upper torso, etc.). In summary, it may be necessary to redefine coding definitions for which poor reliability or clinically unacceptable information is obtained.

Regarding *validity* it has been stated that the goal of the definition process is to select behaviors from those observed that represent the behavioral dimension(s) the coding system seeks to describe. To employ our coding system for "aggressive" behavior as an example, the final pool of items included in the coding manual should be representative of aggressive behavior in the home, and should exclude behaviors unrepresentative of this dimension. A logical implication of this conclusion is that the codes in the manual should reliably differentiate children labeled as aggressive from those who are non-aggressive as defined by other presumably valid criteria. Lobitz and Johnson (1975) offer an example of this approach to validation.

Because previous studies (e.g., Bugental, Love, and Kaswan, 1972; Shaw, 1971) had found no differences in the coded behavior of children referred for treatment (labeled "deviant") and control groups of nonreferred children, Lobitz and Johnson decided to replicate this approach, but they used more sophisticated procedures for matching the two groups (i.e., age, socioeconomic status, number of siblings, etc.). Using the Behavior Coding System (Patterson et al., 1969), families reporting a problem child (referral group) and families reporting no problematic children (nonreferral group, paid to participate) were observed by independent observers for 45 minutes preceding dinner for five consecutive weekdays. The authors found that "referral" children displayed a significantly greater proportion of deviant behavior (a summary of 15 behaviors from the BCS that parents labeled as deviant; Adkins and Johnson, 1972) and high-intensity deviant behavior, as well as a significantly lesser proportion of positively valenced behavior, than did "nonreferred" children. In addition, the behavior of "referred" and "nonreferred" parents differed significantly, with "referred" parents showing more responsiveness to the children's negative behavior and using more commands. Thus, the BCS was found to discriminate between deviant and nondeviant family members, suggesting its validity as a measure of family problem behaviors.[4] Similar findings for the BCS have been reported by others. Patterson, Cobb, and Ray (1972) found significantly different rates of approriate and inappropriate behaviors between boys labeled (by the school) as "major behavior problems" and "normal" controls. Reid and Hendricks (1973) found the BCS's "Negative Coercive Score" (a series of negative behaviors, i.e., disapproval of others, destruction of property, ignoring others) to significantly differentiate "aggressive" preadolescents from normals in the home. Their "coercive" rates were 75 and 30 percent respectively.

As Lobitz and Johnson (1975) point out, the between-groups (criterion and control) approach to validation of an observational assessment instrument must ensure that groups are matched on potentially important variables like age, sex, socioeconomic status, and other dimensions relevant to particular populations. Nor can the possibility that the criterion group (the group labeled "aggressive," "deviant," etc.) will display more problem behavior because of the demands or expectancies of the situation (to look "good," "bad," justify seeking of treatment) be overlooked.

Another validation approach compares scores computed from observational protocols (e.g., total frequencies, standard scores derived from frequency data) with other measures of the same behavioral dimension or construct. Paden, Himelstein, and Paul (1974) correlated the "total appropriate" score (various socially appropriate behaviors) on the Time Sample Be-

havioral Checklist (TSBC) with three other measures of social functioning for a group of psychiatric residents. The significant correlations between these measures reflect the "convergent validity" of the TSBC (as well as of the other measures). *Convergent validity is the degree to which different measures of the same dimension (or construct) agree (correlate).*
While most often employed to validate measures of presumed personality traits (and the trait constructs themselves), the multitrait-multimethod procedures developed by Campbell and Fiske (1959) have been used to validate observation assessment instruments (Mariotto and Paul, 1974; Cone, 1977). This procedure requires the BCA's employing multiple measures (e.g., observation, self-report, questionnaire assessment, ratings by significant others, physiological measures) of at least two different behavior modes or dimensions. All scores are correlated and placed within a correlation matrix.

To illustrate this, let's imagine that we wish to validate our hypothetical observation system of child aggressive behavior. We include another measure of aggressiveness: parent self-reports (provided on a rating scale), to permit an assessment of convergence across two independent measures of aggressive behavior. We also include both an observational and self-report measure of another (and different) behavior dimension: "child compliance to parental requests," and administer all measures to a group of 30 families. The scores for the 30 families on all measures are correlated producing the correlation matrix shown in Table 7-2. We will employ this matrix to illustrate the multitrait (in this case, multi*mode*)-multimethod approach to validation. In order to determine whether our observation system validly measures aggressive behavior, two classes of validity must be assessed: *convergent validity* and *discriminant validity* (Campbell and Fiske, 1959).

Table 7-2
Multimode-Multimethod Matrix

		AGGRESSIVENESS		COMPLIANCE	
		Observation of Family	Parent self-ratings	Observation of Family	Parent self-ratings
AGGRESSIVENESS	Observation of Family				
	Parent self-ratings	(.95)			
COMPLIANCE	Observation of Family	/.30\	[.33]		
	Parent self-ratings	[.08]	/.43\	(.92)	

Convergent validity—How well do aggressiveness scores derived from our observation system agree with some other measure (in this case parent self-report) of aggressive behavior? Table 7-2 shows a correlation of $r = .95$ (see parentheses) between our observation and self-report measures of aggressiveness suggesting high convergent validity. High convergence ($r = .92$) is also shown for the observation and self-report measures of compliance. Although a validation of our observational measure of aggressiveness is the primary goal, it is obvious that validity information is obtained for all measures employed. While convergence is shown, this finding must now be evaluated in the light of other relations shown in the matrix which permit us to assess discriminant validity.

Discriminant validity—Just as it is important to assess precisely *what* behavior dimension an observational system measures (converges with), it is also important to assess what it does *not* measure. Thus, an observational measure of aggressiveness should not converge (correlate) with a similar or different measure of some irrelevant (distinctively different) behavior dimension. This is called discriminant validity (Campbell and Fiske, 1959; Wiggins, 1973) and is assessed in two major ways.

First, it seems logical that the correlations between different measures (observation, self-report) of the same behavior already discussed should be greater than the correlations between different measures of *different* behaviors (e.g., correlating an observational measure of aggressiveness with a self-report measure of compliance: different measures *and* different behaviors) if in fact our instrument measures what it is intended to measure. Thus, same behavior–different methods is greater than different behaviors–different methods. If this is not true, then our instrument does not show discriminant validity and has little clinical utility as a measure of child behavior. Table 7-2 shows these *different behavior–different method* correlations to be .08 and .33 (shown in brackets). Convergent validity coefficients are shown in parentheses and are much higher (.95 and .92 for aggressiveness and compliance respectively). Our observation system thus meets the first criterion for discriminant validity.

A second, more stringent requirement for discriminant validity "is that correlations between variables presumably measuring the same trait (behavior dimension) exceed correlations between different traits (behavior dimensions) which happen to be measured by the same method" (Wiggins, 1973, p. 408). If the behavior dimensions (aggression, compliance) are distinct and seemingly independent, we would expect significantly less convergence for these *different behavior–same method* analyses than for the same behavior–different method analyses described before. If this is not true, then our findings suggest that the common *method* employed (observation) is more responsible for the convergence displayed than characteristics of the behavior(s) assessed. This is called high method variance and reduces the discriminant validity of our instrument. Table 7-2 shows the results of the *dif-*

ferent behaviors–same method analyses (in triangles), and it is clear that these correlations ($r = .30$ and $r = .43$ for observation and self-report methods, respectively) are much lower than for the same behavior–different methods correlations shown in parentheses.

In summary, our multitrait (actually, multibehavior)-multimethod analyses reveal that our observation instrument shows both convergent and discriminant validity (these findings reflect positively on the self-report measure employed also).

One or more of the foregoing avenues of validation should be employed in evaluating a formal coding system, and of course, could be similarly employed with any assessment instrument.

Footnotes

[1]The term "independent" in this context means that the observer is not an active participant in the stream of behavior in the setting at the time ovservations are carried out. His task is exclusively that of observer, independent of setting events. In contrast, it should be noted that setting "participants" (e.g., staff, family members) frequently employ observational methods to encode the behavior of others as a part of their ordinary in-setting responsibilities. Participant observation will be discussed at length in Chapter 8.

[2]To enhance the accuracy of the parents' report, all parents might be asked to self-monitor problem events for some period of time prior to problem definition along the lines suggested in Chapter 6.

[3]Previous sections of this chapter suggested methodological options which might be useful in collecting these preliminary data.

[4]This approach assumes that observers employ the coding system in identical fashion across the two family categories, thus reducing variability attributable to method. The possibility of observers being influenced by the "demand" suggested by comparing families labeled deviant versus nondeviant is obvious. Chapter 10 offers suggestions for minimizing the effects of observer expectancies.

8

THE SETTING

After the BCA has decided on procedures for recording behavior, he must specify the setting in which clients will be observed. In many cases, it may be desirable to observe client behavior in the natural environment, interfering as little as possible with that setting. Although this would seem the ideal setting for observational procedures, there are a number of reasons why observations in a natural setting may be of limited usefulness. Often important behaviors do not occur with sufficient frequency for the observer to detect and encode them (Patterson and Harris, 1968). For example, the expected frequency of a fight breaking out between adolescents in a treatment cottage may be one or two times per week. An independent observer would have to spend considerable time in the setting to ensure his presence when the behavior occurred. Similarly, an observer might spend two hours each evening in the home of a married couple without observing the verbal arguments that the couple reports occur on a "frequent basis." Often it is important for the BCA to observe directly the characteristics of a behavior or an interaction as it is occurring, and observations in the natural environment may not permit this.

As an alternative, the setting can be modified so that targeted behaviors are more likely to occur (Weick, 1968). For example, the setting could be rearranged to evoke certain classes of behavior so that they may be observed and evaluated as a basis for treatment planning (e.g., increase the frequency of competitive games to evoke aggressive/assertive responses). Other alternatives involving modified settings or the use of clinical analogues of the natural setting are also available to the BCA who wishes to increase the predictability of the target and/or reduce the costs of assessment. If the setting is modified or contrived, however, one might question the degree to which resulting behavior can be compared to the client's ordinary behavior. This chapter will define those observational settings that are available, and discuss some of the important issues suggested within and across setting variants. Setting will be defined rather broadly to include *the physical characteristics of the environment, persons or objects present, as well as controls exerted by extrinsic persons*.

The "Natural" Setting

As mentioned before, the client might be observed in his ordinary or "natural" surroundings. The "natural" environment could be a home, school, place of employment, recreation area, or any other setting in which targeted client behaviors are known to occur as suggested by interviews with the client, staff reports, and the reports of informants close to the client. It would seem that the *ecological validity* of behaviors observed should be greatest in the natural environment. By *ecological validity*, we mean *the relation between behavior independently observed and the way behavior would occur in its natural "stream" if an observer were not present.* (Barker and Wright, 1955).

As an example of observations made in a natural setting, Patterson and his colleagues (Patterson, Cobb, and Ray, 1973; Patterson, 1974; Jones, Reid, and Patterson, 1975) have used the Behavior Coding System or BCS (Patterson, et al., 1969) described in Chapter 7 to record ongoing behavior in the homes of children described as "oppositional." Families who participate in the intervention program are required to permit observers to come into their homes at regular intervals prior to, during, and following treatment. The observer is trained to remain as inconspicuous as possible in the setting, and to attempt to limit interaction with family members. It should be noted that these researchers have found it necessary to alter the natural setting in a number of important ways. First, family members are asked to restrict themselves to certain rooms. If members were permitted to move freely about the house, it would be impossible for a single observer to follow and record the behavior of each and every member without also moving, thus increasing the probability that the observer might interfere with ongoing behavior. Also, some members might become isolated in particular rooms, thus limiting the possibility of interaction between family members. By limiting family members to two rooms in the home, the possibility of family interaction is increased and the practical problem of placing the observer in the setting is also dealt with. Another consideration is that many American families are dominated by the television set which may be tuned to favorite shows from the time family members arrive home in the evening, through dinner, and on into the night. If family members are watching TV, the possibility for verbal interactions is markedly reduced; therefore members are asked that the television set not be in use when the observer is present, thus further modifying the natural setting. Other researchers have imposed similar controls on the setting to facilitate observations (Eyberg and Johnson, 1974; Nay, 1974; Lobitz and Johnson, 1975). Once such modifications are made (even if for very practical reasons), the observer is not recording behavior in a natural environment at all, but in what might best be called a controlled natural setting, that is, *certain controls have been exerted over the participants' ordinary, ongoing behavior.* Ecological validity would seem to be reduced in direct proportion to the degree such controls are imposed.[1]

As we have seen, it may be very difficult to make observations in a natural setting without modifying ongoing behavior. Purely "natural" observations require that the observer be somehow embedded in the setting, so as not to "stand out" in any way, and that no modifications be imposed on client behavior or on the setting itself. If a nurse recorded the behavior of a group of psychiatric patients five minutes during each hour *in* the process of performing her usual duties, these observations might correspond to the "natural" definition. If, however, clients were asked to remain in the day room during that period, desks and chairs were rearranged to increase the possibility of interactions, or any other modifications were made, these observations would be considered to have occurred under "controlled" conditions.

Important Issues

It has been emphasized that the BCA may wish to *maximize* the impact of observation procedures on the self-monitoring client's behavior, as these "reactivity effects" are often in line with therapeutic goals. In contrast, the very nature of independent observational assessment suggests that the impact of the observer on setting behavior should be minimized as much as possible, particularly if generalizations about ordinary setting behavior are to be made from the data obtained. In presenting observational formats to neophyte student or staff observers, or to clients who are to be observed, I have often been asked about the "artificiality" or "unrepresentativeness" of behavior observed under these conditions. Common sense and our own experience tell us that our behavior will be affected by the presence of someone who is observing us, particularly if that individual is a stranger or if the outcome of such observations may have an impact on our lives (e.g., will be used to evaluate us). Given this, it is interesting to note that very little well-controlled research has addressed the issue of reactivity (Kent and Foster, 1977) or the manner in which specific observational variants (methods, observers, characteristics of setting and observees) interact to provoke such reactivity. While potential reactivity effects have been employed to call into question data collected by independent observers (e.g., Kent, 1976), no adequate study of reactivity over long-term observations has been performed (Reid and Patterson, 1976).

Earlier studies addressing this issue are plagued by limited periods of observation (White, 1972) or methodological inadequacies (Patterson and Harris, 1968). A few more recent investigations, while not treating reactivity in the interactional fashion suggested above, are worth noting.

Assuming that mechanical recording procedures would yield less reactivity and faster adaptation to the presence of an observer, Johnson and Bolstad (1975) sequentially alternated observer-collected and audiotape data-recording procedures over a period of six nights for a group of families. They found no significant differences in the frequency of three summary behavior categories ("child deviant," "parent negative," and "parent commands" derived from the BCS) across the two recording methods. Testing for the effects of observation conditions as well as changes associated with the passage of time, the authors concluded that "there was no evidence in these data to suggest differential reactivity to the observation procedures, and no evidence for adaptation to the observational procedures" (p. 184). Unfortunately, the authors did not report a separate analysis for each target behavior (e.g., physical negative, disapproving tone, cry, whine, yell, verbal negativism, tease, and demand attention) that contributes to the summary statistic (e.g., "child deviant"). Perhaps differential reactivity effects would have been shown for these individual categories. Also, specific targets occurring at a very low rate across sessions may not have been detected in the daily 45-minute observational period employed by the authors even though reactivity had occurred. In addition, the authors themselves point out that there is no evidence to suggest that audiotape recording evokes less reactivity than the presence of observers, which limits its usefulness as a measure of "natural" occurrence. Finally, family members were aware of the exact time at which recordings were being made, perhaps masking any change attributable to reactivity due to controls family members imposed on themselves in response to the "demand" evident in the situation.

Using a somewhat similar approach, Hagen, Craighead, and Paul (1975) compared the behavior of staff members in a psychiatric ward setting by using a comprehensive time-sampling checklist approach (see Paul and Lentz, 1977) under conditions of observer presence and absence. Under observer-absent conditions, the staff's verbal behavior was monitored with concealed microphones. Audiotaped protocols were later scored for direct comparison with observer-present conditions. The authors found no significant differences in the appropriateness or frequency of staff behavior across the two conditions, suggesting that reactivity had not occurred. It should be noted that these staff members had been observed for many months prior to this particular investigation and may have become habituated to the presence of the observers. Also, the staff members were provided with little prior information about observation schedules, which may have reduced their ability to alter their behavior in response to demands or expectancies operating in the situation. In addition, staff members were aware that they could be observed at any time and that observational data would be employed to evaluate their efforts with the patients. This may have promoted constant staff vigilance which may have reduced the possibility of behavioral variability.

Thus, while some investigators have found evidence of reactivity promoted by the observer (Roberts and Renzaglia, 1965; Suratt, Ulrich, and Hawkins, 1969; White, 1972; Patterson and Harris, 1968; Mercatoris and Craighead, 1975), others have failed to demonstrate such observer effects (Johnson and Bolstad, 1975; Hagen, Craighead, and Paul, 1975). Unfortunately, it is difficult to draw conclusions from these findings because of differences in methodology, targeted behavior, history of client exposure to the observers, and observational strategies themselves.

Given the *possibility* of reactivity effects, it would seem that the BCA should limit the impact of the observer as much as possible. A number of investigators (O'Leary, Romanczyk, 1971; Patterson, Ray, Shaw, and Cobb, 1969) have offered recommendations regarding the manner in which observers should behave in natural settings.

1. The observer should "become as neutral a stimulus as possible" (O'Leary et al., 1971, p. 3), and avoid interacting with the persons to be observed. Particularly when observing children, the observer should attempt to terminate interactions instigated by the child (e.g., questions about observer presence) as quickly as possible. Often, avoidance of eye contact (e.g., looking away at some *other* child) decreases the possbility of such interactions. One way of reducing the obvious questions generated by the observer's presence is to ask the supervisory person (e.g., parent, teacher, houseparent) to provide a rationale to the observees for the observer. This rationale should be presented in "matter-of-fact" language and be easy to understand. Children will often accept a simple reason, such as "Mr. X. is here today to see what we do,". More complex explanations are sure to generate questions and concerns.

2. The observer should physically position himself away from ordinary paths of movement, yet· have unobstructed visual access to the setting. O'Leary et al. (1971) recommend permanently fixing the position of the observer's chair at the rear or side of the room to minimize disruption. In the home, placement in a corner of the room (*not* in a chair which facilitates interaction and may be obtrusive), on a set of stairs, or anywhere on the floor which is out of the way may be ideal. A careful survey of the setting prior to observations aids in discovery of an optimal location.

3. The observer should be devoid of stimulus value. Dress or demeanor that is atypical of the setting may increase the observer's obtrusiveness. Kuypers, Becker, and O'Leary (1968) attribute the failure of a classroom token economy program to observers who were loud and boisterous in the classroom.

4. Particularly in institutional settings, the observer should make certain that all rules and regulations as well as informal policies are followed. Review of procedures with administrative personnel *prior* to the onset of observations obviates the possibility of any such violations.

5. Observers should enter the setting at times that are *least* disruptive to ongoing behavior (e.g., prior to the dinner hour, if this is the focus for observations; during ordinary setting "breaks," i.e., between classes). In fact, whenever possible, the observer should be introduced into the setting for some period of time *before* formal data collection begins. This provides an opportunity for setting participants to adapt to the presence of the observer and may reduce reactivity, although no clear support exists for this speculation.

While adherence to these guidelines may not eliminate reactivity effects, it certainly increases the probability of unobtrusive, systematic conditions across occasions of observation.

A number of other problems beset the observer in the natural or "controlled natural" setting. The problem of base rates has already been referred to. Behaviors such as physical and verbal aggressiveness, destruction of property, self-mutilation or some categories of bizarre behavior often occur at a low rate and thus may not be seen by the independent observer who engages in time-limited natural recording. In these cases the BCA may be required to modify the setting to evoke the target, employ a clinic analogue setting, or employ ordinary setting participants as observers. This chapter describes these procedures in detail.

Another problem is that extraneous variables, unusual events, and other conditions may alter the natural environment so that data obtained are not typical of ordinary behavior in that setting. If observations are made immediately following home redecoration, if visitors are atypically present in the setting, or if a particular setting member is sick, observational data may very well be at variance with the characteristics and frequency of ordinary behavior in that environment. Thus, the BCA must be very cautious in assigning the term "natural" to the data obtained. Ensuring a representative and extensive sample of observation occasions (Johnson, Christensen, and Bellamy, 1976; Johnson and Bolstad, 1973; see also Chapter 9) would seem to go far in offsetting these possibilities.

Many natural settings make observing very difficult due to poor lighting or acoustics or objects that block the observer's view. Also, as the size of the setting is increased (e.g., very large rooms or the outdoors), it may be difficult for the observer to remain unobtrusively in one place while scanning the entire setting. Finally, it may be impossible to gain permission to observe in certain school and institutional settings.

The limitations and issues presented so far must be placed in the context of the goals of the observational enterprise. Often much useful information relative to treatment planning is obtained even when relatively few observations are made in the natural setting. For example, information regarding the living environment and community resources available to a family, or the physical layout of a home, classroom or institutional cottage might enable the BCA to devise intervention methods that are practical and make best use of the setting's resources. The manner in which family members spend their time and assign themselves to the setting (e.g., several children sleeping in a given bedroom) or the characteristics of a setting like a classroom (e.g., inadequate space; noisy, disruptive events occurring in an adjacent room; the manner in which the teacher positions herself to accomplish her teaching objectives) are among categories of information that may not be self-reported by the clients and can only be assessed by traversing the natural environment. In addition, when limited numbers of observations are made under standardized conditions over time, behavioral changes within that structure may provide useful information regarding client *mastery* of certain skills, even if the observer is unsure of the frequency with which such skill behaviors are displayed in his absence.

If the BCA wishes to *generalize* beyond the conditions of observation to alternative conditions (e.g., observer absence; behavior of setting members at times other than those specifically observed), then extreme caution seems advisable and the issues previously discussed must be addressed.

Methodological Variant: Observation by Setting "Participants"

Much has already been said about the potential impact of an extrinsic, independent observer on the ongoing behavior of the participants in a natural setting. Given this potential for reactivity, a reasonable alternative is to train someone who is already a member of the setting to carry out systematic observations. The term "systematic" means that the setting observer is *trained* by the BCA to carry out observations in a manner similar to those conducted by the extrinsic observer. This form of participant observation is often termed observation by "significant others" (Romanoff, Lewittes, and Simmons, 1976) and while peers, family and staff members, and others are frequently called upon to collect information that is employed as a part of assessment or therapeutic evaluation (Wiggins, Blackburn, and Hackman, 1969; Katz and Lyerly, 1963), Romanoff et al. (1976) point out that "little empirical attention has been devoted to the accuracy of the observation process per se" (p. 409).

In order to evaluate systematically how accurate a "significant other" could be in reliably detecting changes in the behavior patterns of targeted acquaintances, Romanoff et al. (1976) assigned 55 undergraduate subjects to one of three conditions requiring them to engage in clinically relevant or controlled behavior (no change). Subjects in a first group were instructed to behave in a "depressed" fashion (e.g., speaking slowly and softly, avoding eye contact), while subjects in a second group were trained to display "elated" behavior (e.g., animated verbalizations, frequent smiling and eye contact).

Subjects in a final group were instructed to "behave in a typical manner." Each subject was required to enlist the cooperation of a "significant other" (roommate, friend, spouse, or parent) who had frequent enough contact to be available to observe the subject's behavior for a continuous two-hour period one day each week for three successive weeks. "Significant others" were trained to employ a 12 bipolar-item, seven-point scale (Observer Rating Scale) to make behavioral ratings during this two-hour block of time. Without the awareness of the observers, subjects were asked to behave in a "typical manner" during the first week, engage in the clinically assigned behavior (depressed or elated) in the second week, and again engage in "typical" behavior in the third week. All "significant other" observers were contacted by telephone throughout the three-week observation period to ensure that they understood the task and employed the rating scale appropriately. Results indicated that the "significant others" were able to detect a significant difference in the subjects' behavior in the expected direction for both the "depressed" as well as "elated" groups, while detecting no change in the behavior of the control subjects, in line with the authors' speculations. Notwithstanding a number of methodological problems attendant to this investigation (the goals of the investigation are quite obvious from the methodology as well as the nature of the rating scale and may have influenced the observers to expect certain changes in behavior), the results suggest that various persons in the natural environment may be willing to serve as observers for a family member or close acquaintance. Some advantages of this approach are: the "significant other" may be present at times that are inconvenient or impractical for the independent observer and during which certain (particularly low-rate) behaviors of clinical interest may occur; observations may be much less obtrusive (thus reducing reactivity) when made by a person ordinarily present in the setting with whom the observee is comfortable; and the schedule on which observations are made can be varied so that the targeted client is unaware of observation onset, thus reducing obtrusiveness and potential reactivity. In already being aware of the current characteristics and approximate frequency of the client's behavior, the "significant other" may be better able than the independent and unfamiliar observer to detect certain subtle behavioral changes. The following disadvantages are worth noting: the "significant other" may provoke as much reactivity as an independent observer if the targeted client is aware that observations are being made; because of the personal relationship involved, the "significant other" may not be able to endorse the target's behavior in an unbiased fashion; to attain and maintain reliability, the "significant other" would have to be exposed to extensive and continuous training if multiple and sophisticated categories of behavior were being assessed (along the lines suggested in Chapter 10 for the independent observer); and "significant others" skillful in making such observations with reliability may not be available or willing to serve in this role.

In the light of these issues, it would seem that the BCA should explore the possibility of employing "significant others" as observers, particularly when targeted behaviors occur at low rates or are exclusively elicited by unique person/situation occasions that occur on an unpredictable schedule. Finally, such observations serve as another source of information that may be usefully integrated with data collected by other methods, and if nothing else, this information may be useful for clinical/descriptive purposes in defining targets for behavioral change. It would seem that the "significant other" could employ a *limited number* of behavioral categories requiring low levels of inference with a reasonable degree of reliability. Unfortunately, little empirical data is available to evaluate this speculation.

At a more sophisticated level, a good deal of literature has addressed the role of the "participant observer," particularly in research and program evaluation efforts (Selltiz, Johoda, Deutch, and Cook, 1959; Suchman, 1967; Fry, 1973; Balaban, 1973). As the term is employed in the literature, "participant observation" uses a well-trained observer who is *introduced to* a clinical or research setting to become a member of the setting. In his setting role, the participant observer then employs an observational system relevant to research or evaluation goals over a sufficient period of time for setting participants to adapt to his presence. For example, Fry (1973) describes the use of two participant observers (a sociologist and an anthropologist) in a patient-run drug rehabilitation program in a state mental hospital. The researchers negotiated with the "patients" to permit the observers access to the setting. The observers agreed to the following conditions: "they would actively participate in the activities of the program that were appropriate to their peer-group status; they would be subject to patient discipline while they were on the drug unit; they would wear patient clothing during the period of time they were in the initiate phase of the program; and they would make a sincere effort to complete the entire program" (p. 276). Fry reports that while one of the observers remained less involved in the functioning of the various phases of the drug program, the "more involved" researcher became an active member of the group and "was cut off from informants outside the research population, including staff and administration" (p. 276). Fry points out that this second observer attained a position of trust and status in the patient group and was able to collect information that was "more likely to be valid" than that of the less involved researcher who was, however, able to maintain a greater sense of "objectivity." While not employed as a means of formal program evaluation, data collected by the participant observers were used as a basis for generating hypotheses and for making specific recommendations about categories of information to be gathered in a more formal evaluation program. Fry reports: "Some of these recommendations were adopted, which provided the opportunity to test with quantitative data some of the tentative explanations provided by the participant observation study" (p. 277).

Along similar lines, Balaban (1973) points out some of the potential advantages of teacher-participant data collection. First, information regarding the "phenomenology" of the role being studied is acquired. For example, the teacher-observer could provide important information regarding the demands of teaching, which might be useful in formulating and evaluating teacher-training programs. Second, participant observations might well contribute to an understanding of why a particular program fails, with the teacher-observer providing useful information regarding "the powerful but often unrecognized forces in schools that make it difficult for teachers consistently to act as mature adults" (p. 64), as well as the adaptations of an individual school in response to a newly instituted program. Third, the participant teacher can collect information regarding the attitudes of other teachers and staff in a program by "becoming aware of his own [attitudes] and how they change or remain the same over time" (p. 64). Fourth, such data may reveal changes in the staffs' perspective regarding teaching activities. Balaban states: "For example, one may be evaluating an educational program that is changed from viewing and treating problem students as being 'emotionally disturbed' to conceiving problem children as having 'learning problems' related to perceptual-motor difficulties" (p. 65). Finally, useful information regarding the norms as well as the taboos displayed by staff members in a treatment program may be obtained, and this information may well define limitations for change or avenues of education required for a program to succeed.

It should be pointed out that whenever participant observation is to be employed, the permission of all persons to be observed must be obtained. In addition, the BCA must stipulate how potentially embarrassing information or illegal acts recorded by the participant-observer will be reported (Fry, 1973).

An Ecological Approach

The selection of a "natural" setting as the focus of observations may not be as simple as it would seem on the face of it. All of us function within and across a variety of settings. Behaviors of clinical relevance are often displayed in more than one of these settings so that the BCA is clearly faced with a choice: In what specific settings will observations be conducted? This selection becomes more critical in the light of a good deal of evidence, collected within a variety of disciplines, suggesting that the setting itself may hold important predictive implications for behavior (Barker and Wright, 1955; Lewin, 1935; Raush, 1958).

In an early presentation of his field theory of personality, Kurt Lewin (1935) makes the point that: "the dynamics of [behavioral] processes are to always be derived from the relation of the concrete individual to the concrete situation" (p. 41). Lewin viewed the extrinsic environment, or "foreign hull," as predicting behavior in an interdependent fashion with certain internal processes that form the basis of the individual's "personality." In their classic *Midwest and Its Children,* Barker and Wright (1955) report on a variety of ecological assessment procedures, designed to explore systematically this interdependence of person and situation, that could be applied either to molecular or macro settings (e.g., an entire town). Borrowing from the biological concept of the ecosystem, this approach strongly suggests that the behavior of any one element (e.g., person) in a particular environment is influenced by and in turn influences a variety of other elements in that system in an interdependent fashion. Viewing any one element (e.g., a targeted child or adult) in isolation, without taking into account the impact of other persons present, situations within which the individual functions, or the idiosyncratic characteristics of the individual himself (e.g., his "personality," his repertoire of behavior), is to obtain an extremely limited and perhaps misleading view of that individual. When information collected is to be employed to define goals for clinical intervention or to evaluate the impact of such an endeavor, it makes sense that the ordinary, preintervention relation between person and situation be explored, and that any behavioral change be viewed in the context of that interdependent system.

A report by Raush (1958) illustrates the potential impact of situation upon person. Raush and his associates observed the interpersonal behavior (toward each other and toward adults) of six hyperaggressive boys who made up the total patient population of a special ward in a hospital. Confining themselves to "simple, descriptive, hopefully inferential reports of the interactions that occur within a period of about 10 minutes" (p. 235), the observers recorded the youngsters' behavior across a variety of settings, times of day, and activities. Raush reports that different situations did in fact produce different classes of behavior and frequencies within classes. For example, the observers found that eating situations (breakfast, other mealtimes, the snack period prior to going to bed) provoked considerably fewer hostile interactions than did nonfood settings (structured games, unstructured group activity, arts and crafts sessions). In contrast, structured group play activities (games) resulted in many more hostile interactions than did activities where the roles of the participants were more open, less bound by formal rules, and uninvolved in winning or losing. Raush points out that "although one cannot, for example, arrange two breakfasts a day, there may be possibilities for choice between more and less propitious times and settings if we want to maximize the likelihood of establishing friendly communications with a child. Certainly, more specific knowledge in these areas would be of use in clinical planning of residential treatment. However, there have been all too few studies in this direction" (pp. 236–237). Next, the observers found that while behavioral change within subjects was expected over the year-and-a-half period, the degree of change varied quite considerably for different situations. For example, the children increased their interactions toward one another at breakfast time while showing relatively fewer interactions toward adults. The findings were reversed for the arts and crafts setting. Breakfast thus seemed to become a more social occasion, while arts and crafts took on a task focus for the youngsters. Rausch points out that: "the findings imply that studies of behavioral change must either sample situational variants or explicitly recognize the limitation of their sources of reference" (p. 237). Interestingly, the observers also found that specific situations seemed to have special meaning for certain children. Raush indicates that the behavior of a child was more a function of the *child in the setting* than of the additive contributions of setting and child. Thus, an assessment of the specific "interrelation of the child with the situation" seems to be necessary to understand these effects. Rausch provides an example of the behavior of two children: Dave and Clif.

Dave was a child who had rather little difficulty with adults—in this he was unlike most of our children—but he had a great deal of difficulty in his relations with other children, and this was particularly true in competitive situations. Clif, on the other hand, was considered to be a somewhat schizoid child as compared to the others. On the average, 46% of Dave's interactions with other children were coded as hostile; 42% of Clif's interactions with peers were considered hostile; from these values, Dave and Clif looked rather alike. If, however, we turn to the structured group play setting, we see that Dave's interactions with children were hostile in 71% of the codings—as compared to his average of 46%; in contrast, the proportion of Clif's hostile codings went down in the structured play setting—from the average of 42% to 20% [p. 238].

Raush's finding implies that the specific situation (setting) chosen for observing siblings, for example, might predict which child would be labeled deviant and which "normal." In summarizing the importance of evaluating the behavior of persons using an ecological approach, Raush points out:

People exist, behave, fantasy and think in specific environments, and conversely, for psychology at least, situations exist only in the sense that they impinge on specific organisms. We cannot say that any behavior is caused by internal forces of personality or that it is caused by external forces of situational variables. We shall, I believe, have to ask questions about the variations that personality differences induce, with reference to the specificity of environment, and questions about the variations that environmental differences induce, with reference to the specificity of personality components. The precision with which these problems have to be faced depends, of course, on the nature of the questions one is trying to answer, but the issue is always a ghost in the background, whether or not one attests to its presence in the design of the study [pp. 240–241].

Lichstein and Wahler (1976) present an excellent and more recent example of ecological assessment in the case of an autistic child. To evaluate the view that autistic children behave in a relatively invariant and stereotypic fashion across environments, the authors decided to employ a multivariate coding system (Wahler, House, and Stambaugh, 1976) to observe the child's behavior in three very distinctive settings over a period of approximately six months. A total of 16 child behaviors as well as six behaviors of adults and peers were recorded in the three settings: home, school during a structured morning classroom situation, and school in the afternoon in a less structured situation including play. The authors performed a "cluster" analysis (Cureton, Cureton, and Durfee, 1970) to evaluate which response and stimulus class behaviors covaried (changed together) across sessions, and this cluster analysis was performed for each setting. Among major findings, the authors discovered that a total of 22 clusters occurred across the three settings, and interestingly enough only one of these clusters appeared in more than one setting (none of the response-response clusters appeared in more than one setting, suggesting "that the child's behavior was different in different environments" [p. 43]. The authors also found a great deal of variability in the child's behavior over the 42 days of observation. For example, the occurrence of "sustained noninteraction" ranged from as little as 19 percent to as much as 88 percent of the time across days, suggesting the importance of extensive sampling across days to obtain an accurate picture of behavior. An excerpt from the authors' description of their results provides an excellent illustration of the clinical usefulness of data collected with the ecological approach.

The pathology of this autistic child was most sharply reflected in the categories self-stimulation (S), object play (OP), sustained noninteraction (NI), and unusual self-stimulation (US). These were his most frequently occurring behaviors (along with vocalization (V)). In a sense, however, his pathology was equally reflected by the low occurrence of sustained toy play (ST), sustained work (SW), approach adult (Aa), and approach child (Ac). This pattern fits very well with the classic description of autistic children. However, the fluctuations in behavior both within and across settings [would be] buried by the use of arithmetic means and global, summary descriptions [pp. 47–48].

The authors were able to use their findings to call into question many of the conceptions of autism reported by others.

The preceding examples suggest a number of drawbacks to limited assessment across settings. Failure to sample multiple settings in which an individual functions could lead to a variety of errors in the selection of goals for behavior change and in the evaluations of that change. First, the exclusive focus on any one setting, particularly when a restricted time frame is observed (e.g., observing the same individual in the same setting every day between 3:00 and 4:00 P.M.), might very well produce a sample of behavior that is unrepresentative of that individual's functioning in other settings of equal relevance. In fact, the finding of a person-situation interaction that is peculiar to one setting and does not appear in others suggests a different strategy for intervention (e.g., move that person out of that setting; change that particular setting) than would be the case if the behavior were assumed to be generalizable across all settings. Second, characteristics of a particular setting may change over time. This alone may provoke changes in target behaviors. To assume that a program of intervention is solely responsible for such changes may not be stating the entire case or may even be completely inaccurate. A careful, preintervention analysis of how particular setting components seem to be interrelated with targets of interest may permit the BCA to learn about the relative impact of setting variables on the particular target. If a given targeted behavior is relatively insensitive to changes in the setting, then this may suggest that setting changes over time, as intervention proceeds, may be relatively less important as predictors of the target. In contrast, a behavior that is found to be quite sensitive to setting changes might be viewed with caution if *both* setting changes and intervention occur simultaneously. Third, a frequent goal of clinical intervention is to ensure that behavior change occurring in some specific setting (e.g., a clinical setting, a natural setting) in fact gneralizes to alternative environments in which the client functions. When such generalization is the goal of intervention, the BCA frequently takes steps to ensure that it occurs (e.g., Marholin, Siegel, and Phillips, 1976), and the behavior is then assessed in settings (criterion environments) divergent from the treatment setting. An ecological approach suggests that targeted behavior may change in its characteristics and/or frequency *merely* as a function of changing the setting in which the individual functions (e.g., Raush's example of Dave and Clif). This behavior change, provoked exclusively by the interaction of setting and person, might be inappropriately employed as evidence of generalization or failure of generalization if the investigator has not systematically pre-evaluated all settings in which generalization is expected to occur.

The finding that clinical intervention often fails to generalize or that the behavior of persons seems to vary quite considerably across settings (Lichstein and Wahler, 1976) becomes much more understandable when an ecological point of view is adopted. The foregoing suggests that multiple situations, times, activities, or other relevant phenomena should be sampled in a more comprehensive fashion if a representative view of an individual's behavior is to be obtained. This is particularly important when the BCA wishes to generalize findings obtained in a particular setting to alternative settings, targets, or persons.

The Clinical Natural Setting

Often, it is impractical or impossible for the BCA to traverse the natural environment to make systematic observations. While some investigators have employed teams of persons to serve as behavioral observers (Patterson et al., 1973), many clinical and research settings cannot financially provide for staff members who serve as full-time data collectors.[2] Systematic observation of client behavior in the clinical setting obviously decreases the cost of such observations and may make it possible for the a BCA to employ observational methods on a regular basis. One possibility is to attempt to make the clinical setting similar to the client's natural environment. This will be called a "clinical natural" setting.

Let us imagine that a BCA wishes to observe systematically the ordinary interaction of a family in a setting similar to the home. A waiting room could be constructed with comfortable chairs, lamps, a rug, and other materials to make it like a home setting. Using a one-way mirror, videotape camera, or an observer who is physically placed in the setting, observations could be made of the manner in which the family members interact with one another while "waiting" to come into the treatment room proper. When such observations are made, the BCA does not attempt to control the behavior of clients in any fashion, but lets them *interact as naturally as possible within the clinical environment.* Along similar lines, when a child's behavior is the focus for treatment, it may be useful to observe the interactions between parent and child in a playroom setting, when they are asked to act "naturally" and do what they wish to do.

Obviously, behavior occurring in such an environment may be influenced by characteristics of the setting proper, the clients' expectancies as to what the BCA desires, or a host of other variables. To the extent that the BCA makes observations of the client on each occasion in a similar fashion and in the same setting, it might be assumed (since all of these variables are being held constant) that any changes in the client's behavior are due to the treatment proper. Thus, even though behavior might be influenced by the artificiality of the setting, observations conducted in a systematic fashion in the same setting across time may provide a useful record.

One important assumption of this approach is that clients cannot behave beyond their repertoires. That is, it seems improbable that an individual could radically change his behavior (e.g., instantaneously learn new skills) even though he is aware of being observed. The parent who has extreme difficulty in obtaining child compliance to frequent commands in the natural environment may very well experience the same difficulties in the clinical natural setting. While the parent may make fewer or more commands than normal in this clinical setting, the strategies employed (e.g., classes of behavior) may be very similar to those employed at home. Thus, no matter how much this parent wants to "impress" or show "how bad the child is," it is not likely that he will be able to alter dramatically his ordinary way of behaving. In addition, if the setting is free from distractions by other staff members, other clients, noise, and so forth, clients will often report that they "forgot" that observations were being made as they became caught up in their ordinary patterns of behavior.

The advantages of clinical natural recordings are obvious. The BCA can ensure that the observational setting is identical each time observations are made and extraneous variables often present in the natural environment are thus limited. It may also be easier to audio- or videotape client behavior if necessary. In addition, the clinical setting permits multiple treatment agents to observe how the client interacts with important others, which may not be possible, due to practical limitations, under natural conditions. Staff members who cannot take the time to drive out into the community to make a naturalistic observation may very well be able to observe clients behaving in the clinical setting. Thus, the expertise of many observers may be exploited in defining and interpreting what is occurring. The clinical natural setting offers a useful option to observations made in the natural environment, and might artfully be used in combination with naturalistic observations to ensure a comprehensive view of client behavior.

The BCA should be certain that clients are aware that observations are being made when this approach is employed. Observing clients in a waiting room, playroom, or some such setting without their knowledge would seem to be an unethical practice. The BCA may wish to inform clients on each and every occasion prior to such observations, or obtain the clients' permission for random observations of their behavior in the setting over time.

The Clinical Contrived Setting

It has already been emphasized that certain potentially important problem behaviors occur at such low rates in the natural environment that the observer is unlikely to witness them. Of course the same would hold true for the clinical natural setting. We have already mentioned that the natural setting may be structured to some extent, as in limiting clients to certain rooms, turning off television, and so forth, but still no specific instructions are provided for clients as to how to behave, what to do, or the like. Because the BCA is often in the unfortunate position of having to collect as much assessment information as possible in a brief span of time, clinic setting variants have been developed that enable the BCA to evoke important problem behaviors so that they may be observed and carefully evaluated. Most of these approaches attempt to simulate important aspects of the natural setting in the clinical setting so that client responses may be monitored and encoded in some fashion. While many such approaches are available and often idiosyncratically employed across clinical settings, it is only in recent years that categories of the clinical contrived approach have been cataloged (McFall, 1977; Nay, 1977). Discussing these various approaches as "analogues" of behavior in the natural environment, this author reviewed the recent literature and found that most contrived situations fall within one of the following five categories: (1) paper-and-pencil analogues, (2) audiotape analogues, (3) videotape analogues, (4) enactments, and (5) role-play analogues. While it is beyond the scope of this text to evaluate thoroughly the literature relating to these approaches, each will be defined and relevant examples will be presented. A brief discussion of their advantages and disadvantages for assessment will follow.

The *paper-and-pencil analogue* requires the respondent to write or describe verbally how he would respond to some situation presented in written form. Often, the client is asked to describe what he would say and/or do in response to a stimulus scene or endorse (e.g., yes/no; multiple choice) one of several prelisted response alternatives. The stimuli usually depict some event in the client's life situation that is relevant to assessment. For example, in determining the characteristics of a client's fear of heights, a written stimulus like the one below would be presented along with instructions that the respondent is to describe what he would say and/or do in the situation.

You are walking into a medical arts building for an appointment with your dentist and you notice that you are quite late for your appointment. A directory placed on the wall shows you that the dentist's office is on the ninth floor of the building. To reach that floor you have two alternatives: an elevator located nearby or a door leading to many flights of stairs. Please describe what you would say to yourself and/or do in this situation. [Spaces provided for response.]

In training groups of mothers to employ "time-out procedure" (brief isolation contingent on a problem behavior) with problematic children, the author (Nay, 1975) employed a number of written analogue items in a paper-and-pencil test of subjects' knowledge of the procedure. The subject was asked to circle the appropriate response alternative. For example:

You have just sent your child to time-out. He stops crying and calls out: "Mom, I'm sorry, I'll be good now." You should:
   a. Go in and tell him you understand, but that he must remain in time-out for the full time.
   b. Ignore it.
   c. Tell him that since he knows what he did wrong, he can get off the chair—but only if he's good.
   d. Let him get off the chair, but say nothing.
   e. None of the above.

Appropriate responses were preselected by a panel of judges familiar with the time-out approach, so that scoring was merely a matter of rating client responses using a response-scoring key.

Obviously, any situation could be presented in written form with instructions for the client to respond in writing or verbally. When open-ended responses are permitted the scoring becomes more difficult, in which case responses should be submitted to more than one scorer so that reliability (agreement) can be obtained to predefined criteria. A main advantage of the written analogue is that it can be administered to large numbers of clients with little cost in assessment time. The major disadvantage is suggested by the nature of the task: it is difficult to determine how a client's written responses of what he would do correlate with his actual behavior in the natural situation. The degree of correlation between written and *in vivo* responses should obviously be assessed in validating the analogue; however, this is rarely reported in the literature. This approach primarily taps the client's knowledge (e.g., of how to respond appropriately) and phenomenal view of how he would approach various life situations, and the interpretation of the data should be qualified by this.

The *audiotape analogue* presents situations similar to the paper-and-pencil approach; however, the situation is presented on audiotape. Typically, a narrator introduces a scene on the tape—for example: "Your boss calls you into the office and very thoroughly berates you for something that you know you have not done wrong. You try to tell him of his mistake, but he takes offense and begins to call you names and question your parentage." This is followed by an actor making a verbal statement appropriate to the scene—Boss: "I just don't know what's the matter with you, I can't depend on you anymore. I'm not going to tolerate this kind of behavior and I want you to know that your job is questionable at this time. What do you have to say for yourself?" In this example, perhaps calling for an assertive response from the client, an auditory cue, such as a tone or statement, then instructs the client to make a verbal response appropriate to the situation. Importantly, the client is not asked to describe what he would do, but to respond verbally to the actor on the audiotape as if the situation had actually occurred in the natural environment. Thus, the audiotape approach attempts to elicit a segment of client verbal behavior which may be either directly observed or tape recorded for scoring later. For example, Goldstein, Martens, Hubben, Van Belle, Schaaf, Wiersma, and Goedhart (1973) presented 50 interpersonal situations on audiotape to groups of psychiatric residents to assess their skills in dealing with social situations. The instructions and an example item are presented below:

We've asked you to come in today for a routine investigation in which every patient will participate. It will be important for you, but we will benefit from it as well, because it will give us information about the effectiveness of our methods. In a moment we will describe several everyday situations. We would like you to respond to each description by telling us what you would say if you were in such a situation. We ask you to tell us what you would say. An example of such a situation would be: It is Friday afternoon, 5:00 and you are about to go home from work. Your boss appears and says: "We've just received some work we didn't expect. It must be completed. Everybody will have to work overtime." The tape will then say: "What is your answer?" When you hear that, we ask you to say in two or three sentences what you would say in reality [p. 34].

In describing this approach, the authors point out that the responses obtained "do not speak to the issue of overt, patient behavioral change in his real life environment" (p. 4), and emphasize the need to correlate audiotape analogue responses to responses in the natural environment to similar situations. More recently this approach has been employed by Arkowitz, Lichtenstien, McGovern, and Hines (1975) to depict relevant "dating" scenes and Nay (1975) to evaluate parental responses to a "problem" child. It could be a most efficient and inexpensive way to obtain a sample of client verbal responses to virtually any stimulus situation relevant to assessment.

Two major advantages of this approach are its flexibility in administration (clinical or natural settings) and the fact that an overt sample of behavior is elicited. A major disadvantage is the exclusive presentation of auditory stimuli. Nonverbal communicative behavior as well as the characteristics of a setting may provide cues to the respondent as to what is an appropriate response, and these cannot be displayed on an audiotape (e.g., the facial expression of stimulus person, public vs. private settings). Finally, it is an empirical question as to whether verbal responses elicited by audiotape stimuli are consonant with those elicited by similar stimuli in the natural setting.

The *videotape analogue* is similar to the audiotape format; however, both a video and audio presentation are made to the respondent, followed by instructions for him to make verbal and perhaps nonverbal responses. In employing this approach, some relevant situation in the natural environment is first chosen (e.g., a child engaging in problematic behavior). Then a script is written which ideally attempts to simulate that situation or set of stimuli. The script may be taken from observational data gathered in the setting so that the simulation can be as consonant with the natural environment as possible. Actors are then chosen to portray relevant persons (e.g., child, spouse, peer, patient) and trained to speak and behave in accordance with the script. Special effects (e.g., multiple cameras, dissolves) might enhance the quality of the production; however, excellent videotape analogues may be made with simple camera-recorder combinations. Typically, a narrator introduces each scene (audio only or audiovisual) followed by actors in the scene proper. The client is then instructed to make a verbal and/or nonverbal response to the person on the videotape. Ideally, presentation of scenes should be preceded by example items which provide the respondent with the opportunity to practice this rather unusual task. The following is an example of script material which might be employed to produce a videotape analogue directed at assessing the competence of staff members in using a treatment program in an institutional setting.

(Audio only) *Narrator:* We appreciate your time in completing these instruments for us today. This time, instead of having you answer questions by writing the answers, we are going to take a look at what you would actually say and do in response to a variety of situations involving patients. On the TV screen you will first hear a narrator describe an everyday kind of situation, then you will see a patient actually behave in that situation. You will notice that when the patient talks to you, he or she looks right at you. Try to think of the patient on the screen as being physically here in the room with you. When you hear a tone, like this [tone], please say exactly what you would say to the patient if you encountered the same situation on the ward. You will begin each scene by standing; however, if you would ordinarily sit down in responding to the patient, you may sit in the chair by the screen as part of your response. Before we begin, let's try a couple of practice scenes so you can get used to talking to the patient on the screen.

(Audio and video) *Narrator* [appears on the screen, seated, facing the camera]: Let's see if you can be comfortable in talking to me. I will ask you a few questions, and you answer them by talking *directly* to me, as if I am in the room with you, okay? What is your name? [tone; five seconds. Time is provided on the running videotape for the respondent to make a response.] Do you feel a bit nervous about doing this? [tone; five seconds for response.] What are your favorite responsibilities here at the hospital? [tone; five seconds for response.] Do you have any questions about what you are to do? [tone; five seconds if "no"; if "yes," the tape is rewound and the instructional portion with examples is repeated.]

(Audio: narrator's voice; video: shows scene in day room, with woman seated; no one else is present) *Narrator:* Now that you've practiced with me, let's have you try with a patient. Mrs. Edwards has been diagnosed a "depressive." She rarely speaks with anyone and most often prefers to remain alone in her room. Notice how she rarely looks up to see what is going on around her. Imagine you are walking into the day room now as the scene begins and you notice that after a while she looks up to you as if to speak.

Mrs. Edwards [begins looking down at floor; at the cue from the director looks up at the camera, glances away, then returns her full-faced attention to the camera, moving her lips slightly—does *not* speak]. [tone; 30 seconds—"Stop".]

While the production of a videotape analogue may not be feasible in settings lacking necessary electronic equipment, this approach obviously offers a more natural stimulus to the respondent, since both nonverbal and verbal behavior may be displayed as well as certain setting characteristics. To the extent that the videotape accurately simulates the natural setting, the validity of responses to the scenes would seem to be enhanced. Particularly when client responses are videotaped, the data obtained may not only be useful for assessment, but may be reviewed with the client at a later time as part of a "videotaped feedback" (Bailey and Sowder, 1970).

Among disadvantages, it is costly to produce a videotape, as the visual presentation demands that the criterion (natural) environment be duplicated as closely as possible. Inaccurate depictions of the natural setting may make the stimuli "unbelievable" for the client, leading to an invalid record of responses. Perhaps the audiotape analogue that forces the client to imagine how the setting and persons appear (in line with his own cognitive set) promotes a more accurate record for clients who possess well-developed imaginations. Thus, parents hearing a child's voice on audiotape may be able to imagine that the child is their own, whereas a visual depiction of the child makes it very clear that the scene is simulated by an actor. Finally, the questions in regard to all of the analogues discussed so far also apply to the video-tape format: Is it an accurate simulation of the natural setting, and does it provoke responses consonant with those provoked by *in vivo* stimuli? To date, there is no empirical basis for answering these questions.

The *enactment analogue* requires the respondent to interact in the clinical setting with stimulus persons or objects which ordinarily exist in the natural setting. The BCA's role here is merely to monitor client responses. The most common example of this approach is the Behavioral Approach Test (BAT) originally employed by Lang and Lazovik (1963) to evaluate the approach responses of fearful clients to feared stimuli. For example, a client afraid of snakes might be asked to approach a snake physically in the clinical setting until anxiety is elicited. This category of analogue has in itself become the object of evaluation efforts (Bernstein and Nietzel, 1973; see Borkovec, Weerts, and Bernstein, 1977) and numerous investigators have developed BATs relevant to particular categories of feared stimuli.

Among non-BAT analogues, parents may be asked to interact with their children (e.g., in play or in a task) as they typically do at home (Herbert, Pinkston, Hayden, Sajwaj, Pinkston, Cordua, & Jackson, 1973; Toepfer, Reuter, and Maurer, 1972); married couples may be assigned a topic similar to those ordinarily discussed (Carter and Thomas, 1973; Eisler, Hersen, and Agras, 1973), or all the members of a family may be asked to discuss certain topics and perhaps reach a consensus (Alexander, 1973). Virtually any stimulus array which could be duplicated in a clinical setting might be the focus of an enactment. Williams and Brown (1974), for example, constructed a realistic tavern atmosphere in a hospital setting and provided alcohol to a population of alcoholics and normal drinkers to determine the manner in which each consumed alcohol. These authors went to great lengths to simulate the lighting, props, sound, and other atmospheric conditions found in local pubs in an attempt to depict the natural setting accurately.

For most enactments, a formal scoring system is developed to evaluate the behavior dimension(s) of interest. For example, with a BAT, the relevant data might be the number of feet the client moves toward a feared object or the number of minutes the client remains in a feared setting (e.g., a dark room). Obviously, when social interactive behaviors are involved, a variety of verbal content, nonverbal, and paralinguistic behaviors can be systematically observed and encoded either directly or from videotapes displaying client responses. This approach is perhaps the most straightforward of the analogues in that the actual stimuli are presented in conditions that simulate a more normal situation.

The major advantage of this approach is that the client is exposed to a standard stimulus and responses are scored according to a predetermined format. Enactments can thus be administered prior to, during, and following treatment as a measure of behavior change, making them suitable for research purposes. The most prominent disadvantage of the enactment is that certain stimuli cannot be reproduced in the clinical setting. For example, if a client were afraid of crossing bridges or swimming, it might be very difficult (if not impossible) to duplicate such stimulus situations. In such cases, the BCA may be forced to observe the client's behavior in the natural setting, or present such stimuli to the client imaginally in the hope that the imaginal stimulus will evoke responses similar to the actual stimulus. Second, data obtained in an enactment are limited by the degree to which natural stimuli are accurately duplicated. For example, most BAT administrators merely present a snake or small animal to a client in a clinical office or laboratory setting; obviously certain natural stimuli that may come to control the behavior (e.g., stimulus control) are not present, thus limiting the validity of the findings. Because this approach has been employed more than any other contrived format, investigators are beginning to evaluate the enactment itself, and the conditions (e.g., expectancy to perform, demand characteristics) that may affect performance.

Finally, the *role-play analogue* requires the client to visualize or *covertly rehearse* stimuli under standardized conditions or *overtly role play* criterion situations with staff members and/or other clients portraying relevant persons. The idea of this approach is that it may not be practical or feasible to reproduce the natural setting and furthermore important persons in the client's life may be unable or unwilling to perform in an enactment. In addition, the BCA may wish to expose the client to a situation that does not typically occur in the natural setting to see how the client will respond; to catalogue the client's repertoire of skills. Thus, the role-play is not limited by the actual characteristics of naturally occurring stimuli and much flexibility is possible. Role playing has been employed to assess certain social skill behaviors, specifically assertive behavior (Eisler, Hersen, and Miller, 1973; Hersen, Eisler, and Miller, 1974; Serber, 1972) as well as avoidant behavior in social situations (Borkovec, Wall, and Stone, 1974; Goldfried and Trier, 1974). As an example of this approach, Eisler, Miller, and Hersen (1973) have developed the Behavioral Assertiveness Test which evaluates the responses of subassertive clients to each of 14 interpersonal situations calling for assertive responses. Typically, a staff member role-plays a stimulus person of relevance to the scene. The following two scenes are representative of this analogue approach.

Narrator: "You're in a crowded grocery store. You pick one small item and get in line to pay for it. You're really trying to hurry because you're already late for an appointment. Then, a woman with a shopping cart full of groceries cuts in line in front of you."
Woman (actor): "You don't mind if I cut in here, do you? I'm in a hurry" [p. 298].

Narrator: "You're having lunch with a friend. Suddenly she asks you if you would lend her thirty dollars until she gets paid next week. You have the money, but were planning on spending it on something else."
Friend (actor): "Please lend me the money; I'll pay you back next week." [p. 298].

With each scene the client is asked to respond as he ordinarily would, and the authors code each of eight behavioral components of assertiveness (duration of looking, duration of reply, latency of response, loudness of speech, compliance content, request for new behavior, affect, and overall assertiveness). Responses are assessed by behavioral observers who observe through a one-way mirror adjacent to the assessment room.

An advantage of the role-play analogue is that almost any stimulus situation can be presented by having the client imagine the stimuli or by presenting him an overt role-play involving setting participants who portray relevant roles. Also, this approach can be used in any setting and does not require special equipment.

The degree to which client behavior in response to role-play scenes approximates behavior in the natural environment probably depends on the similarity between role-play stimuli and natural stimuli, the client's ability to role-play and "get into" the scene, and the instructions provided ("respond as you ordinarily would"; "respond as you'd like to respond;" etc.). However, these suggestions remain speculative due to a paucity of research directed specifically at this approach.

In summary, investigators are increasingly employing clinic-administered analogues due to the reduced costs of assessment and ease and standardization of administration of these approaches. While the Behavioral Approach Test has been most widely employed, a variety of other analogue options are available and should be considered when observations in the natural setting are not practical or feasible. It is difficult to evaluate the relative efficacy of each of these analogue categories because few investigators have evaluated them as the primary focus for research. Thus, it is not clear whether the time-consuming procedures of enactment or role-play will provide a more valid and reliable sample of client behavior than approaches involving paper and pencil or media presentations. It is also important to note that few investigators have attempted to validate analogue measures by correlating analogue data with client behavior elicited by natural (criterion) stimuli (Nay, 1977), and only a very few investigators report test-retest or internal consistency measures of reliability. It is hoped that this potentially important avenue of assessment will receive more systematic attention in the immediate future.

Footnotes

[1]It seems reasonable to assume, in the absence of research addressing this issue, that the specific nature of the controls would interact in some fashion with characteristics (e.g., ordinary locus, perhaps rate and duration) of each observed target to predict validity within a multivariate coding system such as the BCS.

[2]There is some evidence to suggest that the demands of achieving and maintaining acceptable levels of observer accuracy (reliability) with multivariate coding systems require "professional" observers (Paul and Lentz, 1977; Redfield and Paul, 1976).

9

SAMPLING

Once methods are selected and a setting has been chosen for observing the targeted behavior, an initial question is: How often and according to what schedule will the setting be sampled? Ideally, observations should be made on a continuous basis, so that every incidence of a target is noted in some fashion. Unfortunately, this approach is as costly and impractical as it is ideal. Just as the experimenter chooses a representative sample of subjects from the population he wishes to generalize his findings to, the BCA must sample the target so that its detected incidence is representative of its actual frequency. Two strategies for sampling are available: *event sampling* and *time sampling*. In *event sampling, the occurrence of the targeted behavior exclusively determines the observer's behavior;* that is, the observer only makes an endorsement if one or more preselected "events" occur. If the events of interest fail to occur, no endorsement is made. This is a simple and straightforward procedure; numerous variants have been employed to sample a wide range of targeted behaviors (Wright, 1960). In *time sampling, time as well as the incidence of a particular behavior determines the observer's response.* The observer systematically attends to and records ongoing behavior according to a predetermined time schedule. As Wright (1960) points out: "This closed procedure fixes attention of observer and analyst upon selected aspects of the behavior stream as they occur within uniform and short time intervals. The length, spacing, and number of intervals are intended to secure representative time samples of target phenomenon" (pp. 92–93). For example, observations might be made only during the last five minutes of each hour throughout the day, for one minute out of each five-minute time block, or every six seconds for one hour each day for some set number of occasions. The methodological variants of time sampling are numerous and, as might be imagined, the particular schedule employed has important implications for the representativeness of data collected as well as the practicality of various recording methods.

Time sampling has been most frequently employed in research and clinical investigations where a targeted event must be described discretely and according to well-standardized procedures. In addition, time sampling itself has become the focus of a number of excellent methodological critiques (Arrington, 1943; Wright, 1960) as well as research investigations (Powell, Martindale, and Kulp, 1975; Repp, Deitz, Boles, Deitz, & Repp, 1976). It is, however, unfortunate that little systematic research has been performed to assist the BCA in relating specific parameters of time sampling (e.g., schedule, interval of observation) to specific assessment goals (Boyd and DeVault, 1966).

For each sampling approach, a description of sampling methodology will be followed by a discussion of the advantages and disadvantages of the procedure and other important issues suggested by the literature.

Event Sampling

Most event sampling strategies are directed toward merely encoding the frequency of preselected targets ("specific" recording, see Chapter 7) occurring within a global time period (e.g., one hour, across the day). Most often the observer is merely required to make a slash mark, "X," or other endorsement indicating presence or absence of the event. Thus target categories might be listed vertically on the left-hand side of a recording sheet, with the observer required to make an endorsement next to the observed target as it occurs. Or, the observer might employ a mechanical means of endorsing the event.

O'Brien, Azrin, and Bugle (1972), for instance, employed both mechanical and written methods to determine the frequency of crawling and walking responses in a population of retarded children (aged five to seven years) in a day-care nursery school program. The authors defined crawling as "uninterrupted movement across the floor for at least three seconds with a knee in contact with the floor," and walking as "uninterrupted movement across the floor for at least three seconds but with the soles of the feet contacting the floor" (p. 132). Viewing the children's locomotive behaviors through one-way mirrors in two separate rooms, two independent observers were instructed to code a crawling or walking event by depressing one push-button switch when the child walked and another when the child crawled. The switches activated timers and counters in another room. To augment these observations, five different teachers were instructed to note instances of crawling or walking as well as the time of day on a standard recording sheet. The recording sheets were placed in a number of readily accessible locations in the setting. The teachers were trained to estimate three seconds by covertly counting, "one thousand-one, one thousand-two, one thousand-three," and since two or more teachers were usually present, the one physically closest to the recording sheet was instructed to do the recording. The precise definitions of behaviors employed by the authors combined with a straightforward and simplistic recording procedure are hallmarks of the event-sampling approach. As might be expected, the authors report very few disagreements between the two independent observers using the event system, or between an independent observer who was consistently present and the teachers' recordings. By requiring the event observer to write down the precise time at which a particular target is endorsed, the BCA can go back and readily compute reliability between multiple and independent observers. When behavior is not linked to time, which is unfortunately often the case with an event sampling system, it becomes very difficult to assess whether or not multiple observers are recording the same event at the same time. For example, if the two observers in the O'Brien et al. study were to event sample for a period of two hours, without noting time of incidence, there might be very high agreement between observers regarding the total number of events observed, but a remarkable lack of reliability in their observation of specific incidences. Chapter 10 discusses the assessment of reliability in event sampling in more detail.

In another example of a "specific" approach to event sampling, Mahoney, Van Wagenen, and Meyerson (1971) observed children in a school setting for a period of three and a half hours each day for a minimum of five days. During this time, records were kept by the staff members of the number of toileting responses. In addition to noting the incidence of toileting, the adequacy of the child's toileting behavior was rated on a scale from 0 to 10, and these data were recorded on a chart and posted in a conspicuous setting. Both the O'Brien et al. (1972) and the Mahoney et al. (1971) studies indicate one of the major advantages of the event approach, particularly in settings where staff members or other indigenous persons, such as parents or a spouse, are present on a continuous basis. While such persons might not be able to employ a more sophisticated time sampling procedure in addition to carrying out their everyday responsibilities in the setting, they may be able to make the simple incidence ratings required by the event approach. Thus, event sampling readily lends itself to observations by significant others or participants (see Chapter 8) and is often the sampling procedure of choice when it is impractical or unfeasible to employ independent observers.

While the focus on a specific targeted behavior within a preselected category-checklist-rating scale approach is frequently preferred because of its simplicity and precision, many investigators require the observer to note information of interest other than the event itself. For example, the "nonspecific" narrative description typical of specimen recording, described in Chapter

7, permits the BCA to collect information regarding behavior that is an antecedent or consequence of the event, as well as times, locations, persons present, or other conditions that may hold controlling properties. Wright (1960) emphasizes the need for a more comprehensive description of behavior. He states: "Possibly the greatest limitation of event sampling is that it breaks up the larger continuity of behavior" (p. 108). He cites an excellent example of a comprehensive event sampling approach in summarizing the work of Dawe (1934). Dawe event sampling the quarrels that occurred among preschool children in a nursery school setting during free play hours over a period of four autumn and winter months. Subjects were 19 girls and 21 boys, aged two to five years. Dawe watched the children from a central spot on the playground or from a doorway between two of the main rooms. She attempted to reposition herself at the time of a quarrel, so that multiple categories of data could be collected on prepared forms as each event occurred. The forms provided space for recording: (1) the *name, age,* and *sex* of every participant; (2) the *duration* of the quarrel; (3) *what the children were doing* at the time the quarrel began; (4) the *topic* quarreled about: contested ownership, violence, interference with activity, or other social stress; (5) the *role* of each participant: precipitator, main aggressor, retaliator, sheer emotor, objector, or passive recipient; (6) specific *motor and verbal accompaniments*; (7) the *outcome* of the quarrel: yielding to force, voluntary yielding, compromise, interference by child spectator, or intervention by a teacher; and (8) the *aftereffects*: good cheer or resentment. Dawe found that of 200 quarrels observed at the rate of three to four per hour among the 40 children, the average duration was 24 seconds, with only 13 lasting more than a minute. While the length of a quarrel was nearly twice as great for outdoor as for indoor quarrels, those stopped by the teacher were not significantly shorter than those settled by the children. As might be imagined, boys quarreled significantly more often than girls, with rare intrasex quarrels ending with some form of compromise much more frequently than intersex quarrels. Retaliative acts increased with age; however, the absolute number of quarrels declined with the age of the children involved. The vast majority of the quarrels (197) included motor activities such as pushing or striking. While yielding to force was the most common outcome of the quarrel, quick and cheerful recoveries significantly outnumbered resentful aftermaths (about 3 to 1). Wright (1960) has made the point: "Here are data gathered by recording unitary behavior events as they happen, one by one, in the naturally occurring behavior streams of children; and it is submitted that these data are splendidly intelligible and useful" (p. 105). I would wholeheartedly agree with Wright's evaluation, and underscore that a more comprehensive description of behavioral events produces a much more representative depiction of behavior as it occurs, as well as providing information that may be eminently useful for both clinical and research purposes. In summary, then, while the major focus of event sampling is on the incidence of the target, methods of endorsing the behavior and its referents are limited only by the BCA's creativity, practical limitations posed by the sophistication of observers, and the setting itself.

It should be noted that many of the mechanical recording procedures presented in Chapter 7 are suitable for event sampling. The observer might depress a wrist or electronic counter, make a tear in a 3 x 5 card, transfer a coin from one pocket to another, or employ any other mechanism that permits a frequency count. In addition, audio or videotape media can be used to obtain a complete record of behavior within a time frame, and these taped records may then be event sampled by observers at a more convenient time in one of the ways outlined above.

Noteworthy *advantages* of the event-sampling approach include the following. When low-rate behaviors are of interest, event samples made by persons ordinarily present in the setting offer a useful alternative to time-sampling approaches that restrict observation times and may thus miss the rare occasions of the event. Event sampling thus permits an expansion of the observation period in an economical and efficient fashion. Event sampling is flexible enough to accommodate virtually any sort of recording method from specimen recording to "on-off" record-keeping systems employing symbols, check marks, ratings, and so forth. Time sampling systems may not permit this kind of flexibility in record keeping because of the abbreviated and restricted observation intervals often employed. However, event sampling is quite easy to use, and staff members, teachers, parents, and other indigenous persons may be quickly trained as observers. Wright (1960) points out that the most distinctive advantage of event sampling is that it "structures the field of observation into natural units of behavior and situations" (p.107).

Among significant *limitations*, it is frequently difficult to establish reliability across multiple observers, particularly when event data are not linked to specific times within the behavioral stream of events. Event sampling may break up the continuity of behavior as much as time sampling, particularly when limited categories are employed (e.g., the checklist). Finally, because the observer is not cued in any way to attend systematically to behavior at specific intervals, it may be difficult to maintain an optimal level of attention over long periods of time.

Time Sampling

Time sampling *requires the observer to make observations according to a systematized time schedule* which may be very broad in scope, requiring few observations each day or per hour, or quite compressed, requiring the observer to make separate observations and recordings every five or ten seconds. The observer does not have to be present on a full-time basis, and if the time sample is representative, a comprehensive view of the target may be obtained while drastically reducing observer time.

Before discussing time sampling procedures proper, we will define certain key operations. The *observation interval* is defined *as the specific period of time during which the observer actually looks at behavior in the setting.* The *time period within which the observer makes his recording of behaviors observed* is termed the *recording interval,* and of course the recording interval immediately follows the observation interval. This recording interval is fixed at a period of time that allows the observer to make the notations called for by the particular coding system.[1] *The total time period within which the observer views (observation interval) and records (recording interval)* is termed the *observation occasion.* Thus, an observation occasion of one hour could be composed of sixty 30-second observation intervals each immediately followed by a 30-second recording interval. The sequence might look like this:

observation interval—recording interval—observation interval; etc.
(30 seconds)   (30 seconds)   (30 seconds)

The observation interval should remain fixed across all observations, so that observations take place under standardized conditions. It would be difficult to compare data gathered during a one-minute observation interval with data gathered during a three-second observation interval, since the observer would obviously be asked to summarize across much more behavior within the one-minute period. Also, if the observation interval is varied, the observer would constantly have to shift his observational set, increasing the difficulty of the task. Similarly, *the recording interval should be fixed at some duration of time that permits the observer to record observations carefully using whatever recording format has been chosen.* Varying recording procedures also makes the observer's task much more difficult and could be likened to varying the instructions for administering a psychological test each time it is given. This introduces method variance that decreases the interpretability of findings. In contrast, the length of the observation occasion may be varied without reducing the standardization of method by which behavior is detected and endorsed. As pointed out in Chapter 6, selection of occasions during which clients will be observed may, however, affect the representativeness of data collected. By preselecting invariant occasions (e.g., each day the setting is observed from 10:00 A.M. to 11:00 A.M.), the BCA *cannot generalize findings to alternative times* of the day when factors not present during the observation occasion may alter the characteristics and frequency of the target. By extending the observation occasion, employing multiple occasions within the day, or by employing a random sample of occasions (if possible), the BCA enhances the generalizability of findings and ensures a more comprehensive view of client behavior.

The interval of time between occasions of observation is termed the *inter-occasion interval*, and this may vary in terms of hours or even days, depending on the manner in which the BCA wishes to sample clients within and across days. Behaviors may be related to the time of day (or even day of the week) in which they occur. If observations are made right before lunch, immediately after lunch, immediately after physical exertion on the playground, or at the end or the beginning of a class period, the behavior of a population of youngsters may vary a good deal due to the effects on behavior of hunger, fatigue, physical exertion, or structure of classroom task. In addition, certain extra-setting phenomena may influence behavior on a given occasion. In the classroom for example, it may be that the windows face out on the playground and from 11:00 A.M. to 11:50 A.M. other classes play outside, distracting students and promoting disruptive behavior. Observations made during this period would provide a distorted view of the class, and would probably not be representative. Such time-behavior relations are as relevant to adult populations as they are to child populations, and can be detected by conducting observations at multiple and varied times during the day, thus reducing the interoccasion interval.

Once the BCA has information regarding the frequency of certain behaviors over times within the day, specific times might be singled out for observation due to the rate or characteristics of client behavior at those times. Along these lines, Kubany and Sloggett (1973) argue that "there certainly is no basis for assuming that the 20- or 30-minute daily observation period (employed by many investigators) is a random sample of the total population of behaviors of concern" (p. 341). To obtain a random sample of child behavior across times in the classroom day, the authors trained a teacher to employ an approximately random schedule for using a three-category recording system. Rather than fixing an interoccasion interval, the teacher was given the option of employing a four-, eight-, or 16-minute variable-interval (VI) schedule, determined by the time a "problem" student was in the classroom during the day. By variable interval we mean that the interoccasion interval (time between observations) is randomly varied around a four-, eight-, or 16-minute interval of choice. If the student was only present for a limited period of time, the authors recommended that the four-minute VI schedule be employed. The teacher was provided with a kitchen timer as well as a schedule sheet. This sheet is shown in Figure 9-1.

The teacher was asked to select a particular student to be the focus for observations, to choose one of the interval options, and then to record the behavior displayed by the student in the appropriate column on the recording sheet. The numbers running from top to bottom of the sheet indicate the timer setting the teacher was to use to ensure the variable-interval schedule around the time listed at the top of the column. Thus, if the teacher chose a four-minute schedule, she would begin by setting the timer for two minutes, and upon hearing the tone at the end of that period, would record the symbol

Date_____
Student_____
Teacher_____
Starting Time_____
Activity_____

COMMENTS	FOUR	EIGHT	SIXTEEN
	2	12	12
	5	2	8
	7	10	28
	1	4	2
	3	6	24
	6	14	6
	4	8	24
	6	2	6
	4	10	30
	1	14	12
	2	8	16
	5	10	4
	3	6	8
	7	4	30
	2	12	28
	1	4	6
	7	12	24
	3	14	16
	4	2	12
	5	6	2

Figure 9-1
Schedule sheet for 4-minute VI observation schedule. From "Coding
procedure for teachers" by E. S. Kubany, and B. B. Sloggett.
Journal of Applied Behavior Analysis, 1973, *6*, 339–344.
Reprinted by permission.

that best represented the student's behavior. The teacher was provided with the following directions:

When the timer bell rings, the teacher glances at the student and identifies what he is doing *at that instant*. Is he: (1) "on-task" (A)—that is, doing what the teacher wants him to do; (2) "passive" (P)—not doing what he should be doing, but not disrupting others; or is he (3) "disruptive" (D)—e.g., out of seat, talking without permission, or making other noise. The teacher enters the appropriate code symbol—either "A", "P", or "D" in the space next to the number representing the time interval just passed. The timer should then be reset without delay [Kubany & Sloggett, 1973, p. 340].

In comparing data obtained under four-minute variable-interval sampling (five observations made each 20 minutes) with a more continuous schedule employing observations every 15 seconds (80 observations made each 20 minutes), the authors found high correspondence of results; however, no statistical analysis was performed. While this finding is certainly limited by the characteristics and rate of the targeted behaviors observed for that population of subjects, it does suggest that variable-interval sampling of an occasion may produce data representative of behavior displayed within the entire occasion. The authors emphasize that this procedure permits an indigenous observer to collect data throughout the day on a systematic interval basis, so that the entire range of daily times can be randomly sampled. They conclude that finding "different patterns of behavior at different times of the day might provide insights about reinforcing stimuli or sources that maintain appropriate behavior" (p. 341). Other advantages of their recording approach include limiting of the observer's effects on the environment (the teacher is ordinarily present in the setting and can make observations with less potential reactivity than an outside observer), as well as the savings realized by not employing extrinsic observers. The manner in which the choice of a fixed or variable interoccasion interval affects the representatives of observing low- versus high-rate and/or duration events has not been systematically explored in the literature. Unfortunately many multivariate (multiple-target) coding schemes employ the same observation, occasion, and interoccasion intervals even though the rate and duration of targets as they naturally occur may vary considerably. Thus a fixed sampling methodology may adequately sample certain categories of behavior while poorly sampling others.[2]

Methodology

As in event sampling, virtually any recording methodology could be employed in time sampling, limited only by the length of the recording interval. *Specific* recording procedures (see Chapter 7) are used most frequently because they make it easier to establish high levels of reliability (given a finite number of categories) and permit a more systematic appraisal of the data in quantifiable terms. *Nonspecific* methods require the observer to employ specimen recording or some other narrative approach (often augmented by taped media) to describe comprehensively behavior that occurs within the observation interval. As might be imagined, the former approach often results in "memorized symbols, checklists, rating scales, or graphic recording devices" (Wright, 1960, p. 98), while the latter approach is defined by the observers' vocabulary and verbal descriptive skills. Time sampling methods will be discussed in the context of specific recording procedures.

When employing a preselected set of coding categories, the BCA must decide how the observation interval will be sampled. That is, how frequently or for what duration must a target occur within the observation interval to be endorsed by the observer? Second, will each separate behavior category be endorsed upon occurrence, or will the observation interval be summarized to produce one category that best describes the interval? In addressing the first issue, Powell, Martindale, and Kulp (1975) define three strategies for interval sampling: *whole interval time sampling, partial interval time sampling,* and *momentary time sampling.*

When the *whole interval approach* is used, a targeted behavior must be exhibited *throughout* the entire observation interval to be scored. This is obviously a rather stringent criterion, and the BCA must ensure that the selected observation interval is one that represents the average duration of the target. That is, if a BCA were interested in recording a very abbreviated behavior such as head nodding, an abbreviated observation interval would be required (e.g., two to three seconds). If a longer observation interval were employed, it would be impossible for head nodding ever to be recorded by the observer, since the behavior is completed in a period more abbreviated than the observation interval itself. For these reasons this approach is rarely employed.

An alternative, the *partial interval approach*, provides observers with more flexibility in that the target must occur only for some predetermined period of time *within* the observation interval to be encoded, and this time may be selected with specific targets in mind. Thus, given events of different durations, a criterion of "must occur for one-third (e.g., three seconds) or more of the observation interval (e.g., ten seconds) to be endorsed" could be employed. Here, events lasting from three to ten seconds will be observed in a much more representative fashion because the observer is provided with a range time in which behaviors will be endorsed, and this range allows for the ordinary variability in duration frequently seen across targeted events. The least stringent partial interval approach merely requires that the target *occur* within the observation interval to be endorsed. This is by far the most popular of interval approaches employed (Patterson et al., 1973; Lewinsohn, 1974; Mariotto and Paul, 1974; O'Leary et al., 1971; Paul and Lentz, 1977). The Behavioral Coding System (BCS) described in Chapter 7 will again be used as an example (Patterson et al., 1969). Employing a partial interval sampling approach, the observer focuses on one family member in the home (denoted by a number), and writes down any scorable behavior that occurs within a 30-second observation interval (signaled by auditory tone). Observers learn to pace themselves so that a recording is made about every six seconds, as the observer moves from left to right across the recording sheet to the end of the 30-second observation interval. When multiple behaviors occur within the same six-second period, the BCS provides instructions that certain code categories are to have precedence over other codes (a hierarchy). Libet and Lewinsohn (1973) use a similar coding system to observe the interpersonal verbal behavior of persons diagnosed as "depressed." Employing a series of coding categories that represent potential actions (e.g., a verbal statement) as well as reactions (e.g., criticism, disapproval, ignoring), observers record *all* scorable verbal behaviors that occur within a 30-second observation interval (signaled by an automatic timer that delivers an auditory and visual signal every 30 seconds).

Lastly, Powell et al. (1975) have defined *momentary time sampling* as requiring the targeted behavior to be assessed at regular or irregular periods of time, with the behavior scored if it is exhibited at the *moment* of observation. Rather than a separate category of sampling, this approach seems to be merely an example of the whole interval sampling approach where the interval is restricted to an extremely abbreviated period of time (e.g., one to two seconds), enough time for the observer to look up and observe the behavior. The Behavioral Checklist (TSBC) developed by Paul and Lentz (1977; as reported by Mariotto and Paul, 1974; Redfield and Paul, 1976), uses a two-second observation interval to sample the behavior of psychiatric patients in a residential setting. The TSBC samples a total of 71 behavioral characteristics of residents across seven major categories. As described by Redfield and Paul (1976), the TSBC includes the following categories of behavior.

The TSBC is an observational assessment instrument in which all residents' (patients or ex-patients) behavior is coded in behavioral classes with seven categories describing an individual resident's (a) physical location (e.g., bedroom, hallway), (b) position (e.g., walking, lying down), (c) awake-asleep status (i.e., eyes open, eyes closed), (d) facial expression (e.g., smiling with apparent stimulus, neutral with no apparent stimulus), (e) social orientation (e.g., alone, with staff), (f) concurrent appropriate behaviors (e.g., talking with others, watching TV), and (g) inappropriate behaviors (e.g., talking to self, posturing). Scores derived from the TSBC include relative frequency of behavior per observation, within each of 71 behavioral classes, and 6 composite scores representing linear combinations of rationally grouped behavioral items. Composite scores are: Hostile Belligerence, Cognitive Distortion, Schizophrenic Disorganization, and two global indices: Total Approrpiate Behavior, and Total Inappropriate Behavior, and a Social Orientation Index [p. 3].

Five observers present on the ward sample the behavior of each resident for one two-second observation interval each hour. For each of the seven behavior categories, the presence or absence of individual behaviors or descriptors is checked. This coding system is marked not only by the high level of reliability reported for observers (Paul and Lentz, 1977; Mariotto and Paul, 1974; Redfield and Paul, 1976), but by the sophisticated manner in which each individual's behavior is sampled. By sampling residents each hour, as well as randomly varying the time within the hour that the two-second observation interval occurs, the authors have ensured that a representative sample of behaviors is obtained. Also, the "momentary" observation interval restricts behavior that the observer must scan, thus enhancing reliability.

In choosing a particular time sampling strategy, the BCA has little empirical data to direct his efforts, although the study by Powell et al. (1975) provides some preliminary suggestions. Powell et al. were interested in defining the degree to which whole, partial interval, and momentary time sampling produced data representative of data obtained under continuous observation conditions. For interval time sampling, the observers viewed a videotape of a secretary performing normal secretarial duties and recorded in-seat behavior. At the end of each interval the observer recorded if the subject was in his seat for: the entire interval, part of the interval, or none of the interval. The variable manipulated was the length of the observation interval. Six 20-minute sessions were conducted with an interval length of 10, 20, 40, 80, and 120 seconds respectively. Thus the number of observations per 20-minute session ranged from a high of 120 to a low of 10. The authors thus obtained a complete videotape record of behavior within each 20-minute period which could then be compared with the recordings the observers made using each of the sampling interval approaches.

Findings for the whole and partial interval approaches will be discussed first. The authors found that when the length of the observation interval remained abbreviated (10 seconds, 20 seconds, 40 seconds), the whole as well as partial interval records showed remarkably high agreement with the continuous record. For 80- and 120-second observation intervals, the authors found that the partial interval approach resulted in a consistent overestimate of behavior frequency, while the whole interval approach resulted in a consistent underestimate. We will examine these results in more detail.

The stringent whole interval criterion (the targeted behavior must occur for the whole interval of 80 or 120 seconds) made it difficult for the behavior ever to be endorsed, and in fact the authors found consistent underestimation. Thus, at 80 seconds, the behavior would not be scored even though it occurred 72 seconds out of the 80-second interval, yielding a 72-second underestimate. With more abbreviated observation intervals the potential magnitude of underestimation is reduced. For example, with a 10-second observation interval, the target would not be scored if it occurred eight seconds out of the total 10-second interval, but the underestimate here would only be eight seconds.

The overestimation of the target with more extended observation intervals is readily illustrated for the partial interval approach. The "partial" approach treats any instance of the behavior within the interval as an occurrence for that *entire* interval. Thus, if a target occurred for only 10 seconds within an 80-second interval, a mark would be made on the recording sheet, and in tallying the data this mark would seemingly indicate that the behavior occurred for the full 80 seconds (a 70-second overestimation). As the length of the observation interval is reduced, a partial interval approach will not so dramatically overestimate the duration of a behavior. Thus, for a 10-second observation interval, an occurrence for even two seconds of the 10-second interval would be scored, but the overestimate here would only be eight seconds.

Since partial interval sampling tends to overestimate a target while whole interval sampling underestimates its occurrence, Powell et al. (1975) attempted to relate these findings to the situation where a no-treatment or baseline condition within an experiment shows a different rate of occurrence for a target than a treatment condition.

> For example, consider a baseline condition (Condition A) where a continuous measure shows the behavior occurring 80% of the time, and following an experimental manipulation (Condition B) the continuous measure shows the behavior occurring 20% of the time. Using partial interval time sampling, there would be an overestimate in Condition A, but this measurement error could not exceed 20%. In Condition B, the overestimate would again be present, but measurement error could range up to 80%. Using whole interval time sampling, this relationship would be reversed. That is, a large underestimation would be possible in Condition A, followed by a much smaller underestimation in Condition B. Indirect evidence in this study supports the above conclusion, in that the observed behavior did occur a high percentage of the time and resulted in consistently greater underestimations than overestimation [p. 468].

Unfortunately, the authors speak of behavior occurring in global terms (80 percent of the time), and do not attempt to relate their findings to such specific characteristics as *frequency* of occurrence as well as *duration* of occurrence per event. It remains to be seen whether the authors' findings can be generalized beyond the low-frequency, high-duration behavior they employed, and specifically how interval length, manner of sampling the interval (partial versus whole), as well as the rate and duration of the behavior come to predict the accuracy with which sampling estimates a targeted event.

For momentary time sampling the authors found that as the frequency of momentary observations increased, the accuracy of their estimation of a continuous record concomitantly increased. Specifically, the authors found that times between momentary samples of up to 120 seconds very accurately estimated the frequency of behavior when compared with continuous sampling. In contrast, 240-, 400-, as well as 600-second intervals between observations poorly represented data derived from continuous measurement. In fact, with

600 seconds or five-minute intervals between momentary observations, discrepancies as large as 74 percent were observed when data were compared with a continuous record. *As for interval sampling, a more continuous sampling of behavior (time between observations is reduced) yields a more representative depiction of the target.*

Cueing Devices

Obviously, the observer must have some means of determining the onset and offset of observation/recording intervals. While some BCAs have merely asked the observer to watch the clock, or provided a stopwatch (O'Leary et al., 1971), others have employed rather elaborate electronic devices for interval cueing. Patterson et al. (1969), for example, built a tiny electronic metronome into observers' clipboards which provided an auditory tone via an earjack to indicate 30-second intervals. A similar procedure has been employed by Lewinsohn and his colleagues (e.g., Libet and Lewinsohn, 1973). Another alternative is to record tones (e.g., "tone-off" cues for observing; "tone on" cues for recording) at appropriate intervals on audio cassette tape, providing observers with tape recorders that enable them to listen to the tape via an earjack. Cassette tape recorders can be economically purchased and have built-in earjacks. For specimen recording, the cueing cassette may be removed, a blank cassette inserted, and detailed verbal records made using the same machine. This approach is quite flexible, and provides a device which may be used for a variety of other purposes relevant to assessment and treatment. In addition, when a two- or three-way jack is inserted into the "auxiliary" or "external speaker" function, two or three observers can listen simultaneously to the same auditory cue so that reliability may be assessed within intervals over time.

A cueing system should be capable of providing discrete information to the observer as to the beginning and end of observation and recording intervals, and should be constructed so as not to interfere with, distract, or in other ways detract from the observer's efforts at viewing setting behavior. When observations are made in the natural setting, rather complicated, large, or bulky equipment tends to draw attention to the observer, which may be contrary to the goals of observation. Certainly an auditory stimulus should not be audible to persons present in the setting. If a mechanical recording device is employed (e.g., tape recorder), a variety of inexpensive mechanisms are available to control onset-offset according to the BCA's desired time sampling schedule (Wolach, Roccaforte, and Breuning, 1975; Johnson, Christensen and Bellamy, 1976).

The following are among major *advantages* of time sampling. Time sampling permits the BCA to relate behavior very specifically to time within and across observation occasions and may assist in defining important time-behavior relations. This becomes particularly important when observations of several observers are employed to assess reliability. It has already been pointed out that event sampling makes it difficult to determine whether or not two or more observers observe and record the same event at the same point in time, and that total reliability figures based on this approach are often inaccurate. By providing a systematic time schedule for observations, the BCA is assured that reliability is assessed for the same behaviors in the behavior stream, and he is in a position to assess changes in reliability by evaluating the beginning, midpoint, and end of the observation occasion.

Wright (1960) points out that time sampling ensures that certain predefined behaviors are observed under the same conditions of observation each and every time they are observed and provides much more precision in methodology than event sampling can. Wright also emphasizes that time sampling is economical in terms of research time and effort and its coding schemes "minimize equivocal judgments and prescribe definite ways to quantify whatever is observed" (p. 99). Finally, time sampling systems enhance the observer's attention to client behavior, given the frequent cues provided for observing and recording, which becomes particularly important when the observation occasion is extended in length.

Significant *limitations* are the somewhat artificial view of a behavior sequence obtained by time sampling, and the real possibility that sampling parameters may very well predict the frequency and/or duration of the behavior observed, apart from its actual characteristics. For example, the time sampling may break up a sequence of behavior by artificially dividing it into a series of events, when the behavior in fact is one continuous event within the behavior stream. If a behavior such as "fighting" is observed for a population of young nursery school children and an average fight from start to finish lasts about 45 seconds, an observer employing a ten-second observation interval and five-second recording interval would record three separate occasions of fighting in the 45-second period, rather than one. It would be impossible, using this time sampling strategy, to determine the actual number of events. In commenting on this problem, Wright (1960) points out:

Time sampling does not honor natural behavior units. Aggressive acts, conversations, quarrels or friendships, virtually all other segments of behavior in the literature of the method can be ever so long or short, with the outcome that the sampling intervals have to be . . . arbitrary in length. The loose respect of behavior for time leaves no other alternative. But with what consequences? . . . One result here must often be the observation of action fragments. A tally per fragment clearly is legitimate enough for incidence problems as long as each fragment represents what is really going on (aggression, affection, cooperation, or the like) in the complete behavior unit. One can seriously question whether it always does, however, and urge as well that the watching of events through their natural courses must generally be good policy for most research purposes [p. 100].

It may be advantageous to combine time sampling measures of incidence with avenues of nonspecific observation which provide a rich description of behavior-in-situation along the lines Wright (1960) suggests. For example, the observer might first record the incidence of behaviors that occur in the observation interval; then provide a narrative description of antecedent and consequent events, the situation in which the behavior occurred, or other information of interest. Obviously the feasibility of this suggestion depends on the length of the interval between observations.

Finally, as the ordinary rate of the target is reduced, the applicability of time sampling is compromised (Arrington, 1943). For very low-rate events, the BCA must rely on event sampling methods, perhaps employed by persons present in the setting on a full-time basis.

Because time sampling strategies are employed so frequently in the literature, it is unfortunate that there is so little systematic and well-controlled research directed toward examining how the frequency, duration, and other characteristics of a target of interest should predict choice of observation, recording, and interoccasion intervals. Knowing this, perhaps the most basic question for the BCA is: Are the target(s) of interest (given typical rate and duration) likely to be detected given the observation, occasion, interoccasion interval of choice, and the sampling strategy selected? Extensive nonspecific sampling of a setting *prior* to choice of sampling parameters would ensure that the BCA has sufficient information to assist in answering this question.

Footnotes

[1]In some cases a demarcated recording interval is not employed, especially when the observation interval is momentary—for example, two to three seconds (Paul and Lentz, 1977).

[2]To offset this possibility, given divergent ordinary rates and/or durations of behaviors to be observed, the BCA may be required to tailor sampling intervals to specific targets or classes of targets (e.g., of similar rate and/or duration).

10

RELIABILITY ASSESSMENT: Strategies and Issues

Regardless of the method chosen for observational assessment, the usefulness of data gathered is limited by the precision and accuracy with which observations are made. Stallings and Gillmore (1971) make the point that the terms "accuracy" and "precision" are often inappropriately defined as synonyms. They support Kendall and Buckland (1957) who offer the following definitions:

In exact usage precision is distinguished from accuracy. The latter refers to closensss of an observation to the quantiy intended to be observed. Precision is a quality associated with a class of measurements and refers to the way in which repeated observations conform to themselves; and in a somewhat narrower sense refers to the dispersion of observations, or some measure of it, whether or not the mean value around which the dispersion is measured approximates the "true" value [p. 224].

In line with these definitions precision shares a common core of meaning with reliability as customarily defined in psychological and educational mea-

219

surement, while accuracy shares a common core of meaning with validity. This chapter will adopt this distinction in presenting the methods and issues suggested by reliability assessment. Following a review of various definitions of reliability and the assessment methods they suggest, the factors that seem to control the probability of attaining reliability in observational assessment will be discussed in the context of observer training.

Definition and Methodology

While most BCAs would agree that achieving acceptable levels of reliability in employing an observation instrument is important, there is a great deal of variability in the methods by which reliability is assessed in published reports. In addition, there appears to be some question of the suitability of more traditional methods of reliability assessment (e.g., as applied to certain measures of personality "traits") for evaluating the precision of data collected by the independent observer (Goldfried and Kent, 1972). By far the most common measure of reliability employed in observational studies is the agreement between two observers who systematically and independently observe the same behavioral events (Weick, 1968; Jones, Reid, and Patterson, 1975; Kent and Foster, 1977). Jones et al. (1975) state:

Classical psychometric theory (e.g., Gulliksen, 1950) dealt with parallel forms, internal consistency and test-retest reliabilities as conceptually distinct indices of measurement precision, and provided separate statistical procedures for the assessment of each. Users of observational data have traditionally been concerned with interobserver agreement as an index of reliability, which is conceptually close to parallel forms reliability in traditional psychometrics [p. 59].

Thus, in reviewing observational strategies, many authors have limited the discussion of reliability to interobserver agreement (Wright, 1960; Bijou, Peterson, Harris, Allen, and Johnston, 1969; Lipinski and Nelson, 1974; Hawkins and Dotson, 1975).

In contrast, a growing body of reports include multiple measures of reliability. For example, interobserver agreement may be supplemented by an assessment of the *stability* of target events across time (similar to test-retest reliability) and within an observational protocol (similar to internal consistency measures), as well as across situations and divergent observational targets (e.g., clients). This multifaceted approach to reliability assessment is best represented by the concept of *generalizability* discussed by Cronbach, Gleser, Nanda, and Rajaratnam (1972) and explicitly related to observational methodology by Wiggins (1973) and Jones et al. (1975). Because of the frequency with which interobserver agreement is calculated in the literature, an initial methodological presentation will deal exclusively with this approach. Next, definitions and methodologies suggested by a multifaceted approach to reliability assessment will be presented, with an attempt to do justice to Cronbach's generalizability approach within the limited scope of this chapter.

Interobserver Agreement

Estimates of interobserver agreement are typically based on the ability of two or more observers to record the same information while simultaneously and independently watching the same behavior-in-situation. In practice, the two observers either position themselves in a similar location in a natural setting or view targeted behaviors via a videotape presentation for some fixed time interval, each employing the same coding definitions. While either event or time (interval) sampling may be employed, the latter is preferred because it ensures that both observers are attending to the same behavior at the same time, particularly when abbreviated observation intervals are employed (e.g., 30 seconds or less). Typically the percentage of observation intervals in which both observers agree (endorse the same behavior) is assessed; however, some investigators employ a correlation coefficient to compare protocols across observers statistically.

The data obtained by two independent observers who employed three coding categories (A = Attends; OS = Out of Seat; and OA = Out of Area) in a classroom setting will be used to illustrate the calculation of interobserver agreement. Let us imagine that the data for observer 1 and observer 2 represent the behavior of five children, collected using a ten-second observe and five-second record time sampling approach. The behavior of the subjects is sequentially sampled.

Subject	Observer 1	Observer 2	Outcome
1	OS	A	Disagree
2	—	—	—
3	A	A	Agree
4	OA	OA	Agree
5	OS	OS	Agree
1	—	OS	Disagree
2	—	—	—
3	OS	OS	Agree
4	OS	A	Disagree
5	A	A	Agree
1	A	OS	Disagree
2	A	—	Disagree
3	—	—	—
4	A	A	Agree
5	A	A	Agree

Thus, for the first observation interval, observer 1 found the child (subject 1) to be out of his seat while observer 2 found him to be attending (disagreement). The next observation interval was directed at subject 2, and both observer 1 and observer 2 failed to endorse any of the behavior categories, presumably indicating that none occurred during that interval. In the third interval, both observers agreed that child 3 was attending, and both agreed on the behavior of subjects 4 and 5 in the next two observation intervals. All five children are again observed in the same sequence two more times. An agreement is thus defined as two or more observers recording the same behavior, whereas a disagreement is defined as two or more observers failing to record the same behavior. Most typically the percent agreement would be computed by dividing the number of agreements by the number of agreements plus disagreements and multiplying by 100.

$$\text{PERCENT AGREEMENT} = \text{AGREEMENTS}/\text{AGREEMENTS} + \text{DISAGREEMENTS} \times 100$$

The reader may note that observer 1 and observer 2 agreed seven times out of a total of 12 paired observations during which at least one observer scored a coding category. By using our formula we can now arrive at the overall reliability for these two observers; that is, the percentage of the time that they agree in their endorsements across the three categories of the coding system. This process is expressed in the following computation.

$$\text{Percent Agreement (Overall Codes)} = 7/12 \times 100 = 58\%$$

An agreement of 58 percent shows that observers disagreed more than one third of the time.

One problem with reports of the overall percent agreement between observers is that it is impossible to determine the reliability with which each specific behavior category is observed. As in the case of overall agreement, the percent agreement for each specific category is defined as *the number of agreements (when both observers record a particular category, such as "A") divided by agreements plus disagreements (when only one observer records that category) multiplied by 100*. For the behavior "attends," both observers recorded "A" on four occasions, while on another four occasions one observer recorded "A" while the other recorded another coding symbol or failed to record (a disagreement). This may be expressed as follows:

$$\text{Percent Agreement (A)} = 4/8 \times 100 = 50\%$$

Performing the same computation for OS:

$$\text{Percent Agreement (OS)} = 2/6 \times 100 = 33\%$$

For OA, both observers agreed on its one occurrence, and the following computation results:

$$\text{Percent Agreement (OA)} = 1/1 \times 100 = 100\%$$

The percent agreement for two coding categories is considerably less than the overall agreement, and in the case of OS, the 29 percent agreement between the two observers is extremely poor. Thus, percent agreement calculations must be made and reported for *each* behavior category as well as across behaviors to ensure that the overall percent agreement does not mask poor reliability for individual categories.

The finding of 100 percent agreement between two observers for OA suggests another possible problem. This reliability estimate is misleading because of the small sample of one occurrence that it is calculated from. In fact, this one agreement could have been reached by chance alone. Sufficient occurrences must be observed and compared to a criterion (e.g., another observer's protocol) before a reliability estimate can be stated with assurance. There are no absolutes as to the number of occurrences necessary for an accurate computation of reliability; however, it would seem that if two observers have 50 or more occasions to simultaneously observe a given behavior, and they agree at some predetermined standard (e.g., 90 percent), then the BCA may feel safe in concluding that the behavior will be observed with reliability.[1]

Because certain low-rate behaviors do not occur with sufficient frequency in the natural environment to ensure an adequate sample for reliability assessment, the BCA may wish to produce a videotape showing large numbers of these low-rate events, have two observers simultaneously code the tape, and assess reliability for these observations from their protocols. The BCA can ensure that all behaviors within the coding manual are similarly represented on the videotape, even if the tape must be produced with the help of "actors" who roleplay targeted behaviors of interest. More will be said about the use of videotapes in observer training in a later section.

An important issue related to such low-rate events is how to handle empty intervals in calculating the reliability coefficient. *An "empty" interval will be defined as an observation interval within which no targeted event is coded by either of the two observers.* The counting of such nonoccurrences as agreements will spuriously inflate the reliability estimate when either total reliability or reliability of each observational category is computed (Repp, Deitz, Boles, Deitz, and Repp, 1976). For example, Bijou et al. (1969) computed a reliability index of 27 percent agreement between two observers employing four categories of behavior over a four-minute period when empty intervals were not included. The reliability index jumped to 76 percent agreement when empty intervals were counted, illustrating the gross distortion in findings produced by the employment of nonoccurrence data.

As a further illustration, the reader is referred to the previous "classroom" example, where the overall percent agreement for the two observers was 58 percent, using the computational formula presented. This formula did not count a nonoccurrence scored by both observers as an agreement. If we now count nonoccurrences as agreements between the two observers, we find that we have three more agreements, or a total of 10 agreements out of 15 paired observations (agreements plus disagreements). If we let "O" signify occurrence agreement and "N" signify nonoccurrence agreement, the following formula would be employed:

$$\text{Percent Agreement (Overall)} = (O + N)/(O + N + \text{Disagreements}) \times 100$$
$$= (7 + 3)/(7 + 3 + 5) \times 100$$
$$= 10/15 \times 100 = 67\%$$

Hawkins and Dotson (1975), in agreement with Bijou et al. (1969), suggest computing two reliability indices. *Scored-interval agreement (S-I) requires that either one or both observers score the interval.* S-I agreement is computed in the manner first described (all intervals in which *neither* observer scored the behavior are ignored). Because S-I assessment is very stringent, shows high variability with low-rate behaviors (e.g., the behavior occurs only once resulting in either 0 or 100 percent agreement across the observers), and may be speciously elevated by extremely high-rate behaviors (e.g., the observers endorse the behavior as occurring in *all* intervals and thus maintain a high level of agreement merely because of the behavior's high rate), the authors suggest that agreement as to nonoccurrence also be assessed. *Unscored-interval agreement (U-I) counts as disagreement whenever one or both observers score the behavior as occurring, with agreement defined exclusively as neither observer's endorsing the behavior within the interval.* With very high- or low-rate behaviors an assessment and comparison of S-I and U-I agreement enables the BCA to ensure that both occurrences and nonoccurrences are detected with precision and provides a more comprehensive view of the manner in which observers are achieving some level of agreement. For training-evaluation purposes, it may be important to know whether poor agreement is due to a failure to detect or to overdetection (both suggest that the coding definition should be carefully scrutinized as to clarity, over- or underinclusiveness, and level of inference called for), and these trends can be specifically related to individual observers. Both S-I and U-I scores should be included when an observation system is described, perhaps also including the mean of S-I and U-I (Hawkins and Dotson, 1975) for summary purposes. Knapp and Loveless (1976) report on a procedure employing acetate recording sheets and different colored pens as a means of simplifying assessment of both S-I and U-I agreement.

In practice, low-rate behaviors are typically assessed within an event sampling format that merely requires observers (often setting participants who are present on a full-time basis; see Chapter 8) to note the frequency of the target within a more extended time period (e.g., one hour). For this approach, reliability may be assessed merely by *dividing the smaller frequency count (made by observer 1) by the larger frequency count (made by observer 2) and multiplying by 100*. Obviously if the sums are identical, the reliability coefficient is 100 percent. A major problem with this approach is that it is impossible to determine whether or not the two observers were observing the same event at the same time, given that only total frequency is reported. Thus, two independent observers could each record five instances of attending behavior for a given child in a 50-minute class period without agreeing on any one incident of attending. For example, one observer may have noted his five instances during the first 10 minutes, while the other observer recorded each of his five instances during the last 30 minutes. While the reliability coefficient is 100 percent, it is obvious that, in fact, the two observers agree 0 percent of the time. The BCA should attempt to synchronize observations of multiple observers within abbreviated blocks of time to ensure that observers are attending to specific targeted persons at the same time, particularly when ongoing behavior is continuous and of moderate to high frequency.

As a final note on the assessment of interobserver agreement, the BCA should realize that both S-I or U-I agreement findings can be speciously elevated by *chance agreements* between observers. Kent and Foster (1977) have emphasized the importance of correcting for chance agreements and suggest that a formula described by Cohen (1960) be employed instead of the formulas so far presented. Given that a pair of observers record the incidence of a particular target behavior, there are four possible outcomes. If "O" signifies recorded occurrence of the target and "N" nonoccurrence, these outcomes are:

Observer 1	Observer 2
O	O
O	N
N	O
N	N

Both observers might agree on occurrence (O,O) or nonoccurrence N,N) or they might disagree (O,N or N,O) in their endorsements. The BCA can tally the frequency of each outcome (OO, ON, NO, NN) for inclusion within Cohen's (1960) formula to assess *Kappa* agreement, corrected for chance correspondence between the observers.

$$Kappa = \frac{\left[OO - \frac{(OO + ON)(OO + NO)}{OO + ON + NO + NN}\right] + \left[NN - \frac{(ON + NN)(NO + NN)}{OO + ON + NO + NN}\right]}{\left[OO - \frac{(OO + ON)(OO + NO)}{OO + ON + NO + NN}\right] + ON + NO + \left[NN - \frac{(ON + NN)(NO + NN)}{OO + ON + NO + NN}\right]}$$

Kent and Foster (1977) point out that the possibility of chance agreements is highest for S-I reliability when the target approaches 100 percent occurrence and highest for U-I reliability when the target approaches 0 percent occurrence. The interested reader is referred to Kent and Foster (1977) and Hartmann (1977) for an excellent discussion of issues pertaining to interobserver reliability indices.

As an alternative to interobserver percent agreement, a correlation coefficient may be computed between the data reported by two observers for the number of intervals in which the target behavior was observed to occur (e.g., across occasions), frequency counts, ratings of the target behavior, or duration measures. While correlation shows whether or not observers co-vary and depicts the pattern of their endorsements, it does not assess the level of agreement. Even though two observers disagree in their numerical scores, a high correlation will result if the relation between their scores remains constant. As an alternative, analysis of variance procedures could be employed to estimate the reliability of scores across two or more observers as discussed by Winer (1962). A significant difference in the scores between observers would indicate poor reliability.

Multifaceted Reliability Assessment[2]

While interobserver agreement is the most frequently employed means of assessing reliability, a number of other approaches, largely developed to assess traditional personality measures, have also been employed and can be justified on numerous grounds.

In arguing for a multidimensional approach to reliability assessment, Dunnette (1966) suggests several sources of potential error when behavior observations are made, and proposes that the estimation of each of these sources requires a separate and unique set of reliability assessment procedures. The first source of error involves *inadequate sampling of content* and occurs when a targeted event is not thoroughly sampled. A category such as "physical aggression," for example, may contain different and unique elements or referents depending on when a classroom of elementary school pupils is observed. While pushing, shoving, and other acts using hands may predominate on a first observation occasion, other referents of physical aggression, such as kicking, biting, and the like, may in fact predominate on a second, third, or fourth occasion. Thus, the likelihood of inadequate sampling is diminished by extending the number of occasions on which the observer views that particular school-age population. To correct for this source of error, Weick (1968) suggests that the "ratings of the same observer watching a similar event at two (or more) different times . . . be compared (this would rule out error of content sampling)" (p. 404).

A second source of error occurs when the endorsement of particular behaviors is predicted more by unsystematic, chance factors than by characteristics of the behavior as discretely defined. Called *the error of chance response tendencies,* this phenomenon occurs when coded behaviors are imprecisely defined or the observer is inadequately trained. This source of error is easily overcome, and a later section will discuss the procedures and issues of observer training in some detail.

A third source of error occurs when the *environment changes* from observation to observation. It is obvious that even minor changes in the environment can dramatically affect the characteristics and frequency of a given target. For example, a child frequently behaves much differently when a parent is present than when absent, and often remarkable differences are observed in a child's responses across the two parents. In addition, certain changes in the environment may physically facilitate certain behaviors while restricting the frequency of others. A child's running behavior, for instance, would be restricted by the size of the setting in which observations took place. This problem may be less important in certain institutional settings, where the physical environment is relatively invariant over time, and more of a problem in certain naturalistic environments. To avoid this source of error, Weick (1968) suggests that "the ratings of two persons observing the same event ... be correlated, a measure that would rule out the errors of change in the person and the environment" (p. 404). This suggestion of course defines interobserver agreement. While the employment of multiple observers assists the BCA in deciding whether or not changes in data recorded are a function of observer or environment/person (given reliable observations), it is obviously impossible to generalize from one observed environment to other, nonobserved environments or from a person observed on a single occasion to a person's behavior across other, nonobserved occasions. To the extent that observations are conducted across multiple environments or across multiple occasions for the same person(s), the BCA is on much firmer ground in assessing the degree of generalizability of data obtained.

The strategy of multiple observations of the same person(s) over different occasions is very similar to the test-retest reliability approach so often employed in traditional personality assessment. What is measured here is the *stability* of observed behavior over time, and the usefulness of data collected to assess behavior change (e.g., from pre- to post-treatment) obviously varies directly with the stability with which the behavior occurs. This is particularly important when the investigator is interested in establishing a baseline (stable state) for targeted behaviors prior to intervention. If a targeted behavior occurs with variable frequency (instability) across observation occasions conducted at baseline, it is difficult to determine whether behavior change following intervention is due to treatment or due to the instability of the behavior itself.

While test-retest stability estimates are frequently reported for measures of intelligence, personality, and the like, this information is rarely calculated for behavioral assessment instruments. Jones, Reid, and Patterson (1975) suggest that the assessment of stability may be directed at the behavior of an individual across time or a particular target behavior across some collection of individuals. In the first case, *intraindividual stability* is assessed by correlating the frequency of each targeted behavior observed on one occasion with the frequencies observed on additional occasions. An excellent example of this procedure is provided by Jones (1972). Employing data gathered for 26 problem boys and their mothers and 20 control boys and their mothers using the Behavioral Coding System or BCS (described in Chapter 7), Jones compared each subject's scores across the 28 BCS categories for the first half of baseline with that subject's scores for the second half of baseline as a measure of baseline stability. Because each subject had been observed on several days, mean scores were computed for each of the 28 behaviors. Because the base rates of the 28 behavior categories varied considerably for each subject, mean scores were transformed into z scores (an estimate of deviation of each score around the common mean across the 28 scores). At this point Jones had generated a z score for each of the 28 categories of the BCS for both the first and the second half of the baseline. Stability was then assessed by correlating the 28 first-half z scores with the 28 second-half z scores for each subject using a standard correlation coefficient. Jones reports: "It was assumed that at least minimal profile stability could be claimed for subjects whose correlations reached conventional levels of statistical significance. Hence, each subject's profile stability correlation was evaluated against an r of .32 ($p < .05$) for 28 cases" (p. 4).

In addition, the author computed the d^2 statistic by squaring and summing the differences in z scores over the 28 BCS categories for first and second half. This correlation assesses similarity between two profiles (groups of scores) in a more thorough fashion (level and scatter of scores as well as shape are assessed, while a standard correlation assesses only the shape of scores). These correlation coefficients as well as d^2 statistics for all subjects are presented in Table 10-1.

This table shows the mean, standard deviation, range of correlations, and similar data for the d^2 statistic. In addition, the percentage of subjects showing a nonsignificant correlation between the first and second half of baseline is reported. It may be noted that a full 28 percent of the subjects showed nonsignificant correlations between first and second half, thus suggesting a lack of stability in their behavior profiles over time. Jones reports:

Even for those subjects whose profile stabilities were statistically significant, many were low relative to what might be anticipated from such observational data. For example, stability correlations of .50 mean that the two profiles have only 25% of their variance in common. And in three of the four samples, the mean correlations were less than .50! Finally, as indicated by the range of stability coefficients from minus to plus 1 standard deviation, the consistency of these subjects' behavioral repertoires varies substantially in these samples (p. 5).

Table 10-1
Descriptive Summary of Findings for Two Profile Stability
Indices in Four Samples

Sample	CORRELATIONS			d-STATISTICS			
	Mean	SD	±1σ	nonsig.[1]	Mean	SD	±1σ
26 problem boys	.42	.25	.17-.67	9 (35%)	1.15	.43	.72-1.58
26 mothers	.57	.19	.38-.76	3 (12%)	1.01	.45	.56-1.46
20 control boys	.37	.23	.14-.60	7 (35%)	1.22	.43	.79-1.65
20 mothers	.41	.24	.17-.65	7 (35%)	1.31	.48	.83-1.79
92 Total Ss				26 (28%)			

[1]The number and percentage of Ss in each sample with nonsignificant stability correlations, i.e., $r <$ .32, $p >$ .05, one-tail. From "Intraindividual Stability of Behavioral Observations: Implications for Evaluating Behavior Modification Treatment Programs" by Richard R. Jones. Paper presented at the meeting of the Western Psychological Association, Portland, Oregon, April 1972. Reprinted by permission.

It is important to note that this procedure does not permit the BCA to evaluate which of the 28 behaviors within the BCS showed more or less stability, as stability coefficients are computed for each subject *across* the 28 categories. For each individual, this can be assessed only by visually scanning the first and second half for each behavior. While rather unsystematic, this approach permits the BCA to get some idea of those behavior categories that show the greatest variability from the first to second measurement. The ideal approach would be to correlate scores representing two different occasions of observation (e.g., first half versus second half of baseline) across a substantial number of subjects *for each specific category* within the coding system. This is the second category of stability estimation suggested by Jones et al. (1975) and might best be termed *interindividual stability.*

Assessment of interindividual stability of specific codes within a coding system is easier to perform than within-subject assessment because the correlation is across subjects and not coding categories (thus removing the problem of different category base rates). A single coding category is chosen, and the scores (means, frequencies, proportions, etc.) for a group of subjects representing two time periods (e.g., day 1/day 2; mean of first half of baseline/mean of second half of baseline) are correlated. Such an analysis is reported by Jones et al. (1975) for a sample of 54 target boys, 54 mothers, and 41 fathers (first half versus second half of baseline) using the categories from the BCS. The results of this analysis permitted the authors to evaluate the stability of specific codes within the BCS, categories of codes (e.g., relative stability of "verbal" versus "nonverbal" categories of behavior; "first-order" versus "second-order" categories of behavior), as well as differences in stability for a coding category across the boys, mothers, and fathers. Table 10-2 shows the reliability coefficients reported by the authors.

Table 10-2
Stability Correlations (First Half vs. Second Half of Baseline) for 18 Behavior Categories in Samples of 54 Target Boys, 54 Mothers, and 41 Fathers

	FIRST ORDER				SECOND ORDER		
	Boys	Mothers	Fathers		Boys	Mothers	Fathers
VERBAL							
CM	.23	.73	.44	TA	.26	.53	.38
CN*	.68	.80	.54				
CR*	.90	—	—				
HU*	.73	.54	.33				
LA	.23	.46	.35				
NE*	.54	.68	.39				
WH*	.63	—	—				
YE*	.74	.45	—				
NONVERBAL							
DS*	.46	—	—	AT	.36	.38	.43
HR*	.16	—	—	NO	.44	.49	.15
IG*	.27	.63	—	NR	.21	.20	.12
PN*	.38	.63	.63	RC	.32	.21	.16
PP	—	.69	.19	TH	.31	.68	.38
EITHER VERBAL OR NONVERBAL							
AP	.02	.48	.15	SS	.29	.05	.06
CO	.67	.37	.38				
DI*	.66	.62	.48				
DP*	.24	—	—				
NC*	.63	.34	.45				
PL	.51	.59	.48				
TE*	.35	.85	.43				
WK	.59	.50	.16				

*Deviant Behavior Categories. All other codes classified as Prosocial Behavior Categories.

—— Insufficient data for calculation of coefficients.

From "Naturalistic observation in clinical assessment" by Jones, R. R., Reid, J., and Patterson, G. R. In P. McReynolds (Ed.), *Advances in Psychological Assessment,* Vol. 3. San Francisco: Jossey-Bass, 1975. Reprinted by permission.

The authors report:

Over all ... these stability correlations suggest moderate levels of behavioral stability for many of the codes in these three samples. Sixty-three percent of the coefficients were statistically significant at the .01 level ... clearly suggesting that most of the interindividual differences in these scores were at least moderately consistent from the first to the second half of the baseline [pp. 71–73].

The reader should note the variability in stability estimates across the observational categories of the BCS, suggesting the need to perform a stability analysis for *each* separate coding category within a coding system. Intraindividual and interindividual stability estimation each hold certain advantages. When the BCA employs a coding system to establish a stable baseline for an individual subject or some grouping of subjects, the intraindividual approach is certainly an improvement over "eyeballing" the data. Jones (1972) suggests that "more stable estimates of behavioral events might be obtained simply by lengthening the baseline period for some subjects until a criterion level of behavioral stability is achieved" (p. 6). He points out, however, that a lack of behavioral stability may be the result of certain "salient clinical characteristics" of the client's behavior and not a result of insufficient behavior sampling. This suggests that for some subjects variability of behavior may itself become a focus for intervention (given that a stable baseline is impossible). To the extent that intervention efforts are aimed at increasing the stability of a client's behavior, treatment has been instigated and the establishment of an unbiased baseline is thus impossible. More is said about the problems of baseline assessment in Chapter 13.

As to interindividual stability assessment, this approach seems most important when the BCA wishes to employ a systematized, standard observation methodology with a population of interest. If individual coding categories do not show stability, their utility as a source of evaluative data is limited. When a particular behavior category shows instability across occasions of observation, the BCA should evaluate: (1) the specificity of its *definition* (is it too imprecise to be employed consistently?), (2) the *methods* for observation (do observers employ the same methods and observation schedule on each occasion?), as well as (3) the sophistication of *observers* (have they achieved sufficient interobserver reliability?) as potential contributors to instability. One major problem is the assessment of stability for low-rate categories of behavior, given the often inadequate sample of behavior (note the blank spaces in Table 10-2). With such low-rate behaviors, instability due to *chance response tendencies* (Dunnette, 1966) becomes more likely as observers are not provided with sufficient occasions to learn to discriminate the behavior with reliability.

A "Generalizability" Approach

Cronbach and his associates (1972) have suggested that the primary goal of reliability assessment is to generalize from observational data to some other class of observations. The BCA may wish to generalize from the data collected by one observer to other observers employing the same coding system. Obviously a coding system that does not permit such generalization is of limited utility (e.g., every observer employs the system in a unique fashion). Likewise, given the idea of stability previously discussed, one might want to generalize from a series of observations made of some subject on a particular occasion to the behavior of that subject on other occasions. This is particularly important for clinical interventions that seek to assess client behavior change across time. Similarly, it is often desirable to be able to generalize from the particular situation in which data are collected to other situations in which the client functions. Wiggins (1973) suggests that generalization from the conditions of observation to other conditions is extremely important if an assessment instrument is to be useful.

Conditions may refer to particular test items, test forms, stimuli, observers, occasions, or situations of observation. In estimating the reliability of a specific set of conditions, we are interested in the extent to which we can generalize from that set to the universe of which our conditions are a sample. The generalization desired may be quite limited, as when our interests lie in the extent to which we can generalize from the ratings of one observer in one set of conditions to the ratings of the *same* observer in another set. On the other hand, the degree of generalization desired may be extremely broad, as when our interest lies in the extent to which we can generalize from peer ratings of "academic competence" to faculty ratings of "academic competence." Note that the latter is traditionally thought of as a "validity" generalization. That is, peer ratings are generally viewed as "predictors" and faculty ratings as a "criterion." Nevertheless, the extent to which one can generalize from one sample of raters to the other falls within the realm of the theory of generalizability [p. 285].

A brief description of a generalizability approach to reliability assessment (Cronbach et al., 1972) will be followed by an example from the literature.

First a *factorial analysis of variance* is performed on data representing such factors as observers, occasions of observations, or persons observed, constituting the "generalizability" or "G" study (Cronbach et al., 1972). Given that subjects' scores on any dependent variable measure (e.g., observation scores) are predicted by the treatments that subjects receive as well as unsystematic sources of error, the analysis of variance design permits the BCA to determine the amount of variability in a subject's score determined by both treatments and such error sources, and to compute a percent of variance attributable to each. Within the factorial analysis, the variance attributable to more than one treatment (or "factor") can be computed. Thus, a factorial design might include the factors of observers (e.g., Observer 1, Observer 2 . . . Observer n); occasions of observations (Occasion 1, Occasion 2 . . . Occasion n); persons observed (Person 1, Person 2 . . . Person n), or levels of other factors of interest (e.g., situations, methods, etc.). The variance attributable to each factor is statistically evaluated in the light of the variance attributable to error, so that a probability statement can be made regarding the degree of significance between levels of each factor. This design would permit a probability statement as to whether observers employed (e.g., Observers 1, 2, and 3) differed significantly in their recording of data, or whether there was a significant difference between scores across occasions of observation. This multifactor design also permits an evaluation of interactions between factors, with

Table 10-3
Three-Facet Design for Estimating Components of Variance Due to Coders
(Regular vs. Calibrating), Occasions (Segment₁ vs. Segment₂), and Subjects
(Boy₁, Boy₂ . . . Boyₙ)

	REGULAR		CALIBRATING	
	Segment₁	*Segment₂*	*Segment₁*	*Segment₂*
Boy₁				
Boy₂				
Boyₙ				

From "Naturalistic observation in clinical assessment" by Jones, R. R., Reid, J., and Patterson, G. R. In P. McReynolds (Ed.), *Advances in Psychological Assessment*, Vol. 3. San Francisco: Jossey-Bass, 1975. Reprinted by permission.

significance estimates provided. Thus, a significant interaction between observers and occasions would indicate that the recordings of observers were in some fashion a function of the occasion of observation. The results of this factorial analysis of variance are then employed to produce *generalizability coefficients* within a "D" or decision study that permits the BCA to determine the degree of generalizability of reliability data obtained to other observers, occasions, or persons.

In performing the "G" study for data gathered using the BCS, Jones et al. (1975) employed three facets: observers, occasions or segments (times that observations were collected), and subjects, within the factorial design shown in Table 10-3.

Performing a separate analysis of variance for a sample of 13 "deviant" boys and 17 "normal" boys for a total of five codes within the BCS, the authors obtained the variance estimates presented in Table 10-4.

Table 10-4 shows the percentage of variability attributable to each of the three main facets of reliability assessment: observers (coders), occasions, and subjects, as well as the variability attributable to the interactions between these facets. In interpreting this table, the reader should note that a high degree of variability attributable to observers would indicate that they varied substantially in employing the coding system, implying a lack of interobserver agreement. In addition, high variability for occasions would reveal

Table 10-4

Variance Component Estimates (Percents) for Two Samples—Thirteen Deviant Boys and Seventeen Normal Boys—and Five Dependent Variables in a Three-Facet Design

Behavioral score sample	PL + NO		TOTAL DEVIANT		CO		TA		NC	
	Dev.	Nor.	Dev.	Nor.	Dev.	Nor.	Dev.	Nor.	Dev.	Nor.
Facets										
Subjects (S)	43.72	27.16	79.44	0.00	.36	37.56	7.96	0.00	81.17	0.00
Coders (C)	.07	0.00	0.00	0.00	2.14	0.00	.23	.04	0.00	0.00
Occasions (O)	0.00	0.00	0.00	0.00	0.00	0.00	0.00	0.00	0.00	0.00
S × C	0.00	1.13	2.84	0.00	0.00	.38	0.00	0.00	5.25	0.00
S × O	52.02	70.02	12.05	81.37	74.98	53.36	85.87	95.10	10.36	54.18
C × O	0.00	.24	0.00	0.00	0.00	.26	0.00	0.00	0.00	0.00
Residual (SXCXO)	4.17	1.25	5.64	18.62	23.53	8.44	5.93	4.72	3.23	45.82

N. B. Percents do not total precisely 100.0 because of rounding in calculations. From "Naturalistic observation in clinical assessment" by Jones, R. R., Reid, J., and Patterson, G. R. In P. McReynolds (Ed.), *Advances in Psychological Assessment*, Vol. 3. San Francisco: Jossey-Bass, 1975. Reprinted by permission.

little stability in the behavior scorres across time. In this case, the slight variability attributable to both observers and occasions across all five of the observation categories for both the deviant and normal samples supports the authors' conclusion that agreement between observers and stability across time were substantial. In contrast, the high degree of variability attributable to subjects as well as the subject by occasion interaction (S × O) merely means that subjects tended to vary in behavior displayed. In most cases, behavior displayed by subjects varied as a function of the occasion or day of observation. Given the situational specificity of many behaviors displayed in the natural environment, this interaction between subjects and occasions of observation would be expected.

Since the greatest amount of variability is attributable to the subjects by occasion interaction, it becomes important to determine the degree of reliability we can attach to observations of a given subject on a given occasion of observation (the "D" study). Jones et al. calculated generalizability coefficients according to procedures suggested by Cronbach et al. (1972), and report: "these coefficients ars analogous to intraclass correlation coefficients, and represent the magnitude of the generalizability of these scores to an assessment situation where data would be collected for an individual subject, by one coder, during each week day of a two-week baseline" (p. 68). Generalizability coefficients were calculated for each of the five coding categories for both the deviant and normal populations, and results showed that only one (NC or noncomply) was appreciably low (.54). For the other behavior scores, the authors conclude: "measurement of these behaviors for subjects in different situations is not greatly influenced by measurement error" (p. 70).

In evaluating the applicability of generalizability theory to reliability assessment of observational methods, Johnson and Bolstad (1973) conclude:

This model is particularly appealing because it provides for simultaneous assessment of the extent of various sources of "error" which could limit generalizability. In spite of the advantages of this factorial model, there are few precedents for its use. This is probably more the result of practical problems rather than a resistance to this intellectually appealing, theoretically sound model. Even if one were to restrict oneself to three sources of variance . . . (observers, occasions in the same setting, and settings), the resulting study would, for the most useful purposes, be a formidable project, indeed. Projects of this kind appear to us, however, to be well worth doing. We can probably expect to see more investigations which employ this generalizability model (p. 56).

In agreeing with Johnson and Bolstad, I would point out that even if the final decision or "D" study is not performed, a multifaceted analysis of variance design is extremely useful in permitting the BCA to determine sources of variability. Thus, knowing that observer protocols vary as a function of occasion of observation, setting, or particular codes endorsed, provides useful information that may assist the BCA in tailoring additional training experiences for observers to ensure adequate reliability.

The Quest for Reliability: Issues in Training and Assessment Methodology

Following a discussion of the selection and training of observers, this section will present a number of issues that the BCA should consider in planning reliability assessment and interpreting findings.

Selection and Training of Observers

While the methods for assessing the maintenance of reliability are often reported in the literature, very few investigators have discussed how observers were selected or criteria that may predict observer reliability. Perhaps the simplicity of many observational strategies causes BCAs to assume that virtually anyone with a modicum of intellectual and motoric skills can master the task of observation. In fact, many diverse individuals (e.g., university undergraduates, housewives, paid or nonpaid volunteers, "participant" staff) have been employed as observers. Skindrud (1972) alone reports the use of a psychometric test for selecting observers. After recruiting "mature women" who were seeking part-time employment, he administered the Employee Aptitude Survey Verbal and Numerical Test and the Minnesota Clerical Test to assist in observer selection. While reported criteria for performance were vaguely stated ("seven of the applicants scored above average" [p. 5]), he implicitly hypothesized that verbal as well as clerical skills might be relevant predictors of observation aptitude. The relations between certain aptitude and perceptual-motor skill measures and time necessary for training or achieving other relevant criteria (e.g., maintenance of reliability over time) remain to be established in the literature, but seem to be worth pursuing. Particularly when the observational task requires highly specific skills (e.g., attention to fine detail, short latency motor responses to stimuli, the ability to summarize verbally some segment of behavior which is perhaps delimited by one's vocabulary), psychometric as well as behavioral measures might be devised to discriminate among potential observers.

Once observers have been selected, most BCAs require trainees to read and thoroughly understand a "coding manual" of definitions they are to employ. Many of these manuals are very comprehensive and explicit. For example, the popularly employed "Procedures for Classroom Observation of Teachers and Children" (O'Leary et al., 1971) includes general instructions to observers (how they should behave, dress, position themselves within an observational setting, etc.), rationale and procedures for assessment of reliability, detailed descriptions of each coding category, and methodological suggestions for employing the coding system in a reliable fashion.[3] Obviously a written description of coding definitions and methods should be explicit and concise, providing numerous examples of how the coding definitions might be employed (see Chapter 7 for examples). Because of the lack of systematization in the manuals (typically unpublished) used to train observers and communicate methodology, the following outline presents components that the manual constructor might include. The reader will note that evaluative data (reliability and validity findings) are ideally a part of the manual.

1. Rationale for the observation system.
2. Description of setting(s) to which it is applicable.
3. Each coding definition.
4. Description of precisely how behavior is sampled.
5. Any rules governing the behavior of observers, e.g.:
   a. Hierarchy of codes.
   b. How coders are assigned to observation days, settings.
6. Reliability methodology and findings.
   a. Description of methods employed to assess reliability.
   b. Reliabilities for *each* coding definition plus the number of observations (*N*) it is based on.
   c. Overall reliability for system.
   d. Any generalizability findings.
7. Validation methodology and findings.
   a. Description of any validation studies performed: subjects, methods, and results should be described in detail.
8. Review of positive features and observed or potential problems of the coding system.
9. Summary of the foregoing.

Following a reading of the coding manual, trainees might be required to complete a paper-and-pencil test to ensure that they have thoroughly memorized the definitions and methods for each behavior. Unless this information assessment is completed, it is difficult to assess whether poor performance during practice sessions is due to the complexity and/or characteristics of the behavior *or* the mere fact that the trainee has not thoroughly memorized the coding deinitions. Many investigators provide the opportunity for individual or group discussion of observation definitions and methods to clarify the material and answer any questions the trainees might have. For example, Kent, O'Leary, Diament, and Dietz (1974) employed four one-hour training sessions for observers to discuss each of the coding definitions in a manual they had studied, and Patterson, Cobb, and Ray (1973) conducted group meetings with a trainer. Similarly, Nay and Kerkoff (1974) distributed coding manuals to trainees five days in advance of the first practice session. Trainees were encouraged to write down questions suggested by the coding manual and to present them in a group discussion.

As a next step, the trainer has the option of permitting trainees to practice observing in the criterion environment (where they will ultimately be asked to record behavior) or of providing a simulation or reproduction of that environment in the more structured clinic or laboratory setting. Many BCAs produce videotapes of the criterion setting and require trainees to achieve predefined levels of mastery *prior to* observing in the criterion environment. Nay and Kerkoff (1974) define a number of advantages of this videotape training approach: such training permits an assessment of reliability of observers to standard, well-defined stimuli; the trainer may stop the tape and provide verbal feedback to the observers to enhance their learning of coding categories; and difficult behavioral sequences can be replayed so that trainees have an opportunity to master problematic coding definitions. Not only have videotapes been employed as media for observer practice prior to naturalistic observation (Patterson, Cobb, and Ray, 1973; Nay and Kerkoff, 1974), but the observation of videotapes has itself beocme the focus of a number of studies specifically addressed to reliability assessment (Kent et al., 1974; O'Leary et al., 1975; Taplin and Reid, 1973; Wahler and Leske, 1973).

In practice, training videotapes show segments of client/subject behaviors also represented in the coding system. In most cases, an attempt is made to assure that *each* coding system category is displayed by clients on the tapes produced. Typically, "source" videotapes are produced in the criterion environment (e.g., classroom, ward, home) under naturalistic conditions. A sufficient sample of source videotapes must be made so that they may be edited to produce final training tapes that include a representative sample of setting behavior. In particular, with the videotape format ordinarily low-rate events can appear with sufficient frequency (e.g., through the employment of "actors" within role-played filmed sequences; i.e., Redfield and Paul, 1976) to ensure that observers master the codes and that reliability is systematically assessed.

To assess reliability, each videotape can be preobserved and scored by "expert" observers under conditions that maximize high reliability, and a "criterion protocol" made up of these responses can then be employed for reliability assessment. The trainee is required to be reliable to the criterion protocol (and thus the "expert" observers who generated it). This approach increases the BCA's assurance of validity as well as reliability, in that the behavior on tape is a standard, unchanging criterion representing the criterion environment. When two observers code in a natural setting, they may show substantial interobserver agreement; however, there is no assurance that behaviors they both endorse actually occurred in this setting. Thus, high reliability does not necessarily predict high validity. In contrast, the BCA knows in advance the specific behaviors displayed on a videotape.

The following represent examples of methods for constructing such practice videotapes. O'Leary et al. (1975) produced videotapes of two children displaying academic and behavior problems in a laboratory classroom. Three expert observers served as "criterion observers" and recorded the presence of four categories of disruptive behavior: playing, noise, vocalization, and orienting. Reliability was assessed within a 20-second observe 10-second record time sampling format. Interobserver reliabilities consistently exceeded .80 for these three observers. On the basis of these criterion recordings, two sets of videotapes were matched for average rate of occurrence of each of the four categories of behavior. Along similar lines, Nay and Kerkoff (1974) trained 24 undergraduate observers to employ a series of 22 coding symbols (Nay, 1974) to assess the behavior of institutionalized adolescents in classroom as well as in cottage settings. "Source" videotapes were first constructed by obtaining videotape footage of ordinary subject interactions in the classroom and cottage environments under conditions designed to reduce the obtrusiveness of the recording equipment. Training tapes were then produced from the source tapes in the following fashion.

Three training tapes were . . . composed of randomly selected sequences of behavior from the source tapes. Each training tape lasted approximately 50 minutes and was composed of intervals of 10 seconds of action and 5 seconds of stopped action. For all scenes . . . the number of girls to be coded by subjects ranged from three to five. Each girl to be coded was pointed out and assigned a number by verbal instructions on the videotapes. Typically, the girl at the left of the screen was assigned the number one, with the others being assigned numbers in order from left to right. . . . All videotapes were independently scored by two judges thoroughly familiar with the coding system. When disagreement occurred for a particular coding interval, it was submitted to the third judge. A scoring manual was devised based upon the judges' ratings [p. 1177].

The periods of "stopped" action coincided with the ordinary recording interval (five seconds) that observers were ultimately asked to use in the classroom and cottage settings. "Stopped" sequences of behavior may be readily produced with a videotape recorder that has a stop-action feature. As source material from one videotape recorder (VT-1) is transferred to the "final" training videotape on a second recorder (VT-2), the "editor" merely has to switch VT-1 to stop-action mode (sometimes called "pause") while VT-2 continues to record the stopped action for a period of time that coincides with the desired recording interval (e.g., five seconds, ten seconds).

Nay and Kerkoff (1974) found that providing feedback to observers about the correctness of obervation codes enhanced the achievement of reliability when compared with a strategy of merely permitting the trainees to practice observing the videotape without feedback. In particular, immediate feedback (after each sequence of behavior was observed and recorded) proved to be superior to delayed feedback (feedback after every ten sequences of behavior were recorded) in enhancing reliability. In emphasizing the importance of providing immediate feedback to trainees, the authors conclude:

Subjects who are presented with informational feedback have the advantage of testing their own conceptions of the coding system against criteria set down by the designers of the system. This kind of ongoing conceptual revision and confirmation process is further enhanced when the informational feedback is received immedi-

ately after the subject codes the behavior. It seems possible that the greater the latency between the responses and provision of feedback, the greater the probability
that the personal criteria responsible for subjects choosing a specific code or a specific behavioral situation will be distorted or forgotten. When no feedback is received, there are no specific external criteria against which to evaluate one's
understanding of the coding system [p. 1180].

The authors also suggest that the videotape itself might incorporate such
feedback to trainees. For example, a sequence of behavior could be presented, followed by a time period for the recording of response, followed by a
verbal statement (on tape) of the correct code. While this method requires a
bit more sophistication in the production of videotapes, it would certainly reduce trainer time and might be particularly advantageous when multiple observers are being trained.

While reliability can be assessed by comparing a trainee's protocol to the
criterion protocol, interobserver agreement may be assessed at the same time
when two or more observers are trained together. If interobserver agreement
is high while the agreement of the observer pair with the criterion protocol is
low, the observers may be developing certain idiosyncratic and characteristic
ways of interpreting the coding system, perhaps by mutual agreement. This
has been termed observer "drift" by O'Leary and Kent (1972). Requiring all
trainees to achieve reliability to the criterion protocol reduces the possibility
of observer drift and ensures that all trainees are employing observation categories in a consistent fashion.

Given that training videotapes provide an efficient and economical way
for trainees to master a coding system, it should be noted that reliability
achieved to videotape criteria may not generalize to the criterion environment. It may be particularly difficult for observers to discriminate the incidence of certain body movements, as well as more subtle paralinguistic
information (e.g., changes in tone of voice), in a taped presentation. Also, repeated observation of videotapes is often not as motivating to trainees as observations made in the natural setting, thus promoting boredom or fatigue.
Thus, it is important that the BCA obtain estimates of reliability in the criterion setting if that is feasible. One approach already discussed is to assign a
pair of trainees to an observational setting and calculate the percent agreement across their two protocols (interobserver agreement) for each coding
category. A major problem with this approach, observer drift, has already
been discussed.

In training 40 observers to employ a classroom coding system, O'Leary et
al. (1971) formed eight groups of five observers. Each of these groups would
ultimately be required to observe a different experimental condition. After a
series of training sessions during which observers computed reliability and
discussed any disagreements with the members of their five-person group,
reliability within groups (intragroup reliability) was found to be about .70.

The authors speculated that members of each of the eight groups might have developed idiosyncratic criteria for employing the coding system, so that while intragroup reliability would be high, intergroup reliability might be much lower. If each of the observer groups observed a separate experimental condition, this would introduce a rather large confounding, as the researchers could not know whether the data produced by a given group were based on characteristics of children in the classroom setting or the idiosyncratic way each group employed the coding system. To check this possibility, the authors had four of these groups observe and code the behavior of two children presented on eight 12½-minute videotapes over a four-day period. During each of the four days, members of each group computed reliability with each other; however, reliability was not assessed across the four groupings. Although each of the four groups observed the same eight videotapes, the authors found significant differences in the ratings of the four groups on seven of nine coding categories. The only two unaffected categories occurred at a relatively low rate. This idiosyncratic way that a small group or pair of observers may come to employ a standard coding system was termed "drift." The authors suggested that one means of reducing drift in a pair or group of observers is to train a new group or pair some period of time after the initiation of a study, and compare the observations of this "new" group to those of observers who have been collecting data for some period of time. If the "new" and "old" groups of observers produce comparable endorsements of the same behavior, the new observers may then be formally employed for data collection. Another strategy, (Nay, 1974), is to require trainees to reach predetermined criteria for reliability across multiple observers. Rather than employing fixed pairs of observers, the pairs change for each reliability assessment so that idiosyncratic responses cannot develop. When a trainee achieves reliability across some number of observers (e.g., 95 percent agreement across five different observers), the BCA can be assured that drift has been minimized and that all trainees are employing the coding system in a consistent fashion.

Another frequently employed approach to naturalistic assessment of reliability is to compare each trainee's responses to those of an expert or "calibrating" observer. This helps to ensure that all observers are employing the coding system uniformly, given that the calibrator employs the coding system in a consistent fashion across trainees. Even if the calibrator exhibits certain idiosyncrasies that diverge from the coding manual definition of behaviors, all of the trainees must achieve reliability to the same idiosyncratic definitions. Certainly the issue of validity is again raised. However, if the calibrator is systematically checked to a criterion videotape (e.g., to a criterion protocol), the BCA can be fairly certain that the calibrator is both reliably and validly (as defined by the videotape sample of behavior) employing the observation system.

Johnson and his colleagues (Johnson and Bolstad, 1973; Eyberg and Johnson, 1974; Johnson and Lobitz, 1974) are among investigators who employ "spot-check" reliability assessments of a calibrating observer as an alternative to continuous assessment. Following the training of observers to pre-determined criteria for reliability in the clinical setting (e.g., 70 percent or better, Johnson and Bolstad, 1973), the observer is permitted to begin the observation of families in the home situation without constant monitoring. Weekly training sessions permit all observers to discuss definitional problems and methodological issues. A calibrator goes into the home with the regular observer once each week to check the maintenance of reliability over time. Johnson and Bolstad (1973) report:

This calibration may occur on any one of the regular five days of observation. Both observers calculate their percent agreement in the traditional way immediately after the session and discuss their disagreements at this time. If they cannot resolve their disagreement on a particular or idiosyncratic problem, they immediately call the observer trainer, who serves as a sort of imperfect criterion coder [p. 25].

The spot check is not without its problems. One might expect that the observer would be more motivated to employ the observation system carefully and systematically when reliability is obtrusively checked by the "calibrator." In fact, a number of investigators have consistently reported that reliability is enhanced when assessment is obtrusive (i.e., the observer is aware of assessment), regardless of whether observers view videotapes (Reid, 1970; Taplin and Reid, 1973; Kent et al., 1974; Romanczyk, Kent, Diament, and O'Leary, 1973) or directly observe within the natural environment (Reid and DeMaster, 1972; Skindrud, 1972). For example, Reid (1970) found that the reliability of observers dropped from a median of .75 when reliability assessment was obtrusive to a median of .51 when observers were informed that reliability would no longer be assessed.

Romanczyk et al. (1973) computed the reliabilities of five trained observers to each of two "assessors" under conditions of either overt or covert assessment. During overt assessment, observers were told that either Assessor 1 or Assessor 2 was performing the reliability assessment, while under covert assessment the observers were not told that reliability was being evaluated (the assessors were merely present and observing within the setting). In addition, as a check on drift, Assessor 1 and Assessor 2 each adopted characteristic and idiosyncratic modifications of certain codes within the nine-category system. For example, for the coding category of "vocalization," Assessor 1 recorded even very soft vocalizations or mouthings, while Assessor 2 recorded only loud vocalizations and ignored such behaviors as humming, whispering, and sighing. The authors found that reliability dropped from an average of .77 with a known assessor to .33 under covert assessment across the eight days of study. In addition, the observers tended to record fewer instances of disruptive behavior under covert reliability assessment and tended to modify their employment of the coding system to conform with that of the particular assessor assigned to compute reliability for that day. Thus, observers tended to record soft verbalizations and mouthings as "vocalizations" with Assessor 1, while requiring loud vocalizations to employ that coding category for Assessor 2, a clear indication of the observer drift phenomenon already discussed. Figure 10-1 shows the frequency of total disruptive behavior computed over the eight days of assessment by the two observers under both overt and covert assessment.

Along similar lines, Taplin and Reid (1973) randomly assigned 18 undergraduate observers to one of three reliability assessment conditions. Observers within a "no-check" group were informed that they would be "put on their own to code new videotape segments" (p. 550), and it was emphasized that reliability would not be assessed following training. Observers within a "spotcheck" group were informed that they would code new segments of video-

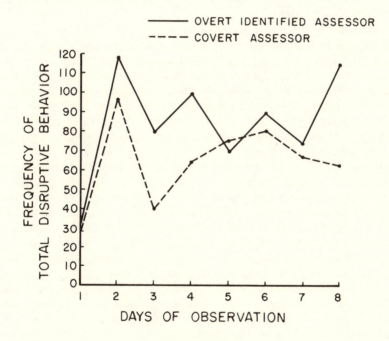

Figure 10-1
Total disruptive behavior computed over eight days of assessment by two observers under overt and covert assessment. From "Measuring the reliability of observational data: A reactive process" by R. G. Romanczyk, R. N. Kent, C. Diament, and D. D. O'Leary, *Journal of Applied Behavior Analysis*, 1973, *6*, 175–184. Reprinted by permission.

tape; however, reliability would only be assessed during certain "spot-checks." This procedure is analogous to employing a "calibrating" observer in the natural environment. A third, "random-check" group was instructed that a random selection of about "20% of their behavior sheets would be checked for reliability against protocols which the E would make some time after observations had been completed" (p. 550). For all observers in the no-check and random-check conditions, the assessor was not present in the room as observers watched and coded the videotapes. The spot-check observers were told to write the words "to be checked" on the top of their behavior coding sheets following the third and sixth data-collection sessions. Observer reliability was found to decrease by an average of 15 percent from training to data-collection conditions, and while there were no consistent differences between the groups, observations made during the spot checks showed significantly greater reliability than mean reliability shown before or after the checks. Similar findings are reported by Skindrud (1972) for data collected in the naturalistic situation.

Summarizing these findings, O'Leary and Kent (1973) state that overt reliability assessment, performed continuously on a spot-check basis, may not reflect the reliability of data generated on a day-to-day basis. In fact, reliabilities of .70 to .80 obtained under overt reliability assessment might reflect actual reliabilities of .30 to .40 under conditions of no assessment. Because observers typically collect data in isolation, with reliability checks made at infrequent intervals due to the high cost involved, the authors conclude that the BCA must be cautious in generalizing from reliability estimates obtained by overt reliability assessment.

O'Leary and Kent (1973) make some rather impractical recommendations for estimating reliability under unobtrusive conditions. They suggest that observers might be monitored continually by an experimenter who is present throughout a study and covertly checks reliability, or that checks could be made via closed-circuit television. Obviously these recommendations are more suited to research studies performed in a laboratory setting than to the applied researcher or clinician. A more practical recommendation is to employ two or three observers to work together in a given setting. Each would be given a schedule of the time period during which he was to observe a particular person (in some group), and these schedules would arrange for occasional simultaneous observation of the same person by two observers so that reliability could be assessed. The authors point out that this arrangement may introduce the problems of overt reliability assessment if the observers discover the periods when they are both recording the same person's behavior. Perhaps by reducing the physical proximity of observers to one another the likelihood of their determining when interobserver agreement is being assessed would be decreased.

A similar procedure was employed by Reid and DeMaster (1972) to assess the interobserver reliability of two observers trained to observe the behavior of 15 preschool children in a free-play setting. Each observation session lasted for one hour during which observers watched ten children for five minutes each. Observers were told that at any given time they would be observing different subjects and that no objective assessment of reliability would be made. In fact, they were required to observe the same child at the same time during the last five-minute observations per day, thus producing a covert check of interrater reliability.[4] As for the previous research findings, the percent agreement between observers fell from 82 percent on the last day of training (overt assessment) to 27 percent on the first day of covert assessment. Other alternatives include checking the observations of trainees to videotape criterion protocols when trainees are informed that reliability "will not be" assessed (unobtrusive), and increasing the frequency of observer training and feedback sessions to further emphasize the need for systematic and precise observations over time.

Jones, Reid and Patterson (1975) conclude that the problem of maintaining the level of observer reliability after or between reliability assessments has not been solved. Reid, Skindrud, Taplin, and Jones (1973) support this conclusion:

Even the use of systematic or random spot checks or partial feedback after each session has not been shown to be effective in preventing rapid observer decay between reliability assessments. Although it is possible that procedures such as initial overtraining or manipulation of observer motivation through contingent, monetary incentives may solve the problem, it is yet to be demonstrated [p. 2].

The authors suggest that one solution to this problem is the discovery of a covariant of observer reliability that could be assessed without the necessity of having another observer obtrusively present. They suggest that the complexity of the observation task might be employed in this fashion. The role of complexity in reliability assessment will now be discussed.

Complexity as a Predictor of Observer Agreement

Complexity has to do with the number of separate behavior categories the observer must discriminate between in endorsing an event and is often assessed using the following formula:

$$\frac{\text{Number of Categories Used}}{\text{Number of Total Entries}}$$

Thus, if a total of 50 behavior events are recorded within a half-hour observation session and all of them fall within five coding categories, the complexity would be $5/50 = .10$. However, if a total of 20 divergent categories were employed to describe the 50 events, the complexity would be much greater (20/50 = .40). Skindrud (1972) obtained significant negative correlations of –.53 and –.65 (both $p < .001$) between observer agreement and a measure of complexity (the percent of unrepeated interactions within each observed behavior segment). Taplin and Reid (1973) found a correlation of –.52 ($p < .001$) between percent agreement and complexity of the criterion protocols employed, while Reid (1973) found this correlation to be –.75 ($p < .01$). These findings have led Jones et al. (1975) to conclude that the relation between complexity and observer reliability is quite strong. Reid et al. (1973) suggest that complexity may be employed as an unobtrusive measure of reliability in the following fashion. If complexity and reliability are highly correlated, the assessment of complexity and provides the BCA with a measure of the change in reliability over time. Given that the reliability of observers seems to decrease consistently following training, but is maintained at a stable level when assessed under unobtrusive conditions, an evaluation of the complexity of protocols across observation periods provides the BCA with an indirect measure of reliability. If complexity is found to increase for particular observation sessions, this provides a signal to the BCA that reliability may have concomitantly decreased and suggests that the observer perhaps should be reassessed within the clinical training environment.

An important implication of this suggestion is that the complexity of behavior displayed by different persons within occasions or the same person across occasions may provoke concomitantly divergent levels of reliability. This suggests that the BCA cannot assume that reliability data gathered when an observer watches one person or one population of individuals is generalizable to another person or population. In addition, since the complexity of an individual's behavior may change over time, the BCA may wish to assess separately the complexity for each person both within and across observation occasions.

Observer Expectation and Biases

Rosenthal (1966) has been prominent among investigators exploring the role of experimenter bias as a predictor of data collected within a research experiment. In earlier studies, Rosenthal and Fode (1963) found that undergraduate experimenters reported faster learning with animals designated "maze-bright" than for those designated "maze-dull" even though there were no real differences in the animals' learning abilities. That such instructions could alter the expectations and thus the behavior of the data collector was further illustrated by Rosenthal and Jacobson (1966). They found that teachers directed more of their classroom efforts toward students who had been identified as "late bloomers" (resulting in higher IQs at the end of the year), even though this group was randomly selected from students in the classroom. A number of investigators have suggested that the findings of "experimenter effects" within the laboratory-oriented research study may have implications for the applied researcher who employs observational data to evaluate treatments. Thus, knowledge of treatment methods employed and/or predicted outcome, or explicit or even subtle communications by the BCA, might alter the recordings of observers to agree with the expectations generated. Whether such expectancies are instigated intentionally or unintentionally, the question becomes: Can such expectations alter the behavior (and thus data) of observers?

Initial studies did show significant differences in data collected when observers were given varied expectancies (e.g., regarding outcome); however, this research suffered from a lack of generalizability due to an inadequate sample of observers (Skindrud, 1972) as well as problems in methodology (Kass and O'Leary, 1970). To evaluate more systematically the role of expectation as a predictor of observer behavior, Kent et al. (1974) trained 20 observers to employ a nine-category coding system in observing videotape presentations of child behavior. One group of observers was informed that they would view videotapes showing baseline (pretreatment) behavior of two children, followed by videotapes depicting the children's behavior following the implementation of a token economy program designed to decrease disruptive behavior. A second group of observers was informed that they would observe baseline behavior followed by a "generalization condition" for which no change in disruptive behavior was predicted. Each of the two children was observed six times by all observers during baseline as well as treatment. Following their observations, the observers were given differential feedback by the experimenters indicating experimental predictions (e.g., change, no change). The authors also administered a questionnaire requiring observers to respond to the question: "What actually happened to the level of disruptive behavior from the baseline to the treatment condition your group viewed? (a) increase; (b) decrease; (c) no change" (p. 777). Results showed that the expectation manipulation produced no significant effects for any of the nine behavior categories or for the total frequency of disruptive behavior recorded. The observers reported behavior change in the direction predicted by the experimental manipulation. Nine of ten observers who were led to expect a decrease in disruptive behavior from baseline to treatment reported that they had viewed such a decrease, while seven of ten observers for whom no change was predicted reported that no change had occurred. Thus, while the actual data collected were uninfluenced by observer expectancy, the observers' interpretations of what had happened were dramatically altered. These findings have implcations for any investigation that requires observers to summarize verbally their findings across observation sessions and suggests that such data be interpreted with extreme caution by the BCA.

Wondering about the experimenter's role in actively reinforcing the observations of a group of observers, as might be the case in certain field-experimental settings (e.g., on receiving data, the experimenter openly makes evaluative comments, approves or disapproves of the data, etc.), O'Leary, Kent, and Kanowitz (1975) decided to further evaluate the role of experimenter feedback as a predictor of data generated by observers. Four "subject-observers" were trained to employ four categories of children's disruptive behavior ("playing," noise," "vocalization," and "orienting") to code a series of videotapes similar to those used by Kent et al. (1974). Three experienced observers served as expert or "criterion observers." During four baseline observation sessions both the criterion and subject-observers independently coded the videotapes. The subject-observers were then informed that four additional videotapes would show the behavior of children following the implementation of a treatment program, and a rationale was provided that "playing" and "noise" would decrease sharply during the treatment phase, while "vocalization" and "orienting" would remain unchanged (control behaviors). Employing a formula to determine the discrepancy between each subject-observer's recording with that of the criterion observer for each day of observation, the experimenter gave the subject-observers extensive feedback directed toward reducing this discrepancy in line with the expectancies generated. Positive reactions of the experimenter included comments such as: "Those tokens are really having an effect on (category)"; "the reduction on (category) is a great example of how children modify only what is specifically rewarded" (p. 46). Negative reactions included: "You don't seem to be picking up the treatment effect on (category)"; "it's strange that you have so many (category)—this treatment always works" (p. 46). The target behaviors of "playing" and "noise" were differentially shaped by the experimenter, while no differential feedback was provided for subject-observers' recordings of the two control behaviors of "vocalization" and "orienting." Results confirmed the experimenter's prediction regarding the role of feedback in altering observational data. There was virtually no change in the recording of control categories of behavior from baseline to treatment, while the two categories of "playing and "noise" decreased in line with the expectations generated. While this study is limited by the small number of observers employed, the brevity of observations over time, and the use of videotape recordings rather than behavior of live children, it clearly suggests that a combination of observer knowledge of predicted effects and experimenter feedback can produce significant biases in observational data. Unfortunately, it is impossible to determine whether the changes produced in the targeted behaviors were due to the expectations provided by the experimenter prior to the observation of "treatment" videotapes or the effects of contingent experimenter feedback across the sessions, or some combination of the two. Placing the findings from the Kent et al. (1974) study in the context of the present findings, the authors conclude:

On the basis of these two studies, it is apparent that the *evaluative* feedback to observers should be eliminated. While the expectation of change itself appears to have no significant effect on observational data obtained using well-defined behavioral categories, one might question any study in which experimenter feedback to the observers is not explicitly avoided. The most conservative stance would be to eliminate all review of incoming data that takes place in the presence of observers [p. 51].

Within most clinical or research endeavors, it would seem highly unlikely that the sophisticated BCA would directly communicate hypotheses associated with treatment outcome or provide feedback or instruction to independent observers. One way that expectancies could be communicated, however, is via the avenue of familiarity with a particular client or client population. Along these lines, an observer who has become familiar with the ordinary characteristics and frequency of a given client's behavior might be less sensitive to atypical behaviors or changes from ordinary frequency than is the completely naive, unfamiliar observer.

Employing a low-inference coding system directed at the behavior of patients within a psychiatric setting (the Time-Sample Behavioral Checklist described in Chapter 9), Redfield and Paul (1976) systematically evaluated the role of familiarity as a factor in instigating expectancies that might bias behavior observations. Four professional observers (average of 2.7 years full-time experience) systematically recorded the behavior of a familiar as well as unfamiliar group of patients. The familiar group had been regularly observed for several years by the observers; thus its members were well known to them. Members of the unfamiliar group were unknown to the observers. The videotapes were equated in terms of the number of appropriate behaviors exhibited by both groups, and were constructed so that patients within both groupings exhibited significant increases in the frequency of appropriate behavior across observation trials. Importantly, half of the familiar patients exhibited noticeable increases in behaviors that were uniquely *atypical* for that individual, with half of the unfamiliar group exhibiting the same increments. The authors found that the observers' reliability remained consistently high (average $r = .95$ with recordings of a criterion observer) over all trials. Regardless of previous experience with the patients, the observers were able to detect atypical events out of line with their expectancies for particular patients. The failure to find an expectancy effect is attributed to the criteria employed in the training of observers (100 percent agreement prior to data collection) as well as to the low level of inference called for by the TSBC. The authors state: "Specifically, observers making relatively inferential judgments may be particularly susceptible to sources of systematic error, while observers trained to make low inference recordings appear less likely to be subject to other influences" (p. 13). Thus the authors postulate that the characteristics of the target to be observed (low versus high inference) may predict expectancy effects.

Given the mixed findings regarding the impact of induced expectancies on observer reliability, additional research is needed to clarify possible interactions between the methods employed to generate expectancies, the targeted behaviors themselves, and characteristics of the observers (e.g., level of reliability, personality variables that may influence conformity or susceptibility to expectancy, fatigue).

Expectancy effects: some practical recommendations. In applied research it is difficult or impossible to assume that observers will not be able to discriminate treatment from control subjects. The questions, concerns, and interactions offered by persons observed provide implicit or explicit information to observers. In addition, changes in the frequencies and/or categories of behavior displayed by persons observed (e.g., as a result of intervention) may suggest the treatments employed and provide clues as to the research hypotheses. Thus, a parent's use of "time-out" procedure or some other formalized intervention on a given occasion of observation is sure to cue the observer that treatment has been implemented and the expected results of intervention may be obvious from the nature of the treatment. This suggests that the BCA may wish to caution observers regarding the possibility of expectancy and observer-bias effects and encourage a high degree of professionalism. In line with this suggestion, Rosenthal (1966) cites evidence that graduate students obtained less-biased data than undergraduates who had perhaps not adopted certain standards regarding an empirical approach to data collection. Johnson and Bolstad (1973) have suggested that observers be debriefed, perhaps via a written questionnaire, regarding the status of persons observed. A questionnaire might ask whether or not the persons are in the process of treatment and what the treatments are, as well as how the observer views the goals of treatment. To the extent that observers remain naive, the BCA can be assured that expectancy effects are held to a minimum (given accurate reporting). They point out that when observers do determine such information, it usually results from an interaction with a member of a family being observed. They conclude that debriefing can be additionally important in reducing avenues by which observers obtain such information about the nature of ongoing treatments, and the questionnaire itself serves as a regular reminder "for the importance of unbiased, objective recording of behavior" (p. 38).

Finally, the BCA should be particularly conscientious about restricitng information to observers regarding specific behaviors targeted for change. While it is likely that observers will discriminate the onset or removal of treatment procedures, it is less likely that they will determine specific categories of treated or untreated (control) behavior events.

Footnotes

[1]It should be noted that the stated optimum level of agreement to be reached in training varies considerably in published reports, with most investigators satisfied

with agreements greater than or equal to 80-85 percent (e.g., Taplin and Paul, 1973; Johnson and Bolstad, 1973). Gordon Paul (Redfield and Paul, 1976) suggests that this criterion is too lenient. In evaluating the employment of highly trained (to 100 percent agreement across coding categories) professional observers, Redfield and Paul note: "professional, highly trained observers apparently are more successful in maintaining accuracy over time than their less well-trained, part-time counterparts, and therefore would seem to be less prone to systematic error which may accompany declining standards of performance" (p. 14).

[2]The material in this section may require a careful reading for those unfamiliar with the concept of reliability. This material is most relevant to the BCA who wishes to construct a formal coding system.

[3]Chapter 8 provides a summary of instructions designed to diminish observer-induced reactivity effects that may be included in a coding manual.

[4]A better procedure would be to space simultaneous observations of the same subject randomly *throughout* the observation period as reliability of observers may change as a function of duration of observation. For example, observer fatigue may tend to lower agreement at the end of an observation session.

UNIT II-D Psychophysiological Assessment

PSYCHOPHYSIOLOGICAL METHODS

Psychophysiology is an old idea but a new science. It is a likely assumption that ever since man began to experience himself as an object of his own awareness, he has had some intuitive notion that bodily changes were, in some measure, related to his moods, his sentiments, his frustrations, his elations. How to relate these dual aspects of human functioning has been a concern of philosopher-scientists throughout the course of intellectual history [Greenfield and Sternbach, 1972, p. v].

Since that statement was made, the potential value of broadening the clinical assessment to include a client's physiological responses to the events that shape his life situation has been underscored by various writers. Textbooks and compendiums of methodologies for psychological, clinical, or "behavioral" assessment have increasingly provided an introduction to psychophysiological assessment methods germane to a comprehensive clinical assessment (Adams, Doster, and Calhoun, 1977; Kallman and Feuerstein, 1977; Hersen and Bellack, 1976; Mash and Terdal, 1976; Lazarus, 1976). But this has not always been the case. For years the development of instrumentation and methodology to assess such physiological phenomena as heart functioning, muscle tension, or electrical activity of the brain has largely come from medical and animal research (Sidowski, 1966; Deifenderfer, 1972; Lacey and Lacey, 1970).[1]

This chapter will offer psychophysiological assessment as another major category of methods that the BCA may wish to include in the clinical assessment. However, this presentation is only introductory, and the interested reader is urged to seek out a more substantive treatment of the methods and issues of psychophysiological assessment (Greenfield and Sternbach, 1972; Brown, 1967; Venables and Martin, 1967). Before proceeding, it may be worthwhile to offer a rationale for the inclusion of any of this material in the present text.

Many clients offer presenting problems that directly involve physiological response systems. The client complaining of high blood pressure (perhaps in response to environmental stress), tightness of the chest, muscle cramps, or nausea is asking the BCA to focus his assessment and intervention efforts directly on psychophysiological phenomena. Without a direct physiological assessment, the BCA would have to rely exclusively on the client's self-report or on any observable indicants of such covert behavior for clinical decision making. Presuming that a bodily insult or disease process is excluded from consideration following a thorough medical work-up, the BCA may well be able to assist the client in gaining control of the physiological response system responsible for his discomfort or dissatisfaction.

Even when a psychophysiological mechanism is not directly implicated in the initial statement of the "problem," the BCA may wish to explore the possibility that a client's physiological response to his environment is partly responsible for his complaint. For example, a client offering vague complaints of psychological "discomfort" or "depression" as a targeted problem may be misinterpreting certain body cues or unpleasant sensations (controlled by physiological systems) as psychological phenomena, or he may be unable to detect the over- or underactivity of a physiological system. Intervention might be directed toward assisting the client to learn certain social skills that will better enable him to address his environment while *also* providing him with the skills to better control his bodily response to life situation events. Thus, while physiological responses are not the exclusive target of intervention, they become one of a variety of targets for which intervention is planned. Obviously, an exclusive focus on only one aspect of the client's behavior (e.g., overt "skills" behavior, tight muscles, or rapid heart rate) might not be successful in altering the other modality, which may lead to an unsatisfactory therapeutic outcome.

Finally, an assessment of multiple behavioral domains and their interrelationships (verbal, motor, physiological) provides the BCA with a much more comprehensive understanding of a client's response to his environment. In addition, physiological assessment provides a kind of validity check on the client's verbal report and other observables that are so frequently the exclusive assessment focus. A client, for example, who verbally reports that he is not fearful when exposed to a previously fearful stimulus, such as a stairwell or unknown animal, may show physiological responses, such as a lack of muscle tension, that tend to validate his verbal report. Of course, self-reports, motor behavior, and physiological responses need not always or even ideally correlate (see Lang, 1968; Smith, Diener, and Beaman, 1974), but in this case the correlation does provide evidence that the client is an accurate self-observer, fully in touch with all aspects of his behavior. In contrast, the client who reports that he is not "tense" while showing high levels of physiological responsivity may be unaware that his muscles are tense or that his heart rate is elevated because he has not learned to survey his physiological state carefully. Such a client might employ global labels (e.g., not "nervous," "uptight") to describe his physical status without understanding how his body is responding to his environment. The BCA would certainly wish to examine further this discrepancy in assessment. In this case, an intervention strategy might be directed toward training the client to be aware of his body (e.g., muscle tension) as a prelude to learning how to control his physiological responses. Finally, it should be noted that in some cases an assessment of physiological responsivity is the only direct measure available to the BCA to assess the target of interest. The client who complains of "anxiety," yet shows no overt behavioral indications of its occurrence, might show differential physiological responsivity across anxiety-provoking situations. In this case, physiological assessment would seem to be imperative.

Perhaps psychophysiological assessment has not been widely employed by the BCA because of the unavailability of instrumentation to many agencies or a general fear that this "highly technological" pursuit is too complex to be mastered or too costly in professional time to be of use. Brown (1972) points out that the instrumentation involved in monitoring something as simple as a client's heart rate vary considerably (from a simple stethoscope to an on-line computer), depending on the *precision* with which the BCA wishes to measure the response (fidelity) and the uses he hopes to make of the information. It should be noted, however, that a simple polygraph, which provides amplification and pen recording of responses, gives the BCA considerable flexibility in monitoring a variety of response systems, and can be purchased at reasonable cost (see Sidowski, 1966, for a comprehensive listing of manufacturers).

Psychophysiological Responses: Possibilities for Measurement

Before the basic methods for measuring psychophysiological responses can be presented, it is important to explore the nature of psychophysiological response systems. Once we obtain a better idea of *what can be measured*, we will more readily understand how we might go about measuring it. In very simple terms, any physiological or biochemical process in the human organism can potentially be reliably detected given the development of a technology for translating that event into a form the BCA can observe.

As might be imagined, some responses, due to their basic characteristics or locus in the organism, are much more difficult for the BCA to detect than others. As a simple example, tactile receptors in the reader's fingertips are capable of detecting the incidence of heart muscle movements or "beats" without the assistance of instrumentation. With the addition of a watch with a second hand or a stopwatch, the reader could easily relate heartbeats to time and compute a heart rate. In contrast, the brain's electrical activity cannot be detected without instrumentation, although the essential nature of these two phenomena (electrical potentials) is the same. While the electrical impulses of the heart and brain can be amplified to drive an oscilloscope (an electronic device that visually shows the pattern of response) or cause simple fluctuations of a pen on chart paper, the heart-rate response offers additional possibilities for purely physical-mechanical detection. You could place an object on an individual's chest and, via film photography, illustrate movements of the object that are directly related to heart movements, thus translating the heart rate into an observable response. This method is unduly elaborate, but it illustrates how the possibilities for measurement are determined by the nature of the physiological response to be measured.

Three major categories of psychophysiological responses can be detected (Brown, 1972), and the measurement methodology for each may vary quite considerably. First, many physiological systems produce *bioelectrical signals*. By "bioelectrical" we mean that *the tissue of interest produces electrical energy that merely needs to be detected by instrumentation*. The detection device most frequently used is an *electrode* (often a metal disc) placed on or near the tissue of interest. The electrode must be capable of conducting the electrical impulses generated by the tissue to the instrumentation so that the signal may be amplified (because physiological impulses are very weak) and translated into some observable output (pen deflections, oscilloscope movements). The heart, for example, generates potentials that may be displayed as the electrocardiogram (ECG or EKG). As already mentioned, the brain produces electrical signals and these may be expressed in the electroencephalogram (EEG). The skeletal muscles offer a bioelectric signal expressed as the electromyogram (EMG). The skin also generates electrical potentials which may be measured as the skin potential (SP). The eye and the gastrointestinal system produce similar potentials which may be detected via electrodes appropriately placed on the body.

A second major category of physiological phenomena, *transduced bioelectrical signals*, are electrical properties of tissue that cannot be measured directly, *but must be assessed indirectly by measuring the response of the tissue to some form of stimulation*. An excellent example is the measurement of skin resistance (SR). Electrical current from an external source is passed from one electrode, usually placed on the hand or forearm, through the body to another electrode that receives the signal so that resistance to this flow of current can be measured. Since skin resistance does not naturally produce a directly measureable electrical potential, this procedure serves as an indirect measurement. Other examples of transduced bioelectric signals include measures of skin conductance (SC) the reciprocal of resistance (how well the skin conducts a flow of current), as well as certain measures of the tissue and blood.

Finally, *physical-biological phenomena* (Brown, 1972) such as pressure, acceleration, or color can be transduced (translated into a signal capable of being measured). For example, the temperature of body tissues or fluids can be assessed by a "thermistor" (a device sensitive to temperature change), blood pressure (BP) can be measured with the mechanical blood-pressure cuff we are all familiar with, and physical movements can be transduced by any mechanical system capable of detecting movement or some product of movement (e.g., sound generated by movement).

In summary, while certain physiological systems generate responses that have only to be detected and encoded, others must be detected indirectly by physically acting on body tissue and evaluating tissue responses, or by physically transducing the physiological response.

As might be imagined, an electrode or other transducer that detects a physiological phenomenon must not, because of its own characteristics, interfere with that phenomenon, nor should it provoke electrical interference that makes the signal difficult to detect. Both Brown (1972) and Thompson, Lindsley, and Eason (1966) present excellent discussions of the characteristics of an ideal transducer.

Once electrical or physical energy is detected and transduced, it must usually be amplified so that it is strong enough to provoke measurable responses in whatever recording medium is selected. Such amplification is similar in some respects to that of a home stereo system, in that the amplifier (in some cases coupled with a preamplifier) modifies the transduced signal into a form capable of being displayed and/or recorded.

The detection of the signal via a transducer might be termed the *input* phase of recording, while the amplification and filtering (e.g., reducing background noise) of the signal are the *throughput*. The final *output* phase involves the display and/or recording of the signal. Here the BCA has numerous options. Most often a *paper-chart recording system* is employed to provide a permanent record of pen movements reflecting changes in the *amplitude* of the signal, as well as its *frequency and period* and *waveform*. Figure 11-1 illustrates these characteristics of a signal.

The *amplitude* of a response reflects its magnitude, and is measured from the peak of the pen's movement as it describes a cycle of the biological signal (e.g., a heart contraction) to a zero potential reference point. Figure 11-1 shows this measurement at A_1, A_2, A_3 and so forth, for both an alternating current (ac) and direct current (dc) signal.

The *frequency* of the signal is the number of complete wave cycles that occur within some unit of time (e.g., one second, one minute). According to Brown (1972), a single cycle or waveform is measured: "from any one point

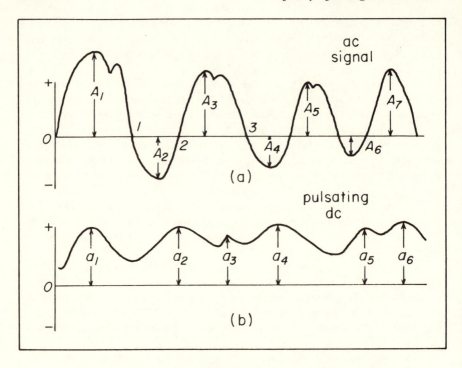

Figure 11-1
Characteristics of an electrical signal. From "Instruments in
psychophysiology" by C. Brown. In N. S. Greenfield and
R. A. Sternbach (Eds.), *Handbook of psychophysiology.*
New York: Holt, Rinehart & Winston, 1972.

on the wave to a succeeding equivalent point" (p. 160). In Figure 11-1 a full cycle occurs from number 1 to number 3—in this case measured from zero reference point. Most signals are expressed as cycles per second (Hz). A 5-Hz waveform would thus contain five complete cycles per second. The *period* of a waveform is the length of time it takes for one complete cycle, and this is most often expressed in milliseconds (msec).

Finally, the *waveform* of a signal is the "generalized shape of a wave" (Brown, 1972, p. 161). Waves could be described as triangular, sinusoidal, or as "spikes."

Other outputs include the *oscilloscope*, which shows an electronic representation of the signal on a televisionlike screen. Oscilloscopic information may be photographed or filmed for later analysis. Another option, the *counter* or *counterprinter*, provides a cumulative count of the number of events (e.g., cycles, heartbeats) or an exact assessment of the time lapse between two events (e.g., time between heartbeats) expressed in numerical form for easy visualization or statistical analysis. Finally, an amplified signal may be audiorecorded on tape using an *FM analogue tape recorder.* It is then passed through an analogue-to-digital (A to D) converter and fed into a computer for statistical analysis or computer averaging of the waveform.

Major Modalities of Psychophysiological Assessment

Heart Functioning

An excellent example of monitoring direct bioelectric signals is found in the assessment of the heart response. Heart functioning is easily monitored with a cardiochronograph, which draws successive vertical lines, one for each heartbeat. A more sophisticated measurement is provided by the electrocardiograph (EKG), which measures electrical potentials that originate in the heart as it contracts. For EKG assessment there are 12 standard body locations on which recording or reference electrodes are placed (e.g., left and right arms and legs, chest). When the electrical potentials detected by these electrodes are amplified, the output is typically printed on a paper-chart recorder as the electrocardiogram and termed the EKG. Figure 11-2 shows an oversimplified example of an EKG waveform.

Note that the peak response (see "a") could be unambiguously observed either on a paper record or on an oscilloscope. The distance between the peaks is employed for timing or counting purposes (e.g., the heart rate or "beat"). While several electrode variants are suitable for EKG recording,

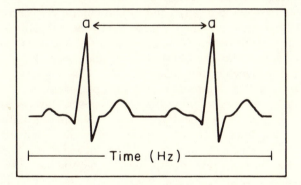

Figure 11-2
EKG waveform. From "Instruments in psychophysiology" by
C. Brown. In N. S. Greenfield and R. A. Sternbach (Eds.),
Handbook of psychophysiology. **New York: Holt, Rinehart & Winston,**
1972. Reprinted by permission.

most are susceptible to artifactual responses produced by client movement under standard measurement conditions. When such movements are impossible to eliminate, the selection of a nonstandard location for recording (which excludes active muscle tissue to the extent possible) is recommended (Brown, 1972). As might be imagined, the attachment of electrodes to various parts of the body makes it quite uncomfortable for the client as recordings are made, and this rather "artificial" situation may very well influence the heart rate (reactivity) or in some other way delimit the client's access to the environment.

With the advent of *biotelemetry* equipment, heart rate can now be monitored without disrupting ongoing client behavior. When this approach is used, the electrodes are attached to a transmitter, which may, for example, be worn on the client's belt, and which sends a record of the client's EKG to a receiver, which can be positioned away from the client or even hidden from view. Transmitted signals are then amplified and recorded in a manner suitable to assessment needs. Norman (1970), for example, has developed a heart-rate and behavior monitoring system that combines a wireless FM transmitter with a videotape camera and microphone in order to record ongoing client behaviors. An evaluation of videotape and EKG records points out potential relationships between overt verbal and motor behavior and heart activity. A similar technique is described by Levine and Grinspoon (1971) who used a telemetry system to monitor heart rate and skin resistance in a population of chronic schizophrenic patients during periods of hallucination and talking. In fact, it is possible to employ "wireless" transmitting equipment to detect and transmit a wide variety of physiological responses, and this approach should be kept in mind if the BCA wishes the client to have free access to his environment as physiological recordings are made.

Heart rate has been typically employed in clinical assessment as a measure of anxiety or stress, presumably mediated by the sympathetic portion of the autonomic nervous system. Some investigators have found increased heart rate when subjects are exposed to stressful conditions (Wellman, Older, and Jones, 1967). Unfortunately, the situation is not all that clear-cut for the EKG or any of the physiological modalities. For example, while one might imagine that exposure to an anxiety-provoking situation will always increase the client's heart rate, this is not necessarily the case. Experimentally provoked anxiety may lead either to an acceleration (Lacey and Smith, 1954) *or* to a deceleration of heart rate (Notterman, Schoenfeld, and Bersh, 1952). In addition, an increase in heart rate in response to some stimulus may not necessarily be related to anxiety, but may merely be an indicant of the orienting response or arousal shown in response to any novel stimulus (Gunn, Wolf, Block, and Person, 1972). According to Gunn et al. (1972), the mechanisms and degree of the heart-rate response are related to the "individual's conscious or unconscious evaluation of the situation, his prior experience, and his previously established reaction patterns" (p. 477).

Importantly, the direction and degree of response to a particular "stressful" experience, as defined by the experimenter, vary considerably across individuals. The work of Lacey and his colleagues (Lacey, Bateman, and Van Lehn, 1953; Lacey and Lacey, 1958) is worth discussing in some detail. These investigators found evidence for what they called "response stereotypy" in the autonomic nervous system. That is, regardless of the characteristics of the stressful stimulus, an individual tends to respond within the same physiological functions (e.g., EKG, SR, EMG) and the entire pattern of the individual's responses tends to be the same from one stimulus to another. Thus, in stressful situations a given individual might consistently show a much greater EKG response followed by a somewhat lesser SR response (and perhaps very little EMG response), and this pattern would be reproduced whenever that individual was faced with stress. The authors also report individual differences in the degree of response stereotype shown across individuals. While "rigid reactors" seemed to respond to virtually any kind of stressful situation in a rigidly consistent fashion, "random reactors" showed divergent patterns of responsivity across stimuli and across occasions. Lang, Rice, and Sternbach (1972) make the interesting point that the rigid reactor who consistently shows maximal activation within a particular physiological modality such as blood pressure may later develop a psychosomatic disorder involving that particular physiological modality (e.g., hypertension). At present little data support this speculation.

Another line of investigation, which applies to heart rate as well as other physiological modalities, is the possibility that certain emotions yield characteristic physiological responses. For example, Ax (1953) found significant differences in heart rate, EMG, diastolic blood pressure, as well as the number of skin-conductance responses, when comparing the reactions of subjects to experimentally induced fear versus anger. While these findings have been supported by other investigators (Schachter, 1957; Sternbach, 1960, 1968), attempts to show physiological differences when more subtle emotions are compared have been largely unsuccessful (Lang et al., 1972).

An important thing to keep in mind is the individual's *cognitive set* when he is exposed to some particular stimulus situation. By cognitive set, we mean the way that the individual phenomenologically views (interprets) what has happened to him. Even though the BCA may believe that a given situation holds noxious properties, that individual's cognitive view of the situation (which, paradoxically, *could* be that the situation is pleasant) will determine his physiological response. Also, responses to some aversive stimuli may be reduced via a process of adaptation (Deanne, 1969).

In summary, while there may be some replicable differences in responses to anger and fear, two basic emotions that hold quite different implications for the individual and much adaptive significance, generally speaking there are no standard, predictable responses to psychological or physical stimuli. The degree and even the direction of physiological responsivity within a given modality seem to be unique for each individual; thus, an individual's responses must be assessed across time and conditions rather than compared to those of others. Specifically, the BCA would wish to determine a client's EKG under relaxed, nonstressful conditions and employ those responses as a context for interpreting responses to clinically relevant stimuli like fear-, anxiety- or anger-provoking conditions. In many cases, this approach involves establishing a "baseline" (in the absence of presumably arousing stimuli). Often an individual's baseline responses will vary across occasions of measurement and must be redetermined each time a physiological modality is assessed.

Electromyogram (EMG)

As another bioelectric signal, EMG measures the electrical impulse or action potential of nerve fibers which enervate muscle fibers (together called a *motor unit*). Since these action potentials cause the muscle to contract and, thus, move from a state of relaxation to a state of tension, the EMG may be thought of as an indirect measure of muscle tension (or its converse, relaxation). It should be noted, however, that even during relaxation and sleep some minimal level of nerve activity occurs, with this level increasing as the individual becomes aroused and prepares for his daily pursuits. While various methods have been employed to measure muscle tension (e.g., muscle tremor, the hardness of muscles measured by a dynamometer), the EMG has been by far the most popular approach.

Because muscular tension may cause clients discomfort, with many fearful or "anxious" persons exhibiting tension as an adjunctive or primary complaint, the EMG is an important element in the BCA's catalogue of measurement possibilities. While single motor units may be measured with needle electrodes which penetrate the skin and physically touch the unit, surface EMG is measured by metal electrodes placed on the skin and is actually the product of a number of motor units participating in a given motor response. The amplitude of the EMG response is determined by the frequency of neural firing of individual motor units as well as the number of units paticipating. As for EKG, EMG activity is amplified, with the output recorded either as auditory tones (which can be interpreted via computer analysis) or on a paper chart. Figure 11-3 shows a typical paper recording of EMG.

Goldstein (1972) points out that since the measurement of amplitude from EMG recordings is quite time-consuming, investigators usually employ some means of integrating the response. The *integrator* measures total electrical activity as a function of time to show both positive and negative pen movements as movements in one direction, so that the total response can be easily measured. Other integrators provide an immediate numerical read-out of EMG amplitude; however, since this approach fails to discriminate between artifacts and actual electrical potentials, it may produce specious results.

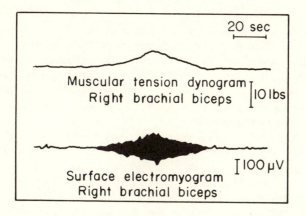

Figure 11-3
A typical paper recording. From "Electromyography" by
I. B. Goldstein. In N. S. Greenfield and R. A. Sternbach (Eds.),
Handbook of psychophysiology. **New York: Holt, Rinehart & Winston,**
1972. Reprinted by permission.

With regard to site of measurement, Voas (1952) found that two highly popular sites, the forearm flexors and the frontalis muscles of the forehead, also show the highest test-retest reliability coefficients across a variety of stimulus conditions.

A good deal of research indicates that clients reporting that they feel "anxious" or "tense" often show more EMG activity than do control subjects not reporting such anxiety (Malmo and Shagass, 1949; Jacobson, 1938). In addition, a few investigators have also found that the site of EMG activity seems to be related to the category of emotion reported by the client. Shagass and Malmo (1954), for example, recorded specific muscle activity patterns and found that forearm tension was associated with conflicts over hostility while lower limb tension was associated with sexual conflicts. This work was replicated by Malmo, Smith, and Kohlmeyer (1956). Unfortunately, in recent years many investigators have failed to find a direct correlation between "anxiety" and EMG; this may be due to a host of factors. For one thing, the specific definition of anxiety employed by clients may vary considerably. For some persons "anxiety" has to do with certain thoughts or other cognitive phenomena; other clients would report anxiety only if some level of physical tension were experienced. Thus, the BCA must be very careful to identify precisely what a particular client means when he uses a global term such as "anxious" or "uptight."

Noble and Lader (1971) have stated that it may be difficult to obtain a consistent relation between "anxiety" and EMG because different muscles yield different results for different kinds of stressors. As with other physiological measures, they feel it is more appropriate to view the EMG as an index of general arousal than to relate this measure to "anxiety" specifically. In a study of the EMG responses of 34 depressed patients receiving electroconvulsive therapy, these authors found a rather low relation between anxiety and EMG, although depressed clients did show greater levels of muscular tension. Recent investigators (McGuigan and Pavek, 1972) have found a significant relationship between certain covert phenomena, such as thoughts and imagery, and EMG responses.

Like other physiological measures, the EMG response may diminish over time, while the stimulus remains constant, because of adaptation. In addition, the electrical activity pattern may change independently of changes in the actual tension of muscle groups. A number of investigators have shown that clients can learn, by receiving feedback about the level of tension within a muscle group, to relax that muscle. This is true even for single motor units (Basmajian, 1963; Green, Walters, Green, and Murphy, 1969). The potential clinical importance of this phenomenon is obvious.

Electroencephalography (EEG)

When electrodes are attached to certain areas of the scalp, oscillating electrical potentials can be recorded. The observation that these potentials seem to vary with different states of arousal has generated an important body of research, first directed at the global differences between sleep and wakefulness. Four predominant frequencies of electrical activity have been examined. Alpha or alpha wave activity (8–12 Hz) characteristically occurs during wakefulness when the individual is relaxed, with an immediate cessation (blocking) if the person is stimulated by a light source, sound, or other intrusive stimulus. Alpha seems to produce a very pleasant, relaxed feeling in the individual. When provided with immediate feedback, such as a tone, which indicates alpha and asked to "clear the mind" and attempt to concentrate on "keeping the tone on," many individuals can readily learn to maintain the alpha state, along with the concomitant relaxation and pleasant feelings. It should be noted that such *biofeedback* training has been used to permit individuals to gain control of a variety of physiological responses, such as EMG, EKG, and blood pressure, and may hold important potential for clinical intervention (see Blanchard and Epstein, 1978). Beta activity (20–36 Hz) occurs when the person is awake and highly aroused. As the individual becomes relatively less aroused and eventually sleeps, the EEG pattern changes markedly, with the frequency of brain waves decreasing as arousal decreases. As the individual moves through theta (4–8 Hz) to delta activity, activity, (4 Hz and lower) we would say that the individual is asleep. Furthermore, EEG records may reliably differentiate between periods of dreaming and nondreaming during sleep (see Cartwright, 1978).

With the advent of the A-to-D computer and highly sophisticated procedures for displaying EEG activity, several investigators have found differences in EEG patterns among various client populations. In some instances, significant EEG differences have been found between schizophrenics and normals (Itill, Saletu, and Davis, 1972; Lifshitz and Gradizan, 1972). Others have found that while no differences exist under ordinary, nonstimulating conditions, certain client populations, such as epileptics or psychotics, show EEG responses to particular stimuli which are markedly different from those of normals (Stevens, Lonsburg, and Cole, 1972; Kamp, Schryer, and Van Leeuwen, 1972). Levy, Issacs, and Behrman (1971) successfully differentiated between elderly depressed and senile patients in 16 out of 17 instances based on EEG responses to light stimulation. Others have found characteristic differences between certain neurological categories of child populations (e.g., dyslexic) and normals (Sklar, Hanley and Simmons, 1972).

Using biotelemetry procedures and multichannel EEG-recording methods, Porter, Wolf, and Penry (1971) have reported reliable recordings and little signal loss or distortion when subjects are behaving freely up to 60 meters away. For example, Hanley, Rickles, Crandall, and Walters (1972) used a computer spectral analysis of waveforms to evaluate instantaneously the EEG pattern of a freely moving 48-year-old, chronic schizophrenic male. With "on-line" computer analysis, EEG abnormalities can be detected immediately if the computer is set to pick up preselected abnormal EEG patterns. Combined with the biotelemetric techniques reported by Porter et al. (1971), this would allow the BCA to receive immediate feedback about important EEG patterns while the client is behaving in a natural setting (Sterman and Friar, 1972).

Skin Responses

A variety of characteristics of the skin—resistance (SR), conductance (SC), and impedence (SI)—have been assessed as purported measures of emotionality, stress, or arousal (Edelberg, 1972). As SR and SC are by far the most frequent, they will be the focus for this discussion.[2] In assessing skin resistance (its reciprocal is conductance), two metal electrodes are attached to the client's skin, usually at the palm of the hand or the sole of the foot. A small electrical current is transmitted between the two electrodes so that the skin behaves as a resistor. By assessing the amount of voltage that the skin permits to be conducted across the electrodes, resistance can be calculated by employing Ohm's law [current flow (I) = voltage (V)/resistance (R)]. With appropriate amplification, conductance and/or resistance can be displayed permanently on paper using a paper-chart recording system or can be viewed via an oscilloscope. If the subject is exposed to any one of a variety of external stimuli (e.g., a sudden noise), a rapid decrease in measured voltage, which indicates decreased skin resistance, will be measured about two seconds later. This transient response has been called the galvanic skin reflex (GSR) or psychogalvanic reflex (PGR). Internal events, such as thoughts or sensations, can also provoke a GSR and in some cases the relationship between covert phenomena and SR/SC is of clinical importance. Resistance typically returns to baseline in a short period (within 30 seconds), with reflex changes amounting to between 5 and 50 percent of the baseline response. Resistance is most often expressed in terms of its reciprocal—conductance, which ranges from 10,000 to 500,000 ohms cm^2, with measured resistance depending on the temperature of the skin (resistance increases as temperature decreases by about 3 percent). Drops in temperature also increase the latency of the electrodermal response.

Because the baseline levels of SR/SC are quite variable across clients, it is important that accurate baseline measures be taken under neutral conditions so that any fluctuations due to particular stimuli of clinical relevance (e.g., imaginal presentation of fear-provoking scene) may be compared to the base level. Under baseline conditions conductance is very low and following the presentation of some arousing stimulus, increases in conductance occur with a latency of one to two seconds. While there is no evidence that stronger stimuli will shorten latency, the amplitude of SR/SC responses may decrease with repeated stimulation as the client adapts to the stimulus. Importantly, demonstrable diurnal fluctuations in skin conductance occur, conductance being much higher in the morning. Also, the physical state of the individual may alter baseline conductance levels. Figure 11-4 shows an example of an electrodermal response to external stimulation.

Regarding the relation between skin responses and "emotionality," it is apparent that *any* stimulus that generally activates the individual may alter SR/SC (Woodworth and Schlosberg, 1954). Also, emotional states reported subjectively by clients are often not reflected in SR/SC changes, so electrodermal activity *may not be thought of as a direct indicant of emotionality*, but only of the level of arousal accompanying many emotional reactions. In addition, both pleasant and unpleasant stimuli may elicit comparable changes in conductance level, further complicating an interpretation of SR/SC responses. Because SR/SC may be radically affected by any stimulus altering the level of arousal, such confounding of stimulus factors must be minimized by controlling the clinical setting in which SR/SC is measured.

The foregoing suggests that changes in SR/SC must be interpreted with caution because of the host of variables affecting a client's response. In addition, SR/SC measures appear to have no real diagnostic value since most studies are unable to differentiate such populations as neurotics, psychotics, or sociopaths, based on electrodermal criteria. Among the notable exceptions to these findings is the work of Gruzelier and Venables (1972) who compared SR responses to an 85-decibel tone in 20 normals and 80 heterogeneously classified schizophrenics. While all 20 of the normals responded to the tone

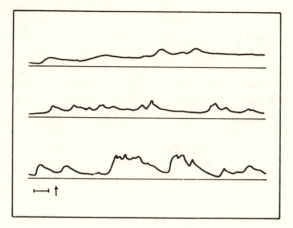

Figure 11-4
Electrodermal response to external stimulation. From "Electrical
activity of the skin" by R. Edelberg. In N. S. Greenfield and
R. A. Sternbach (Eds.), *Handbook of psychophysiology.*
New York: Holt, Rinehart & Winston, 1972. Reprinted by Permission.

with an increase in SR which later habituated, roughly half of the 80 schizophrenics did not respond at all, while the other half showed higher levels of conductance than normals, more variability in baseline response, higher response amplitude, and shorter latencies of SR responses. In reviewing the utility of SR/SC as an index of arousal for schizophrenics and normals, Depue and Fowles (1973) found no consistent differences between the two groups. At the present time, the possibilities of employing SR/SC as an assessment device to discriminate patient populations seem to be limited by these inconsistent findings in the literature.

Other Psychophysiological Measures

While physiological assessments of blood pressure, forearm blood flow, respiration rate, skin temperature, and other similar phenomena are not employed as often as the measures discussed above, their measurements would be performed in similar fashion. A transducer is attached to the targeted site of the body, information is fed into equipment capable of amplifying the targeted response, and this response is then fed into equipment capable of displaying or making a permanent record of clients' responses. Schwitzgebel and Schwitzgebel (1973) and Rugh and Schwitzgebel (1977) have completed a rather thorough listing of psychophysiological measures that the BCA may wish to explore.

The abbreviated presentation given in this chapter is not meant to demean the importance of psychophysiological measurement. The BCA interested in psychophysiological assessment should carefully consult the handbooks published by the manufacturers of potentially employed instruments (see Sidowski, 1966; Sommer, 1974) in addition to the handbooks mentioned earlier. More and more psychological journals are carrying reports of measurement and treatment applications of psychophysiological responses. Psychophysiological measurement seems to provide an invaluable index of certain targeted events and will increasingly be employed by BCAs as a standard assessment tool, with physiological response modalities often becoming the focus of intervention efforts.

Footnotes

[1]A compilation of the physiological response systems and measurement methodology frequently addressed by the researcher can be found in two excellent textbooks of physiological psychology (Thompson, 1967; Grossman, 1973).

[2]It should be noted that when measured under conditions that significantly reduce artifacts (e.g., intermittant contact between electrodes and the skin), electrical skin potentials (SPS) can be measured in the absence of external electrical stimulation.

UNIT III
Clinical Decision Making

12

ORGANIZING
THE ASSESSMENT
TO FACILITATE
CLINICAL
DECISION MAKING

Chapters 1 and 2 provided the reader with a description of aspects of the client's behavior, life situation, resources and motives that might be a part of a comprehensive clinical assessment. All of these schemes encourage the BCA to focus attention upon something other than the client's verbal report; to expand the assessment to include written methods, direct observation of the client's behavior in relevant settings and, sometimes, assessment of psychophysiological systems. Other chapters offered a variety of methodological options across these major methods domains. The multitude of themes and variations presented suggests that there is no one way of carrying out a com-

273

prehensive clinical assessment, but rather, many strategies, each of which may be defensible in different circumstances. That the author or the reader is comfortable with a particular theoretical orientation should, however, have little to do with the manner in which assessment data are organized, regardless of content. The question may be raised: is there a strategy for organizing assessment data which maximizes the probability that the BCA will obtain a comprehensive view of the client and his life situation? It is hoped that the present chapter will provide not only such a strategy, but also a way of thinking about the *process* of the clinical assessment as it is planned and orchestrated, as a picture of the client unfolds and goals are selected that increase the likelihood of successful therapeutic outcome.

The basic ingredients of the clinical assessment will first be defined and discussed. The term *modality* will be employed to mean *any aspect of the client or the client's life situation that is to be the focus for information gathering*. Thus, modality refers to *what* is being assessed. Obviously modalities might vary quite considerably within a given theoretical orientation. For example, the reader will recall that Lazarus (1976) encourages the BCA to assess the modalities of: *behavior, affect, sensation, imagery, cognitions, interpersonal functioning* and *drugs*. In Chapter 2 I offered: *description* of potential targets, *conditions* of occurrence, *historical information*, client *resources*, and client *motivation*. For each modality, specific pieces of assessed information will be referred to as facets. For example, in the modality termed "description," this author would have the BCA assess the client's attributions, overt and covert referents of the target, current frequency, duration and intensity of the target; while the modality of "conditions of occurrence" includes facets of location, activities, times, and self- or environmentally mediated antecedents and consequences. Similarly, the modality of "client resources" includes cognitive and intellectual abilities or deficits, physical abilities/handicaps, social skills or social skill deficits, person support, physical surroundings, financial resources and task and vocational skills.

In summary, the clinical assessment is focused upon certain modalities, each of which present an aspect of the client's behavior-within-life-situation, and each modality can be subdivided into facets to be assessed, depending on the interests of the BCA. It is implicit that the modalities and specific facets chosen for assessment must predict the range of possible methods available to the BCA.

Table 12-1 employs the categories of information found in Chapter 2 as an example of the modalities and their facets that might be a part of the clinical assessment.

The reader is referred to the outline at the end of Chapter 2 for a more thorough description of each modality. Obviously, Table 12-1 could just as easily have illustrated any one of a variety of assessment schemes as the BCA selects different modalities for assessment.

Table 12-1
Information Modalities for a Comprehensive Assessment

MODALITY	MAJOR FACETS
Description	Client's self-statement Referents: Overt and covert Current frequency Current duration Current intensity
Conditions of Occurrence	Locations Activities Time Antecedents: Overt and covert Consequences: Overt and covert
Client resources	Cognitive-intellectual abilities and deficits Physical abilities and handicaps Social skills and social-skills deficits Person support Physical surroundings Financial resources Task and vocational skills Other resources of specific relevance
Client motivation	Assess relevant categories of client's behavior (e.g., keeping appointments, completion of assignments, etc.)

Chapters 3 through 11 of this text presented a multitude of *methods*, some or all of which might be suitable for the assessment of the modalities just discussed. These methods were organized into *four major methods categories: interview, written, observation, and physiological,* and within each, a variety of facets were presented. *A methods facet would be a specific variant of one of the major categories.* Thus, the employment of a behavior problem checklist would be a facet in the written methods category, while the use of specimen recording and self-observation would be examples of facets in the observation methods category. A word about the categorization of methods is called for. Within the literature, methods have been defined using a rather confusing variety of criteria. The *person* who uses the method may define the method category, such as for "self-monitoring" or "participant observation" procedures. In other cases, specific *operations* required by the method define it. The "checklist" requires a checking-off operation on the client's part; hence the

Table 12-2
Multiple Criteria for Defining Observation Methods

Operation	Information Supplier	Setting	Sampling
Mechanical (e.g., Wrist Counter; Movement Transducer, Audio/Video Recording) [M]	**Client** [C] **Significant Other** [S]	**Natural** [N] **Clinical Natural** [Cl]	**Continuous Record** (e.g., specimen recording) [CR]
Product (e.g., Trace, Erosion, Archive, Task Product) [P]	**Independent** (e.g., BCA, Trained Observer) [I]	**Contrived Clinical** [CC]	**Time Sampling** [T]
Written (e.g., Checklist, Symbol System) [W]	**Instrumentation** (e.g., Camera) [Ins]		**Event Sampling** [E]

descriptive label. A "rating" system requires the client to rate statements of some sort. The *setting* of the assessment may also define a method. "Naturalistic" observation methods or "clinic analogues" are examples. Finally, the *strategy employed to sample* some aspect of the client's behavior may be used as a descriptive label (e.g., "time sampling"). Because varied criteria are often employed together (e.g., a "self-observation" method obviously describes the information supplier as well as the characteristics of the instrument), it may be helpful and conceptually appealing to organize the methods facets presented in previous chapters using multiple criteria. As an example, Table 12-2 shows *operations*, the *information supplier*, the *setting* and *sampling strategy* as criteria for defining variants of observation methodology. Each combination of the four criteria thus defines a unique methods facet available to the BCA who wishes to employ observation methods.

Using a slash (/) to separate each of the four criteria, the combination M/C/N/E describes a common variant of self-observation, while M/I/CC/CR describes the audio- or videotaping of a client in a clinical environment designed to approximate his ordinary life surroundings. Table 12-2 illustrates the variety of methods facets available in each observation category and provides a precise way of describing a particular facet. Obviously, some or all of these four criteria could delineate methods facets available for interview, written or physiological methods domains.

Let us suppose that the BCA is interested in assessing each modality and its facets as presented in Table 12-1, using at least one methods facet from each of the four methods categories. A matrix could be formed to illustrate *every combination of modality and method.* Table 12-3 shows such a matrix, using only the *major* categories of modality and method. Each of the cells within this matrix, designated by alpha numerics, represents a unique possibility in planning a scenario for assessment. Take "description of the problem" as an example, as surely this would be a modality included in any clinical assessment scheme. At A_1-B_1, a BCA has the option of employing the interview to obtain the client's view of a problem with a variety of methodological facets available. Without belaboring the point, it is obvious that the BCA could perform an intake interview with the client, with a significant other, or perhaps with a professional who has had occasion to learn about the client. These interviews could occur in a natural setting (such as the home), or in the clinic proper. The methodological alternatives for carrying out this interview (e.g., in terms of the questioning strategies and interview formats; see Chapter 3) offer a wealth of possibilities to the BCA. Alternatively, any one or several written methods (e.g., checklist, rating scale, free response measure) could be used to obtain a description of the client's problems or concerns as illustrated at A_1-B_2. Next, the BCA has the option of employing observation strategies (e.g., mechanical, product or written methods) to observe the client's behavior. Table 12-2 has already revealed the many methods facets that could be brought to bear in this observation. Finally, if an initial description of the problem seems to involve a physiological response system, psychophysiological methods, shown at A_1-B_4, could be employed. Selection of a particular facet of psychophysiological measurement (e.g., heart rate, SR, EMG) depends on the nature of the presenting complaint. Similarly, other cells in the matrix may suggest additional possibilities for assessment.

Table 12-3
Modality-Method Matrix: Possibilities for Assessment

MODALITIES	METHODS CATEGORIES			
	Interview (B_1)	*Written* (B_2)	*Observation* (B_3)	*Psychophysiological* (B_4)
Description of Problem (A_1)	A_1B_1	A_1B_2	A_1B_3	A_1B_4
Conditions of Occurrence (A_2)	A_2B_1	A_2B_2	A_2B_3	—
Past History (A_3)	A_3B_1	A_3B_2	—	—
Client Resources (A_4)	A_4B_1	A_4B_2	A_4B_3	—
Client Motivation (A_5)	A_5B_1	A_5B_2	A_5B_3	—

While the matrix is useful for representing the various method-modality combinations available for the clinical assessment, a later section will show that it may also be employed to organize information collected as the assessment is carried out. We will now turn to a strategy for conducting the clinical assessment, keeping in mind the definitions just discussed.

The Tactics of Clinical Assessment: Some Potential Problems, Some Recommendations

So far this text has merely offered a compendium of options for selecting certain modalities as foci of the clinical assessment along with a review of methods facets that the BCA might select. In training graduate and undergraduate students to carry out the clinical assessment, I have been repeatedly surprised to find that the trainee who proposes time consuming methods of assessment, such as batteries of self-report methods or tests, series of interviews and forays into the client's home to conduct observations, frequently cannot provide a logical justification for his efforts. Perhaps more important, once this wealth of information is collected, students are frequently at a loss as to what to make of the findings; how to "pull together" information representing many combinations of modality and method. This section will present a strategy for planning the clinical assessment, summarizing and integrating findings, and firming up goals for intervention. This strategy will be referred to as a *multimethod approach* to clinical assessment. A discussion of common errors that may restrict the utility (usefulness in making predictions about the client) and generalizability of findings (to alternative settings, times and conditions) will precede a presentation of the major assumptions of a multimethod approach. Then two case examples will illustrate how a multimethod approach might be employed. A final section will offer a series of options for presenting the results of the clinical assessment in verbal and written form.

Clinical Assessment Errors

The process of clinical assessment leading to ultimate intervention involves three major steps: *detection* of certain aspects of the client and the client's life situation relevant to understanding current problems, needs, and ultimate goals; *integration-interpretation*, which involves organizing and summarizing this information so that the BCA understands the client's objectives in the context of those phenomena (client; environment) that have come to control, mediate or limit the client's choices; and, based on the preceding, *selection* of goals for intervention in line with the client's resources. The sophistication with which the first two steps are undertaken places limits upon the likelihood that intervention goals are selected that best meet the client's objectives, and in each of these stages a variety of errors may restrict the reliability or validity of findings. The manner in which each source of error may interfere with the BCA's assessment goals will be briefly discussed.

Detection. A number of unfortunate circumstances or poor choices may restrict the BCA's ability to detect aspects of the client and/or his life situation that contribute to his life problems. Negative outcomes may result from failures in detection or detection of inaccurate or biased information.

Inadequate choice of modalities may restrict in advance the possibility of detecting information that may prove to be central to understanding the client and his life. This unfortunate outcome may have nothing to do with the sophistication of the BCA's data gathering methods; rather, the focus of the assessment may exclude certain modalities of information, perhaps due to the BCA's theoretical assumptions regarding client behavior (e.g., what is *most* relevant is overt behavior or "feelings" or irrational beliefs or interpersonal communications). The author recalls the tale of the blind men who each obtained a much different notion of an elephant using the same method: touching the beast. Each touched a different portion of the elephant's anatomy (trunk, tail, leg, etc.) and, while accurate in his own limited assessment, adopted an incredibly different impression of the entire creature. Analogously, the BCA who adopts a restricted focus toward *what* is to be assessed may conclude with a distorted or inaccurate picture of the client.

Inadequate choice of methods may also reduce the possibility of detecting certain categories of information that could, if detected, modify the BCA's perspective of the client. For example, if the BCA chooses to conduct the assessment exclusively in the clinical interview situation, his view of the client is shaped exclusively by the client's self-report and by the behavior that the client displays across interviews. While some clients are accurate self-observers and may indeed present a true report of themselves and life events, this phenomenological vantage point may be colored by the client's biases (e.g., response sets; see Chapter 5), or the fact that the client just does not attend to aspects of self or situation that the BCA may wish to explore. Similarly, an exclusive focus upon observation methods may provide an accurate account of a client's overt behavior in various life settings, but fail to yield information regarding how the client cognitively views or affectively responds to his own behavior and surroundings, or how those events come to "make sense" to him. In this case the BCA might well be led to focus on overt behavior as a target for intervention, whereas a more profitable strategy might be to assist the client in evaluating his expectations for himself and others, his attributions, feelings or some other domain of private behavior. Furthermore, even if a broad range of methods categories is employed, the BCA's choice of a particular methods facet (e.g., time sampling using a formal observation system) may provide a distorted view of the client-in-situation if that method cannot detect information relevant to the client's life situation.

Method error has to do with the methods themselves; that is, the capability of certain methods to validly and reliably detect the occurrence of events of interest. It should be clear by now that a method that does not meet acceptable standards of reliability and validity (see Chapters 5, 7, and 10) may produce inaccurate and misleading information. Method error is usually discussed in the context of written self-reports, psychometric tests, or observational protocols, but applies to any method of assessment. Examples include physiological measurements taken with inadequate instrumentation, or samples of behavior displayed in the interview under conditions of high reactivity. It is hoped that the emphasis on these issues in preceding chapters will bring them to mind as the BCA selects clinical assessment methods.

Finally, error may be a function of *sources of bias* in the manner in which clients present themselves or the way the BCA perceives information as it occurs. In Chapter 5, it was pointed out that clients often attempt to present themselves in a favorable or unfavorable light or may tend to agree with virtually any kind of statement made by the BCA. Such biases can operate in a consistent fashion across the client's responses to either structured or unstructured stimuli. Chapter 10 noted that the BCA, even if trained to reasonably acceptable levels of reliability in using a particular method, may be influenced by certain expectancies or demands present in the situation, just as the experimenter in the animal or human experimental laboratory may unintentionally distort his findings in line with the experimental hypothesis. A variety of options were offered in Chapter 10 for evaluating sources of respondent or BCA bias, along with strategies for reducing the possibility of the occurrence of such effects.

One or more of the foregoing error sources could restrict the possibility of detecting important aspects of the client's behavior or life situation, or could lead to bias or distortion of what is detected. Attention to each of these sources of potential error in advance permits the BCA to make plans to reduce their probability and to be vigilant for their occurrence. As sources of error are reduced, the picture that the BCA obtains of the client-in-situation will obviously be more accurate.

Integration-interpretation. At this stage of the clinical assessment, information collected by the BCA must be integrated so that summary statements can be made, perhaps within each category of modality. The BCA is now in a position to develop hypotheses as to the phenomena maintaining the client's current behavior or restricting the client's goals. Such interpretations may involve hypothesized motives, needs, or drives, or emphasize functional relationships between the client's behavior and environmental responses to that behavior, depending on the BCA's theoretical orientation. It is obvious that whatever the methodological sophistication of the assessment so far, the manner in which the BCA handles this phase will place limits on the likelihood that the clinical assessment meets its objectives. Thus, the BCA must make certain judgments if a nonactuarial approach to assessment is employed.[1] While individuals no doubt vary in the "art" of clinical decision-making and it is not clear precisely what skills are involved in making accurate clinical decisions, there are certain sources of error that the BCA should always keep in mind.

The *error of congruence* has to do with a bias in favor of perceiving congruence in information collected within and across diverse modalities of information, independent of the actual consistency or inconsistency of the findings. Many psychologists have found evidence that we tend to perceive various parts of a stimulus array as an organized or uniform whole. More to the point, research evaluating the efficacy of certain projective techniques has shown that independent assessors may draw completely different conclusions from a client's responses to these unstructured stimuli. Each assessor is focusing upon information congruent with a hypothesis that emerges from a limited view of the findings or a hypothetical notion brought into the assessment situation. In addition, if discrepant findings are glossed over or de-emphasized, the assessment task is simplified; this may falsely enhance the BCA's confidence in his conclusions. The BCA must guard against *prematurely* forming hypotheses about the nature of the client's behavior, hypotheses that he may later be motivated to defend by ignoring findings discrepant with that conceptualization. Similar to the error of congruence is the possibility of overgeneralization based upon limited findings.

In *overgeneralization*, the BCA may attempt to reach a conclusion about the client's behavior based on limited information. For example, the BCA may wish to make a statement regarding the current frequency and characteristics of some aspect of the client's behavior, although inadequate sampling of occasions within and across days should make it clear that there is insufficient data to draw such a conclusion. In Chapters 6 and 9 the importance of collecting an adequate sample of the client's behavior across occasions for self- and independent observation methods respectively is discussed. Similarly, when data are collected in the interview format, the BCA must be certain that his findings are not based upon idiosyncrasies and situational factors present on a few occasions of assessment (e.g., a single interview), but that they represent a characteristic view of the client's behavior. This can only be accomplished by extending the sample of occasions in which assessments are made. As another example of overgeneralization, the BCA may assess the client's behavior in one or more situations (e.g., clinic, home), and then attempt to draw broad conclusions regarding the client's behavior in a variety of *other* settings. Many BCAs are guilty of overgeneralizing from a limited sample of behavior, as seen *exclusively* in the clinical situation (e.g., the interview). In Chapter 8, options for collecting information across settings reflecting a more comprehensive view of the client's behavior are discussed. Restricted focus with respect to modalities or methods previously discussed might also contribute to errors of overgeneralization. Thus, the BCA who collects observational data and attempts to generalize his findings to aspects of the client's behavior and/or life situation that were not originally the focus of observation would also be guilty of overgeneralization.

Another source of error occurs when the interpretation of a client's behavior-in-situation results either from *inadequate conceptualizations* or *theoretical biases* on the part of the BCA. In the former case the BCA may not have adopted a theoretical framework for understanding how environmental and person events may come to elicit and maintain some aspects of the client's behavior. This is analogous to a driver attempting to make his way across the country without a road map. This certainly does not mean that the BCA must interpret every aspect of the client and his behavior from a particular theoretical point of view, but suggests that the BCA should have some understanding of various theoretical viewpoints which in isolation or in combination may help to explain the client's behavior in his life-situation. Tallent (1976) points out that many BCAs employ inexplicit language, or jargon, to explain phenomena about which they may have little understanding. Focusing on the writing of a psychological report, Tallent states: "The language in which the psychologist *thinks* is also a major issue, influencing as it does both the conceptualization and the presentation of the case. The inexactness and multiple meanings of jargon are well established. When the psychologist thinks in terms of these inexactitudes, can the quality of his writing be any more precise?" (p. 109). In addition, he points out that theoretical constructs are "most useful" and "probably indispensible" in making it possible for the psychologist to understand his client.

At the other extreme is the BCA who is unable to view the client's behavior outside of a particular theoretical orientation. Thus, the BCA committed to a strict operant, functional analytic orientation may see every aspect of a client's functioning as a direct result of environmental antecedents and contingent consequences, and may ignore information not relevant to this theoretical position (e.g., a client's phenomenological view of himself in the situation; the client's values, attitudes, beliefs, etc.). Similarly, an existentially oriented BCA may be so focused on intrinsic events that environmental contingencies present in the client's life situation are overlooked. Blind adherence to any viewpoint, particularly those that restrict inquiry to particular domains of behavior (e.g., exploring the "self" via self-statements, defining irrational beliefs or faulty self-instructions, focusing upon early-life trauma) place unrealistic and impractical limits on human behavior that may be determined by a variety of phenomena and is certainly more complex than this approach would suggest. The BCA should be aware both of his theoretical biases and also that human behavior may be explained from a variety of viewpoints and understood as a result of many phenomena. If the BCA fully understands his own theoretical assumptions, he is more likely to be alert to the possibility of such biasing. The BCA should be willing to listen to and understand alternative points of view, and may even wish to consult with colleagues about a case to obtain another perspective.

Selection. During this phase of clinical decision-making the BCA selects certain aspects of the client, his surrounding environment or both, to be the focus for intervention. The selection of goals for intervention most likely to meet the client's objectives is directly dependent on the extent to which one or more of the preceding categories of error have been present in the detection and integration-interpretation phases. If important aspects of the client's life situation have not been detected or if clinical findings are inadequately integrated or incorrectly interpreted, the BCA cannot be in a position to select goals for intervention that best meet the client's needs. While the BCA may have an extensive armamentarium of proven intervention methods at his disposal, it is obvious that the likelihood that these methods will have a maximally desirable impact on the client depends on the specific targets to which they are applied (Lazarus, 1976).

To reduce the probability of these various sources of error entering into the clinical decision-making process, *a multimethod approach to assessment adopts certain basic assumptions* to guide the BCA's efforts. These assumptions should be generalizable to virtually any clinical assessment task, and form the foundation on which the multimethod clinical assessment is built.

1. While the specific aspects of the client and his surroundings which will be assessed (modalities) do vary depending on the characteristics of the presenting problem and client, theoretical orientation of the BCA and even practical considerations, *as the number of modalities is increased (e.g., overt behavior, physical environment, cognition, feelings, etc.), the likelihood of making errors in detecting important aspects of the client's behavior-in-situation is reduced.* While consonance (agreement) between information collected across the modalities is not necessarily expected (e.g., Lang, 1968; Adams, Doster, & Calhoun, 1977), a lack of consonance (e.g., between client's actual skills and cognitive view of self, between client's self-report and physiological response in the situation, between the reports of others and the client's own view) should be further explored in the assessment, since it may well hold adaptive implications for the client. Assessment of multiple modalities assists the BCA in relating the client's verbal report to other aspects of his behavior and to the specific environment within which the client functions. In addition, assessment of multiple modalities increases the likelihood that the BCA understands the life situation upon which a program of intervention is overlaid, and decreases the possibility of selecting a target for intervention that is unlikely to meet the client's objectives or is beyond the client's resources.

2. For a particular modality, *as the number of methods categories (e.g., interview; written; observation; physiological) is increased, the BCA obtains a more comprehensive view of that modality.* Such a procedure also reduces the possibility of selecting an inappropriate target. Further, assessment using multiple methods increases the BCA's ability to address the question of validity of any one source of information, since information from multiple sources may be systematically compared. Obviously, certain methods are more suitable for assessing particular modalities.

3. Once a particular category method is selected, *the possibility of*

method error (as previously discussed) is reduced as the number of methods facets is increased. Thus, if the BCA is employing more than one written survey of problems (e.g., a checklist) or multiple strategies for observing the client's behavior in a natural situation, the possibility that unreliability or invalidity of any one instrument will distort the BCA's findings is reduced. Discrepancies between data collected across two or more methods facets should cause the BCA to be cautious in integrating and interpreting his findings; in fact, the BCA might wish to carefully examine each of the instruments or methods facets employed to attempt to make sense of such discrepant findings.

4. For a particular selection of method categories and specific method facets, *assessment of the client in situations in which he ordinarily functions (criterion settings) should augment interview or analogue assessments within the clinical environment, whenever possible.* The BCA may thus obtain some sense of the ecological validity of information gathered in the clinical environment, while also viewing the client's behavior-in-setting. A client's verbal report regarding his behavior in natural situations may be evaluated in the light of direct assessments within those environments. In addition, assessment of the client across multiple settings permits the BCA to evaluate whether treatment effects generalize from the clinical to the natural setting when intervention take place in part or exclusively in the clinical environment. Obviously, the BCA's ability to generalize about the client's response to life events is increased by assessment in multiple settings and limited only by the extensiveness of such sampling and the number of occasions in which each setting is sampled.

5. Given selection of all of the above, *assessment across time permits the BCA to evaluate the stability of findings* (the reader will recall that this may also reflect the reliability of methods). As the number of occasions of assessment is increased, the BCA can more accurately define the frequency and characteristics of the client's behavior. This may be particularly important, not only in deciding upon goals for intervention, but in evaluating the efficacy of treatments using one of the single case designs presented in Chapter 13.

a) *Assessments taking place during intervention as well as after intervention permit the BCA to assess the maintenance of intervention effects over time,* an important criterion for any behavior change effort.

A program of assessment that meets these assumptions should decrease the likelihood of one or more of the previously described sources of error limiting the reliability, validity and utility of results. The following two case examples show how a multimethod approach could be practically applied to the assessment of child as well as adult clients. For each case, a matrix is employed to facilitate both the planning of the assessment and the integration and interpretation of findings following the collection of information.

Multimethod Assessment of a Child Behavior Problem

Let us assume that Mrs. X comes to a BCA complaining of her son Billy's "behavior problems"; specifically, she can't get Billy to "mind" her. In an initial intake interview, the BCA determines that Mrs. X is 28 years of age, has been Billy's sole parent for the past three years following a rather bitter divorce proceeding, and is employed as an administrative trainee at a local business between the hours of 8:30 A.M. and 3:30 P.M. each day. Mrs. X is an attractive, bright person who is attempting to establish herself in a career as well as serving in the role of sole parent. She reports that she often resents Billy because of his problem behavior.

Billy is 8 years of age and in the sixth month of third grade in school. Mrs. X reports that she has been having extreme difficulties managing him for the last year. Her major complaint centers around his frequent noncompliance with her requests; also, she has to tell him to do something "again and again", often with unsatisfactory outcome. She thinks that he is also a behavior problem in school, because a recent report card showed a "very poor" conduct grade. His academic grades have fallen in the last reporting period. In addition, she reports that he has recently taken to wetting his bed. She is quite concerned about this and more generally concerned with the arguments and hard feelings occuring as the result of her attempts to "get him to behave."

In this first interview, the BCA attempts to actively listen to Mrs. X, summarizing the content of her statements and reflecting the many feelings that she expresses as a means of clarifying the information offered and establishing rapport. It becomes obvious that Mrs. X is quite frustrated and angry with Billy.

Following the initial intake interview, the BCA provides Mrs. X with a standard behavior problem checklist to obtain a more comprehensive view of the categories of problems she is experiencing with her son, and also to prompt her to remember any categories of problems that she may have overlooked in her initial verbal report. The problem checklist reveals high ratings (indicating a severe problem) in the general categories of "bedtime problems," "noncompliance," "destructiveness," "bed-wetting" and "eating". The BCA reviews each of these areas with the client in a second interview, at which time Mrs. X states that she would like to focus intervention upon Billy's noncompliance and bed-wetting problems before moving on to other areas of concern.

In addition, the BCA interviews Billy in a playroom situation. While interacting with him and attempting to develop rapport, the BCA discovers that Billy is not really sure "why my Mom brought me here," and doesn't feel that there are any problems in the home situation with the exception of his wetting his bed "sometimes." When asked about school, Billy reports that he likes school very much and gets along well with his teacher, Mrs. Caldwell, but that sometimes he finds her to be "mean." The BCA determines on further exploration that she is "mean" when she asks Billy to do something he doesn't want to do. Billy is responsive to the BCA's queries, and because of his excellent social skills is able to establish rapport quite quickly.

The BCA decides that collecting case history information would provide additional descriptive data about this family, as well as some notion of how these problems may have developed and how both parent and child have handled them in the past. The case history, taken with parent as informant, reveals an ordinary pregnancy and nonremarkable physical development of the child. The mother reports that Billy got along well with his peers in a nursery school setting from ages 3 through 5, and adjusted well to kindergarten. In fact, she reports nothing remarkable in the history of the family prior to that time. During Billy's kindergarten year, Mr. and Mrs. X began experiencing marital difficulties which often resulted in verbal fights and, on a few occasions, physical confrontations; however, Mrs. X reports that most of this was "shielded from Billy." The parents received a divorce as Billy was entering the first grade. Mrs. X reports no problems in his adjustment to her as a single parent until the last year. Specifically, she reports that Billy's academic performance showed no change (all "satisfactories," A's and B's) until the current academic year, and that Billy seemed to have no difficulty in establishing close relationships with neighborhood peers or in his interactions in the school situation as reported by his teachers. Mrs. X also reports that prior to the last 4 or 5 months, she experienced little difficulty in managing Billy, and had few problems beyond the ordinary noncompliance one would expect from young children. Focusing on this most recent period in third grade, the mother reports that while Billy showed no difficulty in adjusting to his classmates, he immediately took a dislike to his teacher, Mrs. Caldwell, and reported that he "didn't like her." In addition, Mrs. X reports that Billy became much more defiant at home and began resisting or "putting off" assigned household tasks. Mrs. X reports that she began by attempting to reason with Billy and continues to do so, although this has not been effective. In addition, yelling, spanking, sending Billy to his room, and so forth, have all proved to be "unsuccessful." In fact, she reports that when she spanks Billy he becomes very upset and emotional and often wets his bed that evening. She reports that the bed wetting is a more recent phenomenon that began the previous month, and now occurs two or three times per week. She reports that she has not discussed this with Billy, and has "not known what to do." She is, however, afraid of embarrassing him by discussing it with him. She also reports that a recent physical examination revealed no organic basis for the bed wetting. Finally, the BCA finds that the mother's parents have offered much support for this family, both financial and otherwise, and that the grandfather in particular seems to have an excellent relationship with Billy and interacts with him frequently. Mrs. X and her parents live in close proximity, and the BCA concludes that the grandparents may prove to be an excellent resource when intervention is undertaken.

The preceding thumbnail sketch of this family is based upon two initial interviews (intake and case history); the primary sources of information have been the verbal self-reports of Mrs. X and her son, and her written report in checklist form. The BCA decides to further explore with this parent the conditions that define the noncompliant and bed-wetting behavior (frequency, locations, activities, times, antecedents and consequences) as a means of understanding how the behavior is maintained. To obtain a more comprehensive picture of this behavior in the natural setting, the BCA decides to supplement the parent's report with the teacher's report, using interview methods. This provides a check on the parent's suggestion that the problem may not be isolated in the home, and that the school may be a relevant focus for intervention.

In addition, to obtain a more detailed report from the parent, and to enhance accuracy, the BCA trains Mrs. X to systematically record each time she asks Billy to do something and the result of that request (compliance or noncompliance). Following the description of *what* Billy was asked to do (or stop doing) and the date, Mrs. X is asked to record the settings where her requests occur, the activities that Billy and she are engaged in, and the times of day and antecedents and consequences of the request. In this way, the parent's verbal report within the interview is complemented by a more systematic gathering of information. This task also ensures that Mrs. X is learning to observe her own behavior as well as Billy's, which may prove to be a critically important skill if she is to learn alternative ways of responding to her son and dealing with his behavior.

To supplement the parent's week of record-keeping, the BCA decides to go into the home and observe the family on two evenings between 3:00 and 9:00 P.M. as these are times that Mrs. X reports that Billy's noncompliance is a problem. [At other times during the day, except for the brief period before school, both parent and child are absent from the home.] The BCA instructs Mrs. X to behave naturally with Billy, and attempts to remain as unobtrusive as possible. The BCA makes a comprehensive specimen recording of the interactions between mother and child, noting the conditions of each occurrence of noncompliance in particular. To ensure that no relevant information is lost, the BCA asks Mrs. X's permission to audiotape these sessions. In addition, the BCA decides to observe on two occasions (morning and afternoon) in the classroom to obtain an independent view of the teacher's interactions with Billy. The BCA hopes to place Billy's behavior in the context of the teacher's interactions with other members of the class and to explore characteristics of the classroom setting to see how these may functionally relate to Billy's behavior. Again, specimen recording is selected as a methodology, but due to the large number of students (30) in this class, seating "rows" are sequentially observed to reduce the number of persons the BCA must scan at any one time. While the BCA had the time available to carry out the home and school observations, systematic observations carried out by a trained observer were impossible because of practical limitations in this situation. Thus,

Table 12-4

Matrix Describing Assessment of Child Behavior Problem

	INTERVIEW			OBSERVATION	
	Parent	Teacher	Parent Records	Specimen Record-ing (Home)	Specimen Record-ing (School)
STATEMENT OF PROBLEM	B. won't comply when I ask him to do something (also wets bed).	Won't follow class rules; ignores my requests unless I yell.	Self-recorded # compliances out of total requests (A)—and instances of bedwetting (B).	Total record, com-plicace as a focus. (Two nights be-tween 3:00 PM and 9:00 PM)	Total record, com-plicace as a focus. (Two occasions to-tal for 2 hours each: morning and afternoon)
CURRENT FREQUENCY	"All the time" 2 × /day (for bed-wetting about 2 × /week).	About 3 × /day violates rule. Al-ways ignores my requests.	A = Complied 8 × out of a total of 40 requests (8/40 = 20%) B = 2 × out of 7 nights	Of 14 requests, B. complied immedi-ately with only 3 (3/14 = 22% ap-prox.); little positive interaction.	Of 10 requests, B. complied immedi-ately with only 2 (compliance/request for total class = 4/22 or 18%).
LOCATIONS	At home—worst when in public place, e.g., gro-cery.	On playground is worst. Best if I can get him off to my-self.	Of 40 requests: 36 at home, 2 in car, 2 in store.	Most requests (11) given while B. is in living room with TV on or in kitchen. All 3 compliances oc-curred while B. in bedroom.	Observed only in class.

ACTIVITIES	If B. is watching TV or playing outside—won't. Most likely to comply if with me alone so that I have attention.	Playing with other children worst or competitive games. Best: during math work where each student works alone.	Compliance/ requests: 3/22 while watching TV, 2/10 playing outside, 0/4 shopping, 3/4 alone in room, no TV.	In order of time spent: TV, playing with toy on floor, playing with brother.	For B. Compliance/ requests: 0/6 group reading, 0/1 during lining up, 2/3 quiet work.
TIMES	Usually before school and right before dinner.	Worst right before lunch and in late afternoon. Best during first few hours of day.	Compliance/ requests: 3/5 before school, 2/24 after school (2:30-5:30), 3/11 after dinner (6:00-9:00).	Compliance/ requests: 0/3: 4:00-5:30, 0/2: dinner, 2/4: 6:00-7:30, 1/5: 7:30-9:00. B. seemed cranky right before dinner and after 8:30 PM.	For B. Compliance/ requests: 1/3: 8:30-10:00, 0/3: 10:00-11:30, 1/1: 12:00-1:30, 0/3: 1:30-3:00.
ANTECEDENTS	I call to him—keep calling him until he listens, then ask him.	I ask him politely.	A = "ask him politely" B = "argued before bed on one of 2 bedwetting nights."	M. usually calls to B. from a distance, fails to get B's full-face attention. States requests ambiguously, often as a question.	T. quietly asks B. question; fails to get attention (true of her requests to students generally).
CONSEQUENCES	If he doesn't comply, I ask again—Finally yell or give up and do it myself.	I ask again, then yell or threaten Mr. Edwards (principal).	A = If comply, say thank you; if noncomply, yell, threaten to spank, do it myself. B = None—discuss it but no punishment.	Of 11 noncompliances: 3 M. restated request until compliance, 4 yelled and threatened with spanking, 1 spanked B. and sent him to room, 3 no response.	Of 8 noncompliances: 3 ask again loudly until compliance, 4 compliance, 1 *threaten* with "note to mother" or "principal", 1 no response.

this methods facet was excluded. Other methods facets were excluded for similar practical reasons.

In summary, this case assessment employs three facets of interview methods (intake and case history with parent and intake with teacher), one facet of a written approach (a behavior problem checklist), and three facets of observation procedures (self-monitoring, and independent observations in both home and school situations). The BCA selected these methods from a wealth of possibilities because they could be carried out within a reasonable period of time and would provide a more comprehensive view of the problem than the self-report alone. The entire assessment was carried out over a period of two weeks and at the end of that period, the BCA decided to organize the information by summarizing the findings in a modality-methods matrix similar to that shown in Table 12-3. Table 12-4 presents this matrix as organized by the BCA. The cells of the matrix were completed as the assessment unfolded. The written method—the behavior problems checklist—was omitted from this matrix because it was employed to assist the BCA in obtaining a statement of the problem and did not apply to the other modalities of information. It should be noted that any kind of shorthand written code understood by the BCA could have been used to place this information within the matrix cells, thus reducing writing time.

While this may seem to be a simple and straightforward presenting problem with a rather limited cast of characters, the reader must realize that the information obtained within clinical assessment can become extensive and complicated as the number of modalities and corresponding methods facets is increased. Using a matrix such as that shown in Table 12-4 permits the BCA to organize the information in a way that makes it easy to summarize findings, and permits immediate visualization of data. The matrix may also suggest alternative modalities or methods facets that might be useful, since the BCA can visually note where data is lacking. By sketching out a matrix of this sort ahead of time (which of course defines all matrix categories in advance), the BCA *plans the assessment in a systematic fashion,* assuring that all relevant modalities are assessed, and that proposed methods are suited to the questions being asked, the resources of the BCA and the characteristics of the client. In contrast, unplanned clinical assessment often occurs in a rather haphazard fashion.

Perhaps a detailed look at these findings would be helpful in further illustrating the utility of the matrix for clinical decision making. Each modality facet will be discussed separately, with a summary across the information obtained by the various methods facets.

First, the parent and teacher agree that noncompliance is their primary concern. While they both emphasize Billy's lack of compliance to verbal requests, the teacher also complains that Billy will not follow class rules. That this problem seems to occur across both home and school settings suggests that the BCA may wish to consider intervention in both environments.

An assessment of the current frequency of noncompliance is used to evaluate the extent of the problem, as well as to document a change in the problem following intervention. The parent's report of two times per day appears to be an underestimate if the two occasions of specimen recording in the home are a valid sample of ordinary behavior in that setting. Specimen recording revealed 11 instances of noncompliance out of a total of 14 requests the parent made of the child during the periods of observation. Mrs. X's self-gathered record reveal 32 instances of noncompliance out of 40 requests over the period of one week. This is an average of more than four times per day. Thus, it seems that noncompliance is indeed a problem, and that it occurs even more frequently than the parent initially realized. While the number of instances of compliance is quite low and the mother has a hard time remembering them, the data indicate that Billy did comply on eight occasions. The BCA also notes that Mrs. X spends little time in directly interacting with Billy although the child actively tries to interest his mother in his activities. For example, Billy often asked her a question or tried to get her to comment on his homework. After a brief period of eye contact, Mrs. X would usually turn back to whatever task she had been engaged in and ignore him. On each of six occasions that this occurred, Billy quickly left his mother and went off to his room. In contrast, negative behavior or task requests seem to dominate the interactions between mother and son. Mrs. X seemed very tired on the two occasions of observation, and made verbal reference to this on one of those (she complained about her job and busy schedule).

With regard to bed wetting, the parent's records show that the initial report of about two times per week does in fact seem to be accurate.

In school the teacher reports that Billy "always" ignores her requests (and violates rules about three times each day). Direct observation in the classroom reveals that noncompliance occurred eight times over the two-day period, an average of about four times per observation occasion. It should be realized, however, that each of these observation periods represented one-half of the school day, suggesting that the actual daily rate of noncompliance may be greater. Interestingly, compliance to teacher requests on the part of other students in this classroom also is quite low; only 4 of 22 requests received immediate compliance during the two observation periods. This teacher obviously has difficulty in managing students other than Billy, which suggests that she may need to learn some alternative skills for communicating requests to her students (shifting the focus *away* from Billy as the exclusive target or problem).

The bed wetting is confined to the home when Billy is asleep. Noncompliance occurs at home as well as in public places such as the grocery store. Mrs. X's records indicate that of 40 requests over the week, 36 of them did occur at home, and only 4 in a public setting. The finding that the vast majority of requests and thus noncompliance episodes occur at home suggests that this setting might be the best location to begin intervention. This also suggests that Mrs. X seldom takes Billy into public places, which is something that can be checked with her. Observations in the home reveal that most of the episodes of noncompliance occur when Billy and his mother are in the living room or kitchen areas, where they remain most of his waking hours. Interestingly, all occasions when Billy complied with his mother's requests occurred in his bedroom. The teacher reports his noncompliance at school is worst in the playground and best if Billy is in a setting alone with his teacher. School observations were conducted only in the classroom setting where all of the recorded occasions of noncompliance occurred.

Mrs. X reports that Billy is least likely to comply if he is watching television or playing with friends outside, and most likely to comply if she and Billy are interacting together alone and she has his attention. This is supported by Mrs. X's records, showing that about half of the requests occur when Billy is watching television, and a significant further number occur as he plays outside with his friends in the backyard. Direct observations also reveal that watching television and playing with another child evoke the highest proportion of noncompliance to request. Billy complied with 3 of 4 requests made when the television set was turned off, the house was generally quiet and the mother and child were interacting together. At school the teacher reports that noncompliance is much more likely if Billy is interacting with other children (perhaps as a means of gaining attention), and particularly during competitive games; and he is most likely to comply when he is doing math (at which each student works alone). School observations generally support the teacher's report, with 6 of 8 noncompliances occurring during group reading or when the teacher was lecturing the group as a whole. Only one noncompliance occurred during a quiet, "working" time.

The mother reports the frequency of noncompliance to be "about the same" before school or right before dinner, whereas her record keeping revealed that the vast majority of noncompliance incidents occur between the time Billy comes home from school and the dinner hour. The time between dinner and going to bed is also quite high, while only two noncompliances are reported before school. Thus, the parent's initial report is not fully supported. Observations in the home reveal that the greatest proportion of noncompliance to total requests occurs immediately prior to and after dinner and during the period before bedtime. In addition, two noncompliances over the two days of observation occurred during the dinner hour, a time that the mother did not report as being a problem. These findings would suggest that the period before school is not nearly as likely to be characterized by noncompliant behavior, and that the focus for intervention should probably be during the evening hours. Obviously, the period before school is shorter; this may have accounted for the small number of noncompliant incidents during that time. In school, the teacher reports that the likelihood of noncompliance is highest just before lunch and in the early afternoon. This is supported by the high proportion of noncompliance/requests during the hour before lunch and during the period after 2:00 P.M. observed independently. This leads the BCA to question what is going on during those periods or what the physical status of the child is at those times (e.g., could he be fatigued? hungry? etc.). Such time-behavior relationships are important in provoking the BCA to explore *what* is occurring at a particular time that may be controlling the frequency of a behavior.

Regarding antecedents, the mother's statement that she repeatedly calls to Billy until he listens is supported by observational findings that the mother frequently calls from the kitchen or her bedroom (where she watches TV) without getting Billy's attention or making full-faced contact with him. In addition, home observations reveal that many of her commands are indirect or inexplicit in terms of what she wants Billy to do. Mrs. X's records note that she asks him politely; however, she is quite vague about antecedents. Her records of bed wetting reveal that the one occasion of bed wetting during the week was preceded by an argument between parent and child immediately before bedtime. On this occasion Billy was "sent to bed" because of his behavior.

The teacher also reports that she politely asks Billy to do something. School observations reveal that the teacher's requests are often quietly and indirectly stated as questions. The tone of the request seemed (to the observer) to indicate that the teacher does not expect Billy to comply.

Regarding consequences for noncompliant behavior, Mrs. X reports that she continues to ask Billy to do something if he does not comply at once, and ultimately ends up yelling or giving up and doing it herself. Her records reveal that she yelled on each occasion that Billy did not comply, spanked him on three occasions and sent him to bed on two occasions as punishment. She reports that she does not provide consequences for bed wetting. This agrees with her verbal report. Home observations reveal that Mrs. X continues to make her requests of Billy (on one occasion, seven times), until he finally complies, speaking more loudly each time. Observations also reveal that she employs spanking and assignment to the bedroom as forms of punishment. Generally, this seems to be a quite inefficient means of dealing with the problem.

The teacher reports that she repeats her requests, followed by yelling or threatening to send Billy to the principal. School observations support the teacher's report. Thus, yelling as well as threats of punishment are frequently employed both by parent and teacher with little success in increasing compliance.

A wealth of information has been obtained during the two weeks of assessment. The initial verbal reports of the parent and the teacher have been variously supported, amended, or questioned by information gathered by other methods. It is obvious that extending the number of observations in the home and school, as well as increasing the time during which the parent collects systematic records, would better assure the reliability and validity of information obtained. Chapters 6, 7, 8 and 9 provide a detailed rationale for extending the period of observation, and sampling the setting in a more comprehensive fashion whenever possible.

What do the findings in this case reveal? First, noncompliance is in fact a serious problem for this mother and for the teacher as well. Both mother and teacher have reported that noncompliance is the most serious of Billy's problems, and the mother wishes to change this above all others, suggesting a strong motivation. Noncompliance seems to occur much more frequently in the home than in public places. Billy's behavior in school indicates that he is much more likely to be noncompliant when interacting with his peers in a situation where he may receive a good deal of attention for acting up, and that he is generally much easier to deal with in a one-on-one situation. The findings reveal certain times of the day when noncompliance is more likely, notably just before dinner or bedtime. One hypothesis that might explain this finding is that Billy is likely to be more fatigued after school or before bedtime. The BCA might well explore the possibility of a nap during the school hours or an earlier regular bedtime at home to reduce the child's irritability as well as the probability of confrontations with parent or teacher. The findings strongly indicate that both mother and teacher are apt to be indirect and nonspecific when asking Billy to do something, with requests often being made without their having first obtained the child's attention. This is particularly true for the mother in the home situation; it is highly probable that Billy does not hear the mother's requests on many occasions when she calls out from another room. Finally, it is obvious that both mother and teacher are employing a variety of consequences for noncompliance, none of which are administered in a consistent fashion so that Billy can understand the consequences of his behavior. Physical punishment, yelling, threats, and "room sentences" are variously employed, and in many cases (particularly at home), the mother gives up and fails to follow through with her request. In a very real sense, this child has control of the behavior of the adults who ask things of him, and he has been successful in eliciting yelling and other forms of increased verbal or physical attention by his acts. It must also be noted, if the home observation data are accurate, that Billy receives little affection or attention from his mother as a result of appropriate behavior. Noncompliance and other negative acts are ways that Billy can successfully get his mother's attention. Perhaps if Mrs. X could be encouraged to interact with Billy more frequently when he is not misbehaving, she will better meet his obvious need for affection, and his misbehavior will not be a useful strategy for attracting attention.

With regard to bed wetting, it is interesting to note that when Mrs. X kept systematic records, she found that one instance of bed wetting occurred following an argument (e.g., a situation involving noncompliance). Further parental record keeping would certainly be necessary to evaluate the possibility that reducing such emotional encounters prior to bedtime might reduce the frequency of bed wetting. In addition, there is the possibility that Billy is attempting to punish his mother or to communicate some sort of dissatisfaction via bed wetting.

In summary, information obtained within each of the cells of the modality-method matrix provides a unique view of this child's behavior from the perspective of interested as well as independent parties. This information also provides a data base for evaluation of behavior change once intervention begins, along the lines suggested in Chapter 13.

Multimethod Assessment of an Adult Male

A 28-year-old man complaining of extreme anxiety and "inadequacy" is referred to a BCA by a local physician. The physician reports that a thorough physical examination has revealed no physical basis for Mr. Y's reports of frequent tension and anxiety. A brief regimen of medication with a muscle relaxant has failed to alleviate the young man's "symptoms." The physician asks that the BCA explore possible psychological factors underlying the man's discomfort and the concomitant inefficiency that it is provoking in his personal life. In addition, the physician states that he will be available for further consultation and perhaps collaboration, if the BCA so desires, in the construction of an intervention strategy.

In an initial intake interview, the BCA learns that Mr. Y is "happily married," has two children and is employed by a local retail sales concern as a division manager, with a number of possibilities for future advancement. Mr. Y reports that following his graduation from college three years ago, he decided upon sales as a career. He reports that he is interested in getting ahead in his company for financial as well as other reasons. In an open-ended exploration of the client's reasons for seeking services, the BCA learns that Mr. Y finds it difficult to relax either in the job situation or at home, and reports a "high degree" of physical discomfort because of feeling "uptight" and "anxious" much of the time. Mr. Y reports that it is difficult to clear his mind of thinking about his work and worrying about his success or failure with the company. He often finds it awkward to serve in the role of administrator with the employees that he supervises, and frequently finds it diffucult to provide negative feedback to these subordinates for fear of the "way that they will view me as a boss." He also reports that he has experienced difficulty in social situations, except with his wife or close personal friends, since his high school years. This was pronounced in college, where he frequently avoided situations that might cause him to interact with strangers, particularly with his professors outside of the classroom situation. Mr. Y states that he has "no idea" why he becomes so anxious, can't get his mind off his work, and of late has found it difficult to function at work. Also, he states that he wishes to be more assertive with his subordinates and in making requests of his superiors, but avows that it is "impossible" to change because of the great anxiety he experiences when he attempts to try a different approach. He is most concerned about his future with the company if he is unable to come to grips with his anxieties and is also fearful about how his wife will view him if he fails to receive promotions on a regular basis. Mr. Y reviews his experiences with a number of physicians and specifically with the referral physician, and states that tranquilizing medications have been helpful from time to time, but have not really dealt with the problem. He reports that the foregoing are the major problems in his life and he is generally pleased with his life situation outside of these presenting complaints.

When the BCA inquires about the nature of his feelings of "anxiety" and being "uptight" or about the kinds of things that he worries about, Mr. Y finds it very difficult to be specific. Although he reports difficulty in interacting with fellow employees, he cannot describe specific characteristics of problem situations which cause some difficulty. He also reports that he is not sure how he "comes across" with friends and other acquaintances outside of the job situaton. Finally, Mr. Y wonders whether his selection of a career in retail sales was wise or if some other type of job would be less stressful and better meet his needs.

It is apparent to the BCA that the client's anxiety and his desire to avoid anxiety-provoking situations are central in the client's concerns. The BCA therefore decides to obtain a more thorough description of the referents of the client's anxiety: its frequency, duration and intensity, as well as the conditions which may serve to elicit and maintain discomfort. Because Mr. Y also reports difficulties in social situations, the BCA plans an assessment of the client's resources, with special emphasis on evaluation of his social skills and his motivation to change as a potential delimiter of any intervention effort. The BCA also decides to compile a comprehensive case history to learn how Mr. Y has responded to his environment and life situation in the past and also to learn about the development of the client's "discomfort" over time. Because of Mr. Y's frequent contacts with physicians and his current use of a minor tranquilizer, the BCA decides to collect information from them about the client's current physical condition, and to explore the possible role of medication in intervention.

Additional interviews with the client are obviously necessary to obtain a detailed description of the problem and conditions of occurrence. The BCA also decides to interview the client's wife and to obtain the client's permission to interview significant others who frequently interact with and observe the client. The BCA further decides to have him endorse a symptom checklist that provides descriptions of thoughts, feelings, sensations and overt behaviors that others have experienced accompanying anxiety. This checklist will be used in the interview as a means of further probing the characteristics of the client's discomfort. The Minnesota Multiphasic Personality Inventory (MMPI) is also to be administered to this client; the BCA decides to employ the "critical items" that the client has endorsed as a means of further examining the referents of the problem. Also an idiosyncratic rating scale (Chapter 5) is developed with the client's help in order to systematically and quantitatively rate the current frequency and intensity of the client's discomfort and his motivation to change. The BCA plans to use this scale for evaluation purposes as intervention proceeds.

The BCA is struck by Mr. Y's inability to describe his own behavior, and decides that training the client to systematically self-monitor his behavior-in-situation will be important not only to augment the interview and written approaches, but also as an important skill for the client to develop. The BCA also decides to systematically observe any manifestation of the client's discomfort in the interview situation. To get a better picture of the client in his life situation, the BCA plans to conduct two interviews in the home with both the client and his wife. Once a picture of the conditions which seem to elicit and maintain the client's behavior emerges from all this information, the BCA decides to employ a roleplay clinic analogue that will simulate one or more life situations problematic to the client (e.g., providing negative feedback to a subordinate; asking his boss for a raise). The goal will be not only to evaluate the client's overt response to the simulations but to carefully probe, via questioning, the covert antecedents that seem to precede an episode of anxiety (e.g., self-statements, imagery) as well as possible self-mediated consequences. Because this client reports severe physical tension, the BCA also decides to assess the client's EMG and EKG, two physiological methods facets, as the client is exposed to the analogue situations.

This is only an abbreviated account of the BCA's motives in outlining the various modalities of information to be assessed and the methods to be employed. The BCA decides to formalize his assessment goals using the matrix shown in Table 12-5. The modality facets to be assessed are along the rows of this matrix and the methods facets, along the columns. An "X" within the resulting cell shows specific methods that the BCA plans to bring to bear upon a specific modality. Each cell ("X") in this matrix would of course be filled in with a capsule description of the information obtained, so that the BCA can readily summarize across the row for a modality such as cognitions or overt behavior, and see all the information pertaining to that modality. This permits the BCA to evaluate the convergence or divergence of information collected across the methods facets (e.g., information verbally reported by the client and from the client's spouse as contrasted with observational data).

As in the first case example, it may seem an enormous task to fill in each of the matrix cells with assessment information; however, it is difficult to see how this wealth of information could be organized and summarized without using a systematic approach. Also, if the BCA lays out the matrix in advance, filling in summaries of information as that information is collected, the task is easier and may even aid in clinical decision-making as assessment unfolds. An additional advantage of the matrix is illustrated in Table 12-5. By scanning

Table 12-5
Matrix Describing Assessment of Young Adult Male

MODALITIES	INTERVIEW			WRITTEN			OBSERVATION			PSYCHOPHYSIOLOGICAL	
	With Client	With Spouse	With Other	Symptom Checklist	Individual Ratings	Others	Self-Monitoring	Interview Observations	Clinic Analogue	EMG	EKG
Cognitions	X			X		MMPI items	X				
Sensations	X			X		MMPI items	X			X	X
Overt Behavior	X	X	With Physician	X			X	X	X		
Frequency	X	X	With Physician		X		X	X	X	X	X
Duration	X	X	With Physician				X	X	X	X	X
Intensity	X	X					X	X	X	X	X
Case History	X		With Physician								
Locations	X	X					X				
Activities	X	X					X				
Times	X	X					X				
Intrinsic Antecedents	X						X			X	X
External Antecedents	X	X					X	X	X		
Intrinsic Consequences	X						X			X	X
External Consequences	X	X					X	X	X		
Social Skills	X	X				Assertion Questionaire		X	X		
Person Support	X	X	With close friend					BCA interviews client in home on 2 occasions			
Physical Surroundings	X	X						BCA interviews client in home on 2 occasions			
Financial Resources	X	X						X			
Vocational Skills	X	X	With Job Counselor								
Client's Motivation	X	X				X		X			
Others: Medication & Physical Status	X	X	With Physician								

down a given "methods column" the BCA is in a position to make decisions in advance regarding the relevance of a given method for collecting information across each of the modalities that he proposes to assess. The matrix provides a kind of organizational plan that ensures that each method is employed to its fullest advantage on each occasion of its use. This author has frequently employed direct observation in such natural settings as the classroom or home, only to find that, as a result of poor planning, some information that could have easily been gathered at the time was lost. A series of interviews, a case history, a complement of home observations and so forth can thus be organized to ensure that important information is in fact obtained.

While the results of this assessment will not be described in detail, the reader has been provided with an explicit overview of the BCA's goals in this case. Several modalities will be assessed using different methods; a great amount of information will be obtained. If this clinical assessment is carried out skillfully, the resultant information will enable the BCA to meet each of the four goals for a clinical assessment outlined in Chapter 1. A detailed *description* of the client's problem will have been obtained, along with information that enables the BCA to understand how that problematic behavior (or lack of behavior) is probably maintained (*causality*). In addition, the BCA should now know the client well enough to examine the suitability of potential intervention *methods* in the light of the client's goals, resources and motivation to change. Finally, a data base has been developed which, if employed during and following intervention, could be the basis for a systematic *evaluation* of the process and/or outcome of intervention. The results of the clinical assessment may not only be communicated to the client, but also to others who participate now or in the future in the client's treatment. The next section offers some strategies for such communications.

Communicating Assessment Findings

The process of deciding on goals and intervention methods frequently begins with the BCA's presentation of information to the client following clinical assessments. Some BCAs will wish to offer post-assessment "feedback" to the client regarding the BCA's own view of the problem, while others may feel more comfortable in providing informational feedback on an ongoing basis. At any rate, the BCA and client will at some point decide on goals for intervention. Some writers have called this process of feedback and goal definition, "pinpointing." Specifically, "pinpointing" involves discussing assessment information with the client as a prelude to mutually (if possible) defining goals for intervention. In some cases, Goal Attainment Scaling procedures (Kiresuk and Sherman, 1968; see Chapter 5) are employed in writing down intermediate and ultimate goals, so that the course of intervention can be evaluated by both BCA and client in the light of explicit criteria. In other cases, a variant of the Problem Oriented Record (Weed, 1970) may be used to define each of some number of "problems," followed by a proposed intervention plan. More will be said about the Problem Oriented Record in a later section.

While Chapter 3 has already reviewed a variety of interviewing skills that the BCA can employ in presenting assessment information, actively listening, and clarifying priorities for intervention with the client, perhaps a word should be said here about the communication of assessment findings in written form. The written "report" is not new to many BCAs; psychologists and social workers, for example, have long been identified with a written report of some kind (e.g., the psychological report, social work history). In fact, most human service agencies require the establishment of an archive defining the history of agency involvement and contemporary status of a given client.

It might be useful to briefly summarize the rationale for written record keeping as a prelude to presenting approaches that the BCA may wish to consider in communicating findings. Tallent (1976) defines the report as a "document written as a means of understanding certain features about a person and his circumstances in order to make decisions about, for or with him, and to intervene positively in his life" (p. 10). This suggests that the writing of a report may in itself provoke the BCA to carefully review and organize assessment data as a part of clinical decision-making. Grant and Maletzky (1972) offer the following benefits of well-kept written records. First, they serve as adjuncts to the BCA's memory, providing archives of historical, interview, observational or other information, as well as of previous and current treatment plans. If for some reason a BCA is unable to continue his therapeutic relationship with a client, a well-organized record ensures that a referral BCA has a systematic account of the evaluation of intervention. The written record thus provides accurate, contemporary information not only to the BCA but to others (e.g., for referral, peer review, or teaching purposes). In addition, well-kept records provide a source of information for developing and testing clinical hypotheses, and for program evaluation or research purposes when an adequate data base has been collected. Finally, Grant and Maletsky suggest that a written record serves as a legal document and they emphasize the necessity for well-kept records if the client ever becomes involved with adjudication and/or if records are subpoenaed. Recent court decisions (Wyatt v. Stickney, 1972) have specified that a data base must be provided from which an individualized treatment plan can be developed. Regardless of the sophistication and effectiveness of a treatment strategy, it cannot be legally recognized if it is not documented in writing. Grant (1972) observes:

The court makes it very clear that adequate documentation—the details and progress of that care plan—can only be accomplished by a comprehensive written record. No longer can the record be an incomplete, haphazard, anecdotal, virtually useless and unused accessory to care. The court decision [Wyatt v. Stickney] outlines the necessary contents for a complete record and makes this record the central component for both the provision of care and accountability. If data is [sic] not in the record it [sic] does not exist. If something was done and not recorded, it was not done. Memory and post-hoc assertions are not held to be reliable substitutes for timely, sequential records of the progress of care. (pp. 8–9)

Formats for the Written Report

It is difficult to present an outline of the features that should or should not appear in a report since so many divergent organizational formats have been employed to present the client and his life situation, perhaps because reports are written for a variety of purposes. For example, Chapters 3 and 4 discussed methods and issues attendant on the BCA's initial interviews with a client. Interview, written, observation, and in some cases psychophysiological methods facets may all be employed to define goals for intervention. The outcome of these assessments is often expressed in the form of an *intake report*. A description of interactions with the client (e.g., *a session*), a summary of objectives met "so far," and suggestions for future interactions might be collectively termed the *progress report* or progress "notes." Such reports of progress are usually followed by a report describing the course and outcome of intervention once termination has been instigated by the client, therapist, or both. This *termination summary* often provides a review of intervention methods that were employed to reach each intervention goal, with an in-depth summary of the client's response to that intervention plan. In addition, recommendations for future contacts with the client and scheduling of follow-up assessments may be included. Other reports may present the results of a specific assessment method, such as a report describing an examination of intellectual functioning or the outcome of a psychoneurological "work-up." Or a report might be directed at answering focused questions posed to the BCA by a court, an agency, or some other entity for adjudication or benefit-setting (e.g., for certification of disability) purposes. We might call these *specialized reports*.

Because of this text's focus on the assessment phase of intervention, a brief presentation of approaches to writing the intake report will be presented. A general protocol for intake description will be followed by an introduction to the Problem Oriented Record (POR). The POR was selected because of its popularity and applicability to any intake task, particularly to a setting where more than one BCA will have occasion to carry out intervention. Most intake reports will address in some manner the following information. (This outline has been used by the author in training a variety of BCAs.)

I. *Description of the client:* Identifying information is provided which describes the characteristics of the client relevant to agency requirements. The client's name, age, sex, a brief description of physical appearance as well as a statement of the agency, name of the assessor, and date of the report might be included.

II. *Statement of referral problem(s):* A statement is made of the process by which the client was referred to the BCA. The client may have referred himself or he may have been referred by another professional or agency. Following this, a statement of the referral "problem," couched in the language of the referral source, is recorded.

III. *Brief history of the problem(s):* Here the historical development of the problem is described. A summary of important information derived from the comprehensive case history (across all major developmental periods and categories of information) is ideally focused at the development of the problems that are referred to in section II or that emerge from assessment. Institutional records as well as reports of the client and/or informants may be integrated in this section.

IV. *Assessment data base:* The date of each occasion of assessment, the setting, and assessment procedures employed are recorded. The idea is to provide the reader with sufficient information so that the instruments and specific methodologies as well as the extensiveness of the assessment can be evaluated. An example is provided below.

Mrs. Jones was seen at (agency) on three occasions: an initial intake interview (9/26/80) was followed by two interviews aimed at obtaining a further statement of John's problem behavior and her current approach to it. On 10/3/80, 10/6/80, and 10/8/80, both Mr. and Mrs. Jones were briefly interviewed at their residence. Following each interview, all members of the family were observed interacting under "natural" conditions for the period of 45 minutes. Family members were asked to remain in either the living or family rooms to assure visual access by the observer. No other restrictions were imposed. Observations were made using [*describe method briefly; if a formal coding system or behavior checklist was employed, describe by title*]. In addition, both Mr. and Mrs. Jones were asked to complete the Becker Adjective Checklist on 10/8/80. Mrs. Jones was asked to keep a daily diary that included a description of each time John failed to comply with a request. For each notation, she was asked to include the time of occurrence, situation, how she handled the noncompliance and John's response to her approach. She continues to keep this diary at present.

V. *Integration of findings:* In this section each assessed modality of information is presented, with findings across multiple methods integrated and summarized. The use of the decision matrix previously described is most helpful in examining consistencies and inconsistencies of findings across methods. At this point, the BCA does not draw conclusions or define explicit goals for intervention, but merely presents the findings and attempts to make sense of them for the reader. The example that follows, as well as the integration of findings presented in previous case examples, are illustrative of this procedure.

While Mrs. Jones originally stated that John is a child who is "out of control" and probably "emotionally disturbed," further probing within the interviews shows that most of her troubled interactions with him seem to involve her issuing commands and his failure to comply with them. Arguments and physical confrontations (pushing and shoving when Mrs. Jones attempts to spank John) sometimes follow a repetition of the request and John's repeated failure to comply. This confirms John's report that he wishes his mother would leave him alone and not "bug" him "all the time" with silly requests. In addition, John reported that often he's not sure what his mother actually wants him to do and that it is impossible to satisfy his mom. In observing Mrs. Jones and her son interact in the structured clinical situation it was obvious that Mrs. Jones frequently speaks to her son without maintaining eye contact and was quite vague in providing instructions to him in performing the tasks [to reach consensus on a family issue]. While mother and son began the task by attempting to reach consensus, the interaction ended when Mrs. Jones pronounced that she would have to make the decision because of John's "uncooperativeness." Our observations indicated that John had initially attempted to engage his mother in discussion, turning away and giving up only when he became frustrated with his mother's frequent interruptions. When this family was observed in the home situation, Mrs. Jones issued an average of fifteen commands, many of them repetitions of previous requests, during the hour-and-a-half period of observation. Most of these were directed at asking John to clean up around the house and put things away. John complied immediately on an average of only twice per session, indicating his mother's ineffectiveness in eliciting compliance. It is important to note that Mrs. Jones frequently calls to her son from another room, fails to gain his attention in advance and frequently does not give him the opportunity to comply before issuing another command, which often only serves to infuriate him. John is observed to turn away from his mom and seemingly immerse himself in television or reading whenever a request is made. On a number of occasions he seemed to enjoy provoking his mother to repeated requests and ultimate confrontations. In contrast, John's teacher and a school counselor do not report any difficulties in obtaining compliance from him; thus this problem seems to occur exclusively in the home situation. There are no consistently delivered consequences for noncompliance. Noncompliance can result in Mrs. Jones ignoring John, verbal reprimands, sending him to his room for "isolation," or attempts at spanking.. The attempts at spanking frequently result in John's attempting to physically restrict Mrs. Jones' hand. This often makes both parties quite angry. On one occasion they were observed to strike each other.

VI. *Goals for intervention:* From among the problems described in section V, a series of specific goals for intervention are presented in explicit language. In some cases these goals are prioritized and a rationale presented for this sequencing. For each of the goals the BCA should present a detailed treatment plan taking into account the client's resources and motivation, as previously defined. The nature of this intervention plan will obviously depend upon the BCA's theoretical orientation, the nature of the problem and what is practically possible. These goals can be explicitly defined using the Goal Attainment Scaling approach presented in Chapter 5. It is important that the BCA and client together develop a clear statement of objectives from which a well-defined course of intervention may follow.

The Problem-Oriented Record (POR) will now be presented as an example of problem definition and specification of the treatment plan. The reader may wish to incorporate one or more features of the POR in writing the intake report, or employ the POR in its entirety as a unified system of record keeping and communication.

The Problem-Oriented Record. Originally developed by Weed (1970) to provide a unitary approach to record keeping that can be employed across categories of professionals in medical settings, the Problem-Oriented Record strategy is applicable to virtually any set of conditions within which the BCA wishes to develop, implement and follow up a treatment plan with a client, particularly when more than one BCA will be involved in employing and monitoring intervention strategies. In its original form, the POR is composed of four major components, applicable at different points in the course of assessment and intervention. First, the *data base* includes the body of information that forms the basis for clinical decision making; i.e., all of the information collected across different modalities and with different methods. This data base might include case history information collected from the client or from other sources, a review of systems, physical examination and laboratory work performed in a medical setting, the results of a psychiatric "mental status" examination, the results of psychometric assessments of intellectual functioning, personality, aptitudes or responses to checklists, rating scales and the like, a summary of the results of observations conducted in clinical or criterion settings, notes describing the verbal responses and behavior offered by the client in the interview, and the outcome of any psychophysiological assessments performed. The data base includes the entire body of information recorded in a form understandable to an independent person who might have occasion to read through assessment findings. Obviously the information that forms the data base might vary considerably depending on such factors as the nature of the client, the presenting problem and the setting in which the BCA functions.

The second component of the POR is the *problem list*. According to Grant (1972), the problem list should be a comprehensive outline of medical, environmental, psychological, behavioral and social problems discovered by evaluating the data base. Central to this approach is the comprehensive listing of all problems, each given a number, even though a given BCA may be unprepared or ill-equipped to develop an intervention plan for each. Some of these problems may not be immediately made the focus for intervention, while others may result in referrals to other BCAs, medical personnel, relevant members of the community, and so on, who are equipped to deal with that particular problem. Each problem is assigned a number for descriptive identification purposes, but these numbers do not usually suggest a priority for intervention and have no meaning other than identification.

The third component of the POR is the formulation of an *intervention strategy* for each of the problems on the list. This strategy might include proposals for further assessments when the BCA feels that the problem is ill-defined or insufficient assessment information is available, suggestions for referrals to other persons, or a statement that intervention is postponed for the present. Once a numbered problem is entered into a client's chart or other record, it is assumed that one of these plans will be proposed for it.

Finally, *progress notes* are a means of keeping track of the day-to-day outcomes resulting from implementation of the treatment plan for each numbered problem, and ongoing integrations of these findings. In addition, revisions of the original treatment plan or the development of new plans form a part of the progress notes. Frequently, they are divided into four sections defined by the acronym SOAP. First is *subjective data;* that is, what the client or others say about problems or the outcome of treatment plans. Next comes *objective* findings, derived from observational instruments, or more systematic written assessments on the part of BCAs involved in the case, as well as any unobtrusive measures. Then an *assessment* describes the case monitor's current conceptualization of why subjectively or objectively assessed progress is being made or failing to be made, with the fourth component, *plans*, offering revisions of current treatment plans or new plans to be implemented at once.

Some agencies include a section titled *objectives* which defines specific, behaviorally explicit goals for each of the numbered problems immediately following the problem list, with plans directly related to the objectives. Such a section would ensure a clear understanding, by all BCAs involved with a given client, or precisely how the client's behavior is to change as a precondition for defining the treatment plan. Objectives are particularly important in evaluating the effectiveness of intervention using one of the single case design strategies presented in Chapter 13, and can help to ensure that the client (to the extent possible) as well as other relevant persons are aware of the criteria by which outcome is to be assessed.

As pointed out by Grant (1973) the POR has been adopted as a record-keeping system by many states for use in programs in medical schools and certain state-supported institutions. In addition, the Veteran's Administration began using the POR in all general medical field stations in 1974. Grant states: "The rapid increase in acceptance and utilization of the system and its apparently inherent face utility has begun to prompt interest from a variety of third party payers of health care services. Both government and private third party payers are contemplating making reimbursement contingent upon problem-oriented client records" (p. 6). Discussing the rationale for using the POR, Katz and Wooley (1975) emphasized that all of the client's significant behavioral, medical, social and environmental problems are identified. This is an approximation to "better consumer accountability" in delivering comprehensive care: The POR improves communication among BCAs and others involved in the client's treatment, thus enhancing the ease of "information transfer"; problems previously defined in terms of abstract jargon or terminology derived from a particular theoretical orientation become functionally defined in behavioral rather than abstract, mentalistic or diagnostic terms in such a way that independent parties can understand precisely what is treated and how; the procedure increases the possibility of the individualized care required under certain recent legal decisions (Wyatt v. Stickney, 1972; Morales v. Turman, 1974; see Martin, 1975 and Friedman, 1975); the POR provides useful feedback to BCAs regarding changes in the client's behavior and gives a data base for program evaluation and research purposes. Katz and Wooley encourage different categories of BCAs to modify and improve the record-keeping system to meet their specific needs, while emphasizing the logic of a comprehensive and unitary approach to record keeping. Table 12-6 provides an example of a problem list resulting from the collection of a data base for Mr. Y, the 28-year-old man who complains of "extreme anxiety and inadequacy" described in a previous section.

Table 12-6
Example Problem List for 28-Year-Old
Male Reporting "Anxiety" as Problem

DATE	PROBLEM NUMBER	PROBLEM LIST	STAFF INITIAL
11/17	1	Uncertain as to Mr. Y's medical status and role of minor tranquilizer in his medical treatment.	J.F.
11/17	2	Mr. Y's physical tension and anxiety that seems to be related to either direct interactions or thinking about interacting with his colleagues at work or any stranger. Muscular tension is particularly pronounced in mornings.	J.F.
11/18	3	Deficits in knowledge and skills in providing criticism and negative feedback to subordinates.	J.F.
11/19	4	Mr. Y is uncertain as to suitability of his present job. Does not know what other vocational options are available to him.	M.R.

Table 12-7
Examples of Objectives and Treatment Plans

DATE	PROBLEM NUMBER	OBJECTIVE/TREATMENT PLAN	STAFF INITIAL
11/18	1	To obtain records of recent medical exam. Obtain release of information from Mr. Y and request report from Dr. Milton.	J.F.
11/20	2	To reduce Mr. Y.'s muscular tension as evidenced by a reduction in self-ratings of tension of at least 2 rating scale units and ability to role-play interactions with colleagues without showing behavioral indicants of anxiety (particulary sweaty palms and flushed face). Also to report at least 3 interactions at office that client would rate at 2 units or less. Train in muscle relaxation procedures, then employ systematic desensitization to reduce conditioned anxiety associated with particular colleagues.	J.F.
11/20	3	To provide Mr. Y with multiple options for giving negative feedback and to enhance his skills in doing so. Employ modeling, role-playing and coaching to train client in ways to assert himself in responding. In addition, encourage client to practice relaxation (see Problem 2) in role-played situations. Also, encourage Mr. Y to join social skills group at Valley Mental Health Clinic and make referral if he is willing.	J.F.
11/20	4	Assist Mr. Y in clarifying his goals and current job-related assets/deficits. Referral to CVC for vocational counseling deferred until 10/20.	M.R.

Table 12-7 shows the specific objectives and treatment plans devised to deal with each of the four problems shown in Mr. Y's problem list.

Finally, Table 12-8 gives an example of how progress notes might be recorded for problem number two. The reader will note that the acronym SOAP defines subjective and objective data, assessment and treatment planning respectively.

Finally, potential problems that the BCA should consider in preparing the written report will be addressed.

Table 12-8
Example of Progress Notes For One Problem

DATE	PROBLEM NUMBER	PROGRESS NOTES
11/25	2	Relaxation training was begun on 11/23, 2 sessions of 1 hr. conducted to date
		S—Mr. Y reports that he is able to note a significant difference between tension and relaxation for limbs, facial muscles and neck. Reports that the muscles of the back, chest and stomach are difficult to relax. In addition, he reports difficulty in clearing his mind of anxiety-provoking thoughts.
		O—He is able to perform the exercises correctly at my verbal instructions. Observed facial blushing at least twice during each session. Mr. A. (another BCA) observed Mr. Y practicing the exercises this morning.
		A—Mr. Y appears to be motivated to learn and practice relaxation. He experiences difficulty in relaxing muscle groups of the body trunk, a primary locus of discomfort when he is anxious.
		P—Continue relaxation training until Mr. Y can relax each muscle group on his own within 10–15 seconds. Focus on musculature of the body trunk and increase homework to practice relaxing shoulders, back, chest and stomach to 4 times/day. Praise Mr. Y when he is shown to be practicing on his own. Systematic desensitization postponed at present.

Potential Pitfalls

In offering a variety of models for report writing, Tallent (1976) discusses some problems in communicating information in writing. Tallent polled 1,400 clinical workers, psychologists, social workers and psychiatrists, asking respondents to complete the sentence: "The trouble with psychological reports is. . . ." A large number of respondents criticized the use of jargon, psychiatric/psychological terminology and wordiness. Many of them also noted that reports are often vague or ambiguous. Most of the sample emphasized the need for conciseness, simplicity, and straightforwardness in presenting information. They agreed that many reports are not organized or thought out before they appear in written form; they are often "fragmented. . . rather than being integrated" or "not organized around a central pattern" (p. 45).

Finally, report writers were criticized for frequently offering speculations not clearly backed up by data, and for failing to distinguish between speculative and factual material. One category of report that has been studied by a variety of researchers (Ulrich, Stachnick, & Stainton, 1963; Snyder, 1974) was originally named the "Barnum Report" by Meehl (1954), after the well-known entrepreneur and man of the world, Phineas T. Barnum. The Barnum Report presents a combination of mildly negative, neutral and flattering remarks which are applicable to almost anyone. Tallent (1976) reports that one of his colleagues distributed a Barnum-style report to each of 39 class members in a university course, explaining that the report was "an individual personality analysis which the instructor had arrived at through inspection of samples of the students' handwriting" (p. 55), and thus specifically tailored to each student. Although all students received the same report, each of them accepted it as an accurate reflection of himself with the exception of two students who indicated very slight error. The report was characterized by such statements as: "above average in intelligence or mental alertness," "you have a tendency to worry at times but not to excess," "you are strongly socially inclined, you like to meet people, especially to mix with those you know well," "you are ambitious and deserve credit for wanting to be well-thought of by your family, business associates and friends." It is obvious that these statements would apply to almost anyone; they are ambiguous, vague, over-inclusive and of little utility in providing a clear and concise description of a person's behavior or life situation. The reader is referred to Tallent (1976) for a more extensive discussion of pitfalls faced by the report writer.

Footnote

[1]The reader may recall the issue of clinical versus statistical prediction presented in Chapter 5. A purely statistical approach merely compares the client's responses to a statistical model or to some reference grouping of clients which leads to probability statements based purely upon statistical criteria.

UNIT IV
Clinical Assessment
For Case Evaluation

TREATMENT EVALUATION STRATEGIES

Philip C. Kendall and W. Robert Nay[1]

Mental health professionals who attempt to instigate clinical behavior change should be aware of their responsibilities to assess and evaluate the effectiveness of the methods employed. The term *evaluation* refers to the systematic assessment of a treatment's impact on those behaviors targeted for change. In essence, we wish to describe accurately the relation between variation in the treatment (independent variable) and variation in the target behavior (dependent variable). Such evaluation may compare treatment effectiveness across groups, thus emphasizing the generality of findings, or focus exclusively on the single case, thus emphasizing individual differences.

The single-case evaluation strategy will be the focus of the present chap-

ter as BCAs are more likely to work with single individuals in clinical (not research) settings. Also, the array of statistical and design issues germane to a
discussion of between-groups research is beyond the scope of this text. Our
initial discussion includes clinical vs. statistical significance, and the difference between group and single-subject designs. Both single-subject and group
designs are assigned a role in treatment evaluation. Substantively, eight treatment evaluation strategies or designs appropriate to the single subject are
presented, compared, and evaluated, and some general criteria to evaluate reports of case studies are provided. Accompanying the discussion of some of
the major strategies are hypothetical data, real examples from the authors' experience, and examples from the literature. No attempt is made to criticize
the specific studies cited as examples. Rather, the designs themselves are the
focus of discussion.

Significance: Clinical vs. Statistical

In many areas of research "statistical significance" is the basis of judgment
of reliable effects, no matter how small the actual effect. In the application of
treatment, results which are statistically significant yet not profound enough
for practical, clinical purposes are of limited utility, despite the level of significance (e.g., a statistically significant weight loss of 6 pounds for treated
subjects as compared to a loss of 0.4 pounds for controls, where all subjects
are still very overweight). The essential criterion is the power of the treatment to alter successfully the targeted behavior in question. Therapeutic
goals may require total elimination of some class of behavior (destructive or
self-damaging behavior) or acceleration or reduction to some degree. The degree of change that is desirable is defined by BCA and client within environmental constraints. Single-subject strategies allow for treatment evaluation in
relation to predetermined treatment goals (e.g., a meaningful outcome would
be when the overweight client loses enough weight so that he or she is no
longer overweight according to height-weight charts[2]).

In many respects the attempt to achieve clinically meaningful change is
more exacting. For one, the treatment must provide visible results which are
satisfying to those involved. In addition, the outcome of a single client's treatment cannot be hidden by group averaging, nor can statistical significance be
touted when the effect is so small that it is clinically senseless. It is also more
exacting in that one continuously monitors the data and the treatment program with $N = 1$, which is usually not the case in group studies (Browning
and Stover, 1971).

Figure 13-1 shows that the behavior of three individual subjects, who perform quite differently, can be displayed as a "group average" response which

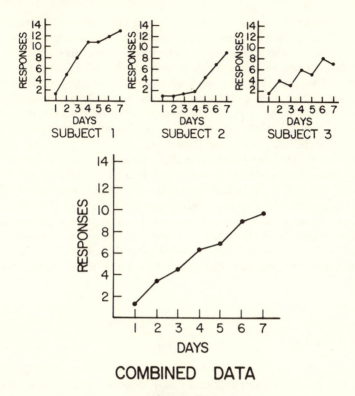

Figure 13-1
Behavior of 3 individual subjects whose "group average"
is unlike any single one.

is unlike any of the individual response patterns. How could a BCA, interested in helping Subject 2, for example, make use of such group data? One of the strengths of the group approach is that the results are applicable to all clients. Yet, as has been noted, some clients may change rapidly and others only gradually, producing an overall statistical improvement which may be misleading when individual clients are considered.

Group vs. Single-Subject Designs

Group studies compare average responses obtained between groups of persons who receive (experimental subjects) and fail to receive (control subjects) some form of treatment. In the single-subject strategy, the comparison is not made between the performance of two or more groups treated differently, but between the performance of the same subject during two or more periods of time in which he may be treated differently. In contrast to the group design, the single-subject design presents all the values of the treatment (the independent variables) to a single subject or single group of subjects. If the single-subject strategy is followed properly, it can demonstrate whether functional control of the target by the treatment has been achieved, and the intensive study of the single case can be a valuable source of hypotheses for later investigation using the group approach.

In the recent literature the letters A, B, C, D, and so on have been used to represent different phases of single-subject designs (see Browning and Stover, 1971; Wolf and Risley, 1971; Barlow and Hersen, 1973; Hersen and Barlow, 1976). "A" denotes a no-treatment phase called baseline and "B", "C", "D" stand for successive treatment conditions. The baseline phase is the initial period of observation in which the pretreatment frequency of occurrence of the targeted behavior is assessed and recorded in some fashion. The treatment phases reflect the frequency of occurrence of the target following the onset of treatment(s).

The B Design

The most primitive strategy, the B design, consists simply of the administration of a treatment technique. No baseline (pretreatment) measures are taken, and the investigator assesses the target(s) only *during* the administration of the treatment program. Since there are no baseline data, the BCA cannot be certain whether observed changes in the client's behavior are a function of the treatment or any one of several uncontrolled factors to be discussed in the next section. Although this strategy is probably superior to collecting no data and at least ensures that the BCA is cognizant of the current frequency of targeted events (perhaps useful for clinical purposes), it is of little practical utility in evaluation.

The A-B Design

This design compares the results of baseline measurements made prior to treatment with data collected during treatment. Wolf and Risley (1971) state, "Originally, the most popular experimental design was the two-stage A-B design. We would measure a behavior during the baseline condition (A) and then watch for a change in the behavior during the treatment condition (B)" (p. 312).

Prior to an evaluation of this design, the "baseline" itself will be considered. The pretreatment frequency of occurrence of targeted behavior illustrates the magnitude of the problem and provides an accurate description of the trend of occurrence of the behavior before treatment is initiated.

Unfortunately, the literature does not provide the BCA with precise guidelines for the number of observations necessary nor recommend an optimum time duration for the baseline. Most writers suggest that the targeted behavior must be stable prior to intervention (Kazdin, 1978), and Sidman (1960) has suggested that stability be defined as variability within a range of five percent. In addition, various writers have suggested that frequent observations should be made to prevent any misinterpretation of random fluctuations within and across days (Kiesler, 1971). In fact, the BCA often notes considerable changes in the frequency of the target across the baseline days. If this is the case, it may be impossible to interpret changes in the targeted behavior once treatment is initiated. For example, imagine the case where the total daily frequency of a target, while fluctuating considerably, gradually diminishes from about ten times per day to about three times per day at the end of the baseline period. Once treatment is implemented, the BCA notes that the frequency of occurrence continues to be maintained at a low level (e.g., about two to three times per day), and thus assumes that his treatment was responsible for the results. This is an example of what might best be called a "continuation" effect; that is, the frequency of the target was obviously changing in a desirable direction *prior to* the implementation of treatment, and continued to do so once treatment was initiated. In this case, it is difficult to know precisely which factor is responsible for behavior change within the baseline, but it is obvious that the BCA cannot clearly attribute the desirable results to the treatment. Any time that the targeted behavior is showing progressive changes in one direction or another during baseline, the BCA should attempt to determine what is responsible for those changes.

Along these lines, Campbell and Stanley (1963) have suggested a variety of phenomena that may cause a targeted behavior to change in the absence of formal treatment. For example, it may be that the reduction in the target just described was due to some life event (e.g., new job; the intervention of a new teacher; the introduction of a more appropriate peer model). Campbell and Stanley have termed this *history* and it is obvious that a variety of phenomena operate in the client's ordinary environment that may cause desirable or undesirable changes in the targeted behavior. Other factors may include behavior change due to *maturation* (Campbell and Stanley, 1963), and it is obvious, particularly during certain developmental periods, that significant behavioral changes can be observed over a period of weeks and months merely due to certain ongoing physiological-biochemical processes in the individual. Along these lines, the ingestion of a drug or the implementation of medical treatment at the same time that a treatment program is implemented may confound the results, making it difficult to know whether the drug or medical regimen *or* the BCA's treatment is responsible for the outcome.

Another factor is termed *instrument decay;* this refers to changes in the methods of measurement at different stages of treatment. These measurement changes (e.g., differences in the way behavior is observed, unreliability) may in themselves be responsible for apparent behavior change, in the absence of any real change on the part of the client. Finally, Campbell and Stanley speak of so-called *regression* effects. It may be that if we observe a behavior on a few occasions we see only extreme levels of occurrence, when in fact, if we were to observe the behavior over many days, the average or mean level of the behavior would be quite different. In our example, initial observations might reflect extreme scores, with behavior change within the baseline merely reflecting regression to the mean. This phenomenon can only be overcome by extending the period of observation to include a sufficient number of data points (e.g., days of data collection). Finally, *transient physical states* may provoke behavior change that enhances or masks treatment effects. For example, if a child were observed during a brief period of time that was also marked by illness, stress, or fatigue, the behaviors observed might very well be quite different from the ordinary behaviors observed in the absence of these physical states. Behavior provoked by such changes in physical status may, unfortunately, occur from baseline to the implementation of treatment, thus speciously indicating that the intervention method was responsible for the change.

A number of these potential problems can be overcome by extending the number of days of baseline data collection and by ensuring that treatment is not begun if extreme instability or trends indicating a reduction or acceleration of the target behavior are evident. It should be noted that the "eyeballing" of results during the baseline period can be supplemented or supplanted by statistical methods. For example, Gottman, McFall, and Barnett (1969) suggest fitting a curve to the data using the method of least squares and then analyzing the structure of the baseline (or the various treatment phases). The interested reader is referred to Glass, Wilson, and Gottman (1973) for a thorough analysis of useful statistical approaches, called time-series designs.

Another problem facing the BCA in establishing a baseline has to do with the ethics of extending a nontreatment period when clients are in need of intervention. Given the desirability of determining whether or not a treatment is effective and the value of gathering an extensive amount of information to assess optimal combinations of targets and interventions, the BCA must also ensure that the client is not asked to experience unreasonable discomfort over extended periods of time. Clearly, when the occurrence of the targeted behavior is potentially harmful to the client or others, the BCA will wish to do everything possible to restrict its occurrence. It should be kept in mind, however, that whenever treatment plans are imposed *outside of* a systematic and comprehensive evaluation of the client's behavior-in-setting, there is the real possibility that less-than-optimal intervention programs will be designed. This unfortunate outcome is also ethically questionable; a violation of the client's right to competently delivered treatment.

As a rule of thumb, the BCA should evaluate the role of the proposed assessment methods within clinical decision making and their potential benefit to the client. If an assessment methodology is primarily employed to further the BCA's research interests (e.g., an innovative assessment approach) and the information to be obtained has little potential utility in the development of an intervention strategy, then clearly the BCA should inform the client of this and ensure that the client consents under fully informed conditions (see Martin, 1975). If, on the contrary, various assessments are likely to contribute to treatment planning and are carried out within a reasonable period of time with full client awareness of what the BCA hopes to accomplish, then a period of systematic, baseline evaluation is not only ethically justifiable, but essential to the client's welfare. Inappropriate selection of targets for change and/or haphazard selection of treatment strategies, both of which may result from inadequate case assessment, do little to further the client's welfare and in fact may contribute to the client's distress. Recent court decisions applying to institutionalized clients have emphasized the need for an "individualized" treatment plan for clients (e.g., *Morales v. Turman,* 1974; *Wyatt v. Stickney,* 1972; summarized in Martin, 1975; Friedman, 1975), and such individuation is clearly the result of systematic and comprehensive assessment.

Issues of the baseline phase aside, the A-B single-case design holds certain

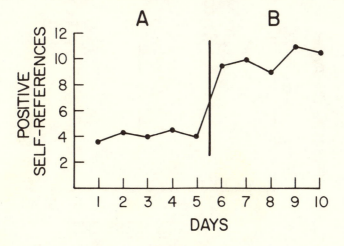

Figure 13-2
Observational data for "depressed" client over five-day
baseline period.

advantages over the B design, while also exhibiting some unique limitations. A case example illustrates this design.

A 28-year-old client displaying behavioral signs of "depression" was unobtrusively observed by a ward attendant over a five-day baseline period. These data are shown in Figure 13-2 (see A phase). Following the initiation on Day 6 of staff social interaction and praise contingent on her positive self-statements, the frequency of positive self-statements immediately increased (see B phase). While it appears that this treatment is "responsible" for the positive change, such a conclusion is not warranted. In fact, any one of a host of factors could be responsible for the behavior change shown from A to B phase (e.g., history, instrument decay). While we can't know for certain *why* the behavior changed, we do know that there was a change from baseline and can document its magnitude. This is important information; certainly the A-B design is an improvement over the simple B approach.

The B-C Design

The B-C design is merely a comparison of successively administered treatments. Hypothetical results of a B-C design are presented in Figure 13-3 which shows a decrease in inappropriate physical behavior with increasing response cost (five- and ten-point losses) for a population of adolescent delinquents treated using the token economy approach. The interpretation that a

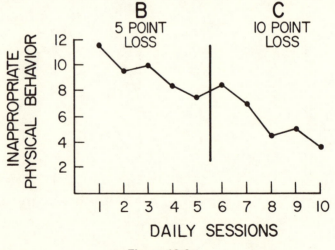

Figure 13-3
**Hypothetical results for response-cost program
within a B-C design.**

ten-point loss is a more effective suppressant than a five-point loss cannot be justified on the basis of the decreasing trend seen in the first phase (a continuation effect). Likewise, it is possible that results shown in both phases are also due to unidentified factors.

Another criticism is that the B-C design is susceptible to uncontrolled order and carry-over effects. Order effects are related to the ordinal position of a treatment within a sequence of treatments. In the example, the ten-point loss could be an effective treatment only because of its being the second treatment in the sequence (e.g., would not be effective unless preceded by a five-point loss). Carry-over effects attributable to earlier treatments in the sequence are also possible. For example, the success of the ten-point loss condition could be due to the potency of the five-point loss treatment which has carried over and continues to suppress behavior. Order and carry-over effects can occur separately or simultaneously.

In summary, this design is extremely weak and is not recommended. It lacks control and precision. With only slight additional thought, the BCA can implement a more sophisticated design.

The A-B-A or A-B-A-B Design

Given that the implementation of a treatment or B phase results in a stable change in the frequency of the target from original baseline or A conditions, the A-B-A design asks: If the treatment is now *removed* and baseline is reinstated, will the target return to baseline frequency? If results are similar to those depicted in Figure 13-4, this suggests that the B condition (treatment) was primarily responsible for the observed decrease in rate of the problem behavior. Note the *immediate* effects of both the installation and removal of the treatment phase. If these immediate behavior changes are not evident, care should be taken in interpreting the results.

Obviously, the employment of additional B and A phases (e.g., A-B-A-B-A-B) adds additional power to this design and increases the likelihood that the treatment is in fact responsible for behavior changes observed.

Kazdin (1978) points out three major variations in this design. The first, already described, withdraws the treatment at the second and succeeding A phases and is sometimes called a "withdrawal" design. A second version examines the importance of the contingencies between the treatment and targeted behavior and is often employed in evaluating behavior modification procedures relying on reinforcement or punishment made contingent on the target. In this case, the BCA continues to deliver the treatment (e.g., positive consequences), but does not make it *contingent* on the target. If the target reverts to baseline frequency, this provides evidence that the *contingent* appli-

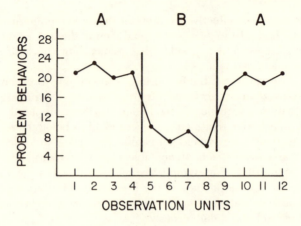

Figure 13-4
Effects of installation and removal of treatment within an
A-B-A design.

cation of the treatment is responsible for behavior change. A third variant alters the contingencies between treatment and target, but in a different manner. All responses *other than* the original target result in the treatment consequences (e.g., praise, token reinforcement). Sometimes called differential reinforcement of other behavior (DRO), the results of this manipulation show the impact not only of withholding the treatment, but of applying it to alternative behaviors. If the target decelerates in frequency while the alternative behaviors accelerate, then the BCA has evidence of the role of the consequences in instigating and maintaining behavior. Obviously this last variant might be unacceptable if the "other" behaviors reinforced are maladaptive or discomforting to the client. In fact, the withdrawal of treatment itself poses a variety of ethical as well as practical problems for the BCA, which will now be discussed.

If the properties and/or length of the treatment condition are such that the newly acquired behavior is powerfully established in the client's repertoire, withdrawal of the treatment may not result in a change in rate. In addition, withdrawal of treatment may allow the client to retrieve undesired habits more quickly and make them more resistant to deceleration or elimination. Another problem with reversals is that it is difficult or even impossible to closely replicate the original baseline conditions (e.g., "Try to treat Mr. X like you did 2 weeks ago"). O'Leary and Drabman (1971) note that a return to the "original" conditions, even when carefully monitored, may be quite different from the conditions which operated prior to treatment. Even if staff are capable of reproducing preintervention conditions, there is still the serious question of whether the clients perceive them as similar. In addition, clients' perception of the second baseline can be markedly altered by carry-over effects from previous conditions (e.g., a "set" to behave in a particular fashion). There are also occasions where reversals are undesirable and ethically questionable; for example, when the target behavior is self-destructive, dangerous, or damaging. Or, staff or family members may not want the undesirable behavior to return. Certainly, *a final B or treatment phase should follow the withdrawal of treatment* if the client's behavior still occurs at an undesirable level (A-B-A-B as opposed to A-B-A).

Nay (1974) reports on a decision *not* to reverse contingencies following implementation of a token economy program with a population of "delinquent" adolescents.

In the present case, the school administrators would not permit a return to baseline, fearing that a reversal might well provoke large-scale destructive behavior among a population of youngsters expecting to be disappointed. The predictable elevation in deviant behavior would be as much a function of subjects' anger at having their first opportunity to experience positive feedback for their efforts terminated as it would of a return to "natural" conditions. Although such a return would no doubt have produced convincing illustrations of high rate inappropriate behavior when points (tokens) were removed, such data would be open to question for the reasons mentioned (pp. 230–231).

There are alternate means available, other than reversals, for identifying the agent of change. Observing a yoked-control subject who receives exactly the same conditions except for therapeutic treatment, might be considered. Still other alternatives include O'Leary and Drabman's (1971) suggestion of sequential introduction of treatment variables, replications with other persons, use of untreated control groups, and some of the design variants to be discussed in later sections of this chapter.

The A-B-A-C-A or Successive Treatments Design

The successive treatments design (A-B-A-C-A) employs a withdrawal following the implementation of each of several treatments. Two reasons commonly offered for this are: first, to assess control of the target by the treatment and second, to compare the relative effectiveness of different treatments. Because the client is exposed to an increased number of phase transitions and compounding of treatments, this design is extremely susceptible to all the criticisms and weaknesses of the withdrawal design already mentioned, including the increasing impossibility of reproducing baseline conditions, carry-over and contrast effects which confound methods and reduce the interpretability of findings, and ethical considerations of the numerous no-treatment phases.

The Multiple-Baseline Design

Many of the single-subject designs discussed thus far have employed the withdrawal of treatment, and for reasons already mentioned this may not be the design of choice. In addition, for certain targets, withdrawal is impossible for practical or ethical reasons.

As an alternative, the multiple-baseline design *sequentially* introduces treatment to: *different targets for the same client, different settings for the same target,* or *different persons in the same setting* (holding the target constant). While a specific behavior, setting, or person receives treatment, other behaviors, settings, or persons remain untreated and serve as controls for the treatment. Each variant of the multiple-baseline design overcomes the objections raised for the withdrawal design provided that the BCA can postpone treatment for the "control" phenomena until stable behavior change is observed for the treated phenomena.

There are many evaluation questions for which the multiple-baseline design is well suited. Often the BCA is confronted with implementing and evaluating treatment in settings that do not permit random assignment of subjects to groups so that formal inferential statistical methods may be employed. Classrooms, cottages, wards, and similar pre-existing settings are often composed of clients who are grouped together for a variety of reasons (age, sex, diagnosis, etc.) which do not meet the standard of random assignment. The multiple-baseline approach permits the BCA to evaluate the effect of treatment for clients across such pre-existing settings. To decide the sequence of treatment, each setting should be randomly assigned to treatment or baseline conditions. For example, Figure 13-5 shows how a self-control treatment could be implemented to reduce aggressive verbal behavior across three self-contained classrooms (cottages, wards, etc.) for a population of normal middle-school students. After a ten-day baseline, treatment is administered to Classroom 1, while 2 and 3 remain at baseline. Notice that by Day 20 (ten days of treatment) Classroom 1 has shown a decrease in mean rate of aggressive verbalizations, while 2 and 3 (still untreated) remain at baseline levels. On Day 21, treatment is now implemented in Classroom 2. By Day 30, both 1 and 2 have shown a decrease while 3 remains at baseline. Finally, treatment is applied to Classroom 3 on Day 30, which results in an immediate decrement in problem responding. Thus, *all* classrooms show behavior change contingent on treatment, and all students ultimately receive the treatment. While unspecifiable factors may feasibly produce the change in client behavior in a simple A-B design, the finding that different groups of clients contingently respond to treatment following random assignment to multiple baselines strongly suggests control by the treatment.

The multiple-baseline design is also suitable for evaluating the effects of treatment for an individual case. Figure 13-6 shows a multiple-baseline design

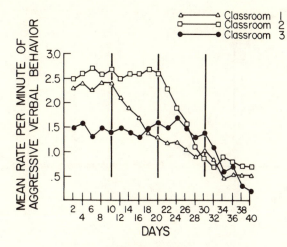

Figure 13-5
Results of self-control treatment across three classrooms
within a multiple-baseline design.

employed to evaluate the effects of verbal self-instructions and response-cost, a treatment for impulse control, across three behaviors displayed by a nine-year-old boy (Kendall and Finch, 1976). The child's impulsive behavior included his switching from one topic of conversation to another, from game to game, and from one rule of play to another. As seen in Figure 13-6, as the treatment was imposed on each target behavior, its incidence was reduced while the other target behaviors (other baselines) were unaffected. The success of the treatment procedure is evident in the change in the target behavior, which occurs only following treatment.

Finally, of course, the BCA may wish to test the efficacy of a treatment across different persons in the same setting; in this case the targeted behavior would remain constant. As for individual behaviors or settings, the persons to be assessed should be randomly assigned to the sequence in which they will receive treatment. Once a treatment effect is observed for the first person, the treatment may then be implemented with the second, leaving the third and other persons to serve as controls. Ultimately, each client in the setting is treated in sequential fashion. One major problem with this approach is that it may be difficult to treat one or more persons in isolation in a setting where multiple persons are present. For example, if we wish to test the effects of modeling fearless behavior on the fearful behavior displayed by a group of children, we could randomly select a given child to be exposed to the modeling while the rest remained untreated. If we perform our treatment (e.g. differentially respond to the "treated" child) in the classroom setting, the other children may also be exposed to the treatment (perhaps incidentally) which eliminates their usefulness as controls. In addition, even if we treat our first

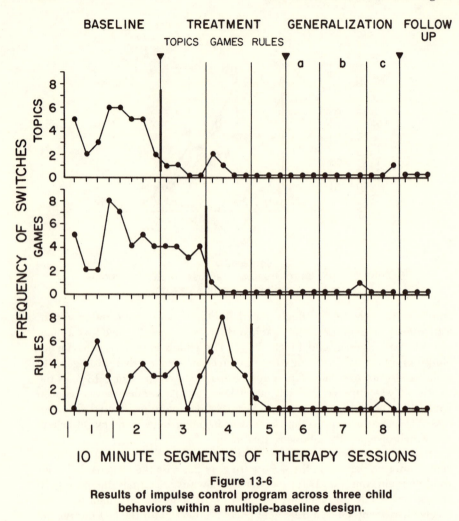

Figure 13-6
**Results of impulse control program across three child
behaviors within a multiple-baseline design.**

subject outside of the classroom setting, placing him back into the classroom
to evaluate the impact of the treatment on his behavior, it is possible that the
other students may learn merely by observing the treated child. This, of
course, reduces their usefulness as controls. In any self-contained setting (e.g.,
a ward, classroom, or even an everyday home situation), it may be difficult to
treat any one person without also influencing the behavior of other persons
present, thus reducing the utility of this multiple-baseline variant.

Methodological Issues Suggested by the Multiple-Baseline Design

The multiple-baseline approach assumes that each of the phenomena ultimately to be treated is independent; that is, that the imposition of treatment on one element (e.g., targeted behavior, setting, person) will not directly affect other elements. Thus, the phenomena should be uncorrelated or unrelated to one another. This is particularly true for the multiple baseline across behaviors. Treatment directed at any one behavior may cause effects that generalize to other behaviors in the client's repertoire. Or, the treatment may increase the client's access to the environment, which may in turn affect the frequency of control behaviors as yet untreated. Thus, the BCA should carefully assess the independence of proposed targets prior to intervention to ensure that they do not seem to be related to one another.

The multiple-baseline design requires that the proposed treatment is relevant and necessary for more than one client behavior, across settings, or across other persons. This may not be the case in a specific situation. Thus, it may be necessary to attempt to alter only one, discrete, circumscribed behavior for a given client. This would effectively eliminate the multiple-baseline approach from consideration (unless *other* persons exhibit similar problem behaviors, function in the same setting, and are willing to be treated, in which case a multiple baseline across persons might be possible).

Another issue, pointed out by Kazdin and Kopel (1975) is that the multiple-baseline approach assumes that all responses, persons, or situations will be affected similarly by a particular treatment, and thus change will be contingent on its application. They point out that this may not be true and that failure of one or more baseline phenomena to change could be indicative of unique person-treatment relationships and not due to the ineffectiveness of the treatment itself. As a well-known example, many parents report the different impact of spanking as a punishment when it is applied to different siblings in the same family (e.g., crying, sullen withdrawal, aggressive behavior, dependent responses). One desirable way of clarifying such possibilities is to increase the number of baselines, thus ensuring that the treatment is applied across a sufficient number of phenomena to yield clear-cut effects (e.g., contingent behavior change for five of six targets). Kazdin and Kopel also point out what may be a faulty assumption of the multiple-baseline strategy: that extraneous events to be controlled for (e.g., those phenomena we previously termed "history" [Campbell and Stanley, 1963]) will affect both treated and untreated behaviors, settings, or persons, while the treatment will *exclusively* affect the treated phenomenon. Obviously an extraneous factor or the treatment itself may have *either* generalizable or unique effects across targeted phenomena. The only way of evaluating these possibilites is to ensure that a sufficient number of baseline phenomena are systematically evaluated and to replicate findings whenever possible.

Finally, the BCA should keep in mind that there is no control for the final behavior to be treated within the multiple-baseline format. Particularly if a restricted number of baselines is employed (e.g., two or three), findings for the final behavior are open to serious question. A simple equation is: the number of baselines being collected (N) minus 1 will yield the number of behaviors with the advantage of a controlled comparison. Noting this in advance, a BCA should plan to provide some other measure of control (e.g., a withdrawal) for the final behavior, particularly if only a few baselines are to be assessed.

Holding the above assumptions in mind, the BCA would do well to consider the multiple-baseline approach when withdrawal of treatment is undesirable and when baseline phenomena can be identified. If the assumptions can be met, problems inherent in this design would seem to be much more readily dealt with than those attributable to the approaches relying on a withdrawal of treatment.

The Simultaneous Treatment Design (A-$\frac{B}{C}$-B- or C or D)

This design is described by Browning (1967) as a solution to the characteristic difficulties of the A-B-A-B design. The A phase again represents the baseline period while B, C, and D are three treatment conditions administered simultaneously and successively in counterbalanced order. The final period, either B, C, or D, indicates that the most effective treatment condition was continued.

This approach is particularly useful when the BCA wishes to evaluate systematically more than one treatment within a *brief* span of time before selecting a final strategy. A withdrawal of treatment is not required and the BCA is not compelled to define and treat more than one targeted behavior. Also, the use of a Latin-square design provides counterbalancing of the order in which the treatments are administered as well as of the BCAs (if more than one) who administer the treatment. Counterbalancing controls for effects that might be due to the sequence or order in which treatments are administered since each treatment proceeds or follows the other treatments an equal number of times.

An excellent case example is provided by McCullough, Cornell, McDaniel, and Mueller (1974). The authors were interested in evaluating the relative efficacy of two popular intervention strategies in increasing the cooperative classroom behavior of a six-year-old boy, Cedric.

Two experimental treatments were compared. The contingencies for Experimental Condition A paired social reinforcement (verbal praise, physical contact) with cooperative behavior, while uncooperative behavior was ignored. The experimenters predicted that praise and physical contact from the teacher would, when delivered following the occurrence of some behavior, increase the frequency of that behavior. This had in fact been observed to occur during the base-rate period. The literature also supported the hypothesis that teacher attention functions as a positive reinforcer for elementary-age children (e.g., Hall, Lund, & Jackson, 1968; Thomas, Becker, & Armstrong, 1968). Withdrawing teacher attention from Cedric for uncooperative behavior was judged to be a potentially punishing consequence. Experimental Condition B paired social reinforcement with cooperative behavior but administered "time out" for uncooperative behavior. Specifically, Cedric was removed from the classroom by either the teacher or the teacher's aide and was alone for two minutes. Both teachers continued to manage their large class while the study was run. The scope of the project was necessarily limited by the classroom demands imposed on the teachers. Thus, no control groups were run to investigate the differential effects that punishment might have had when delivered without any administration of social reinforcement. Time was another important consideration. The teachers wanted to know, as quickly as possible, the best strategy to take with Cedric. The present design, an extinction and counterconditioning program, was constructed to answer their question [p. 290].

Each classroom day was divided into morning (9:00–11:00 A.M.) and afternoon (12:00–2:00 P.M.) periods for data-recording purposes. Following Phase One baseline observations of the frequency of Cedric's behavior, both the teacher and the teacher's aide were trained to administer Conditions A and B. The counterbalanced order of administration is shown in Table 13-1.

Figure 13-7 shows the results of the simultaneous treatment during Phase Two.

Because Condition B (praise plus time out) proved to be superior to Condition A, this procedure was then implemented on a full-time basis in Phase Three. Thus, within a brief period of time, alternative available treatments were systematically evaluated, with the optimum treatment immediately implemented after this evaluation.

A number of advantages of the simultaneous treatment design have already been mentioned. A further advantage is the possibility of statistical analysis of findings using a Latin-square analysis (see Benjamin, 1965). Dis-

Table 13-1
Special Latin Square Design

Time	TREATMENT			
	Day 1	Day 2	Day 3	Day 4
AM	A_{T-1}	B_{T-2}	A_{T-2}	B_{T-1}
PM	B_{T-2}	A_{T-1}	B_{T-1}	A_{T-2}

Note: t-1 = the teacher; T-2 = the teacher's aide. From "Case Report: Utilization of the simultaneous treatment design to improve student behavior in a first-grade classroom" by J. P. McCullough, J. E. Cornell, M. H. McDaniel, and R. K. Mueller, *Journal of Consulting and Clinical Psychology*, 1974, *42*, (2), 288–292. Reprinted by permission.

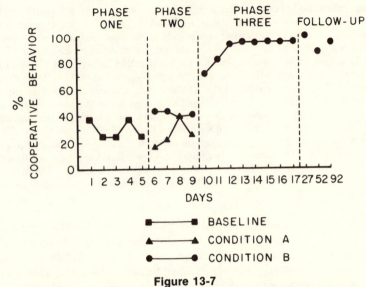

Figure 13-7
**Results of various treatments within a simultaneous treatment
design. From "Utilization of the simultaneous treatment design
to improve student behavior in a first-grade classroom"
by J. P., McCullough, J. E. Cornell, M. H. McDaniel, and R. K. Mueller,
of Consulting and Clinical Psychology, 1974, *42*,
288–292. Reprinted by permission.**

advantages include the planning and coordination required of staff members
in administering a treatment in counterbalanced fashion and the possibility of
carry-over effects. Also, the client may find it difficult to discriminate the different contingencies given that the same staff members administer them,
often for brief periods of time (Kazdin, 1978). It would thus be impossible to
know which specific treatment promoted resulting behavior change.

The Changing-Criterion Design

Initially described by Hall (1971), this design evaluates the impact of
changing treatment contingencies (e.g., number of correct responses that must
be made to earn a reward) on the frequency of the target. If the target
changes in frequency to meet successively different criteria for performance,
this suggests that the treatment is in control of the target. Used frequently to
evaluate the effects of behavior modification contingencies in the classroom
setting (Dietz and Repp, 1973; Hartmann and Hall, 1976), this design could

be employed for any target for which explicit performance criteria can be defined. Hartmann and Hall (1976) present an example of this design in evaluating the math performance of a child who was reinforced (e.g., access to recess, opportunity to play basketball) for his performance. To evaluate whether or not the reinforcers (treatment) actually controlled the student's correct math responses, the authors varied the number of correct responses required to earn a reinforcer over ten treatment phases following an initial baseline period. Figure 13-8 shows the child's performance at each phase (noted by letters).

The authors describe their methodology and results as follows:

During the baseline phase, the teacher gave the student a worksheet with nine division problems. In baseline (Panel A), the number of problems completed decreased from four during the first day to zero. In the first treatment phase (Panel B), the criterion number of problems to be worked was set at two, the next highest whole problem over the baseline mean. The consequences for correctly solving two problems on

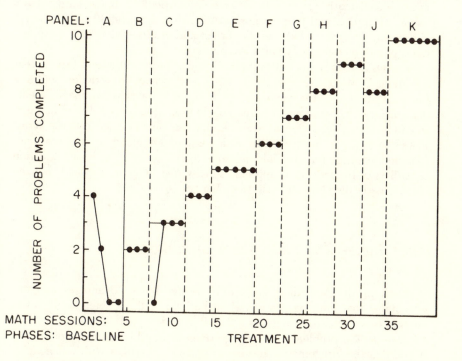

Figure 13-8
Results of a program to enhance a child's math performance within
a changing-criterion design. From "The changing criterion design"
by D. P. Hartmann, and R. V. Hall, *Journal of Applied Behavior*
***Analysis*, 1976, *9*, 527–532. Reprinted by permission**

the worksheet during a 45-min work session included access to recess after the session and the opportunity to play basketball. Failure to complete two problems within the allotted time prolonged math time until the problems were correctly computed. In subsequent treatment phases, identical consequences were in effect and the criterion was advanced by one problem after three consecutive days of performing at the specified level. During the fourth treatment phase (Panel E), the problem criterion level was maintained for five rather than three consecutive days, and during the ninth treatment phase (Panel J), the criterion was dropped one problem, rather than raised one problem. Following this final worksheet phase, the subject was required to solve 10 problems in the math correctly (Panel K) under the same contingency arrangement. During this, as well as prior treatment phases, math performance perfectly matched the criterion rate with but a single exception (Panel C) [p. 528].

Hartmann and Hall (1976) caution that the length of each phase should be sufficiently long for the frequency of the target to "restabilize" at a new and changed rate, the magnitude of behavior change across phases (contingencies) must be sufficiently great to be detectable, particularly if the target shows much variability, and two or more criterion changes should be employed. When correspondence between the target and criterion change is not clear, more phases of criterion change are necessary.

Kazdin (1978) points out that this design is more suitable to targets that are gradually shaped than to those responses that may be instigated within a few presentations of the treatment. He also points out that extraneous events (e.g., history) may confound results. To add to the interpretability of findings, the BCA should decrease as well as increase performance criteria across phases to evaluate the possibility of a continuation effect or historical confounding (e.g., the target would continue to change in a particular direction regardless of the treatment applied). Finally, the BCA must ensure that the client clearly discriminates criterion changes.

The Single-Case Designs: A Summary

Each of the preceding single-case designs holds advantages and disadvantages that must be considered in the light of the specific target(s) and goals of case evaluation. While the B, A-B, B-C, and A-B-A designs offer particularly serious problems from an experimental or ethical vantage point, it is hoped that the foregoing discussions will provide the BCA with sufficient information to make best use of whatever design is selected and to interpret findings with appropriate caution. One or more of the single-case designs is applicable to virtually any evaluation methodology or intervention strategy. When conceived as fundamental to the *planning* of assessment, so that steps can be taken to reduce possible confounds and incorporate a chosen design's features, systematic single-case evaluation becomes practical for all BCAs who wish to move beyond "gut feelings" as the primary criterion for assessing the "goodness" of their efforts with clients. In this age of consumer enlightenment and humanistic values anything less may soon become unacceptable to persons seeking the BCA's services.

Footnotes

[1]This chapter was written as a joint effort. Philip C. Kendall is a member of the faculty of the Psychology Department, University of Minnesota.

[2]These clinically meaningful outcome evaluation criteria (the use of normative data) are much needed in group comparison studies.

References

Adkins, D. A., & Johnson, S. M. An empirical approach to identifying deviant behavior in children. Paper presented at the Western Psychological Association Convention, Portland, Oregon, April, 1972.

Alban, L. S., & Nay, W. R. Reduction of ritual checking by a relaxation-delay treatment. *Journal of Behaviour Therapy and Experimental Psychiatry*, 1976, 7, 151–154.

Alexander, J. F. Defensive and supportive communication in normal and deviant families. *Journal of Consulting and Clinical Psychology*, 1973, 40, 223–231.

Allport, G. W., & Odbert, H. S. Trait-names: A psycho-lexical study. *Psychological Monographs*, 1936, 17, (211).

Arkowitz, H., Lichtenstein, E., McGovern, K., & Hines, P. The behavioral assessment of social competence in males. *Behavior Therapy*, 1975, 6, 3–13.

Arrington, R. E. Time sampling in studies of social behavior: A critical review of techniques and results with research suggestions. *Psychological Bulletin*, 1943, 40, 81–124.

Ax, A. F. The physiological differentiation between fear and anger in humans. *Psychosomatic Medicine*, 1953, 15, 433–442.

Azrin, N. H., & Powell, J. Behavioral engineering: The use of response priming to improve self-medication. *Journal of Applied Behavior Analysis*, 1969, 2, 39–42.

Bailey, K., & Sowder, T. Audiotape and videotape self-confrontation in psychotherapy. *Psychological Bulletin*, 1970, 77, 127–137.

Balaban, R. M. The contribution of participant observation to the study of process in program evaluation. *International Journal of Mental Health*, 1973, 2, 59–70.

Bandura, A. *Principles of behavior modification*. New York: Holt, 1976.

Bandura, A., Blanchard, E., & Ritter, B. Relative efficacy of desensitization and modeling approaches for inducing behavioral, affective and attitudinal changes. *Journal of Personality and Social Psychology*, 1969, 13, 173–199.

Bandura, A., & Kupers, C. Transmission of patterns of self-reinforcement through modeling. *Journal of Abnormal and Social Psychology*, 1964, 69, 1–9.

Bandura, A., & Perloff, B. The efficacy of self-monitoring reinforcement systems. *Journal of Personality and Social Psychology*, 1967, 7, 111–116.

Bandura, A., & Walters, R. *Social learning and personality development*. New York: Holt, 1963.

Barker, R. G., & Wright, H. F. Psychological ecology and the problem of psychosocial development. *Child Development*, 1949, 20, 131–143.

Baker, R. G., & Wright, H. F. *Midwest and its children; the psychological ecology of an American town*. New York: Row, Peterson, 1955.

Barlow, D. H., & Hersen, M. Single case experimental designs. *Archives of general Psychiatry*, 1973, 29, 319–325.

Barrish, H. Saunders, M., & Wolf, M. Good behavior game: Effects of individual contingencies for group consequences on disruptive behavior in a classroom. *Journal of Applied Behavior Analysis*, 1969, 2, 119–124.

Basmajian, J. V. Control and training of individual motor units. *Science*, 1963, 141, 440–441.

Becker, W. C. The relationship of factors in parental ratings of self and each other to the behavior of kindergarten children as rated by mothers, fathers, and teachers. *Journal of Consulting Psychology*, 1960, *24*, 507–527.

Bell, R. Q. Adaptation of small wrist watches for mechanical recording of activity in infants and children. *Journal of Experimenal Child Psychology*, 1968, *6*, 302–305.

Benjamin, A. *The helping interview.* Boston: Houghton Mifflin, 1969.

Benjamin, L. S. A special Latin Square for the use of each subject "as his own control." *Psychometrika*, 1965, *30*, 499–513.

Bernal, M. E., Gibson, D. M., William, D. E., & Pesses, D. I. A device for recording automatic audio tape recording. *Journal of Applied Behavior Analysis*, 1971, *4*, 151–156.

Bernstein, D. A., & Neitzel, M. T. Procedural variation in behavioral avoidance tests. *Journal of Consulting and Clinical Psychology*, 1973, *41*, 165–174.

Bertalanfly, L. V. *Organismic psychology and systems theory.* Worcester, Mass.: Clark University Press, 1968.

Bijou, S. W., Peterson, R. F., & Ault, M. A method to integrate descriptive and experimental field studies at the level of data and empirical concepts. *Journal of Applied behavior Analysis*, 1968, *1*, 175–191.

Bijou, S. W., Peterson, R. F., Harris, F. R., Allen, K. E., & Johnson, M. S. Methodology for experimental studies of young children in natural settings. *The Psychological Record*, 1969, *19*, 177–210.

Blanchard, E. B., & Epstein, L. H. *A biofeedback primer.* Reading, Mass.: Addison-Wesley, 1978.

Blunden, D., Spring, C., & Greenberg, L. M. Validation of the Classroom Behavior Inventory, *Journal of Consulting and Clinical Psychology*, 1974, *42*, 84–88.

Boren, J. J., & Jagodzinski, M. G. The impermanence of data-recording behavior. *Journal of Behavior Therapy and Experimental Psychiatry*, 1975, *6*, 359.

Borkovec, T. D., Fleischmann, D. J., & Caputo J. A. the measurement of anxiety in an analogue social situation. *Journal of Consulting and Clinical Psychology*, 1973, *41*, 157–161.

Borkovec, T. D., Wall, R. L., & Stone, N. M. False physiological feedback and the maintenance of speech anxiety. *Journal of Abnormal Psychology*, 1974, *83*, 164–168.

Borkovec, T. D., Weerts, T. C., & Bernstein, D. A. Assessment of Anxiety. In A. R. Ciminero, K. S. Calhoun, & H. E. Adams (Eds.), *Handbook of behavioral assessment*, New York: Wiley, 1977.

Boyd, R. D., & DeVault, M. V. The observation and recording of behavior. *Review of Educational Research*, 1966, *36*, 529–551.

Brammer, L., & Shostrum, E. *Therapeutic psychology.* Englewood Cliffs, N. J.: Prentice-Hall, 1968.

Broden, M., Hall, R., Dunlap, A., & Clark, R. Effects of teacher atention and a token reinforcement system in a junior high school special education class. *Exceptional Children*, 1970, January, 341–349.

Brown, C. C. A proposed standard nomenclature for physiological measures: A committee report. *Psychophysiology*, 1967, *4*, 260–264.

Brown, C. I. Instruments in psychophysiology. In N. S. Greenfield, & R. A. Sternbach (Eds.), *Handbook of psychophysiology.* New York: Holt, 1972.

Browning, R. M., & Stover, D. O. *Behavior modification in child treatment: an experimental and clinical approach.* Chicago: Aldine-Atherton, 1971.

Bugental, D. E., Love, L. R., & Kaswan, J. W. Videotaped family interaction: Differences reflecting presence and type of child disturbance. *Journal of Abnormal Psychology*, 1972, 79 285–290.

Burgess, E. W., Locke, J. J. and Thomes, M. M. *The Family*. New York: Van Nostrand, Rhinehold, 1971.

Buss, A. H. *Psychopathology*. New York: Wiley, 1966.

Campbell, D. T., & Fiske, D. W. Convergent and discriminant validation by the multitrait-multimethod matrix. *Psychological Bulletin*, 1959, 56, 81–105.

Campbell, D. T., & Stanley, J. C. *Experimental and quasi-experimental designs for research* Chicago: Rand McNally, 1963.

Cannell, C. F., & Kahn, R. L. Interviewing. In G. Lindzey & E. Aronson (Eds.), *The handbook of social psychology* (2nd ed.). Reading, Mass.: Addison-Wesley, 1968.

Carkhuff, R. R. *Helping and human relations: A primer for lay and professional helpers* (Vol. 1). New York: Holt, 1969a.

Carkhuff, R. R. *Helping and human relations: A Primer for lay and professional helpers* (Vol. 2). New York: Holt, 1969b.

Carter, R. D., & Thomas, E. J. A case application of a signaling system (SAM) to the assessment and modification of selected problems of marital communication. *Behavior Therapy*, 1973, 4, 629–645.

Cartwright, R. D. *A primer on sleep and dreaming*. Reading, Mass.: Addison-Wesley, 1978.

Cautela, J. R., & Kastenbaum, R. A reinforcement survey schedule for use in therapy, training, and research. *Psychological Reports*, 1967, 20, 1115–1130.

Cavior, N., & Marabotto, C. M. Monitoring verbal behaviors in a dyadic interaction: Valence of target behaviors, type, timing, and reactivity of monitoring. *Journal of Consulting and Clinical Psychology*, 1976, 44, 68–76.

Chapman, R., Smith, J., & Layden, T. Elimination of cigarette smoking by punishment and self-management training. *Behaviour Research and Therapy*, 1971, 9, 255–264.

Ciminero, A. R., Calhoun, K. S., & Adams, H. E. *Handbook of behavioral assessment*. New York: Wiley, 1977.

Ciminero, A. R., Nelson, R. O., & Lipinski, D. P. Self-monitoring procedures. In A. R. Ciminero, K. S. Calhoun, & H. E. Adams (Eds.), *Handbook of behavioral assessment*. New York, Wiley, 1977.

Cobb, J. A., & Ray, R. S. Manual for coding discrete behaviors in the school setting. Unpublished manuscript, Oregon, Research Institute, 1970.

Cohen, J. A. A coefficient of agreement for nominal scales. *Educational and Psychological Measurement*, 1960, 20, 37–46.

Cone, J. D. The relevance of reliability and validity for behavioral assessment. *Behavior Therapy*, 1977, 8, 411–426.

Cone, J. D., & Hawkins, R. P. (Eds.) *Behavioral assessment: New directions in clinical psychology*. New York: Brunner/Mazel, 1977

Craighead, W. E., & Mahoney, M. J. *Behavior modification: Principles, issues, and applications*. Boston: Houghton Mifflin, 1976.

Cronbach, L. J. *Essentials of psychological testing* (2nd ed.). New York: Harper & Row, 1960.

Cronbach, L. J. *Essentials of psychological testing* (3rd ed.). New York: Harper & Row, 1970.

Cronbach, L. J., Gleser, G. C., Nanda, H., & Rajaratnam, N. *The dependability of be-*

havioral measurements: Theory of generalizability for scores and profiles. New York: Wiley, 1972.

Cronbach, L. J., & Meehl, P. E. Construct validity in psychological tests. *Psychological Bulletin,* 1955, *52*, 281–302.

Crowne, D. P., & Marlowe, D. *The approval motive: Studies in evaluative dependence.* New York: Wiley, 1964.

Cureton, E. E., Cureton, L. W., & Durfee, R. C. A method of cluster analysis. *Multivariate Behavioral Research,* 1970, *5*, 101–116.

Danish, S. J., D'Augelli, A. R., & Brock, G. W. An evaluation of helping skills training: Effects on helper's verbal responses. Unpublished manuscript, University of Pennsylvania, 1975.

Davie, R., Butler, N., & Goldstein, H. *From birth to seven: The second report of the child development study* (1958 cohort). New York: Longman, 1972.

Dawe, H. C. An analysis of two hundred quarrels of preschool children. *Child Development,* 1934, *5*, 139–157.

Deane, G. E. Cardiac activity during experimentally induced anxiety. *Psychophysiology,* 1969, *6*, 17–30.

Deifenderfer, A. J. *Principles of electronic instrumentation.* Philadelphia: Saunders, 1972.

Depue, R., & Fowles, D. Electrodermal activity as an index of arousal in schizophrenics. *Psychological Bulletin,* 1973, *79*, 233–238.

Dietz, S. M., & Repp, A. C. Decreasing classroom misbehavior through the use of DRL schedules of reinforcement. *Journal of Applied Behavior Analysis,* 1973, *6*, 457–463.

Drabman, R., Spitalnik, R., & O'Leary, K. D. Teaching self-control to disruptive children. *Journal of Abnormal Psychology,* 1973, *82*, 10–16.

Dunnette, M. D. *Personnel selection and placement.* Belmont, Calif.: Wadsworth, 1966.

Edelberg, R. Elecrical activity of the skin: Its measurement and uses in psychophysiology. In N. S. Greenfield & R. A. Sternbach (Eds.), *Handbook of psychophysiology.* New York: Holt, 1972.

Edwards, A. A. *The social desirability variable in personality assessment and research.* New York: Dryden, 1957.

Eisler, R. M., Hersen, M., & Agras, W. S. Videotape: A method for the controlled observation of nonverbal interpersonal behavior. *Behavior Therapy,* 1973, *4*, 420–425.

Eisler, R. M., Hersen, M., & Miller, P. M. Effects of modeling on components of assertive behavior. *Journal of Behavior Therapy and Experimental Psychiatry,* 1973, *4*, 1–6.

Eisler, R. M., Miller, P. M., & Hersen, M. Components of assertive behavior. *Journal of Clinical Psychology,* 1973, *29*, 295–299.

Ellis, A. *Reason and emotion in psychotherapy.* New York: Lyle Stuart, 1962.

Eyberg, S. M., & Johnson, S. M. Multiple assessment of behavior modification with families: Effects of contingency contracting and order of treated problems. *Journal of Consulting and Clinical Psychology,* 1974, *42*, 594–606.

Fairweather, G. W., Sanders, D. H., Maynard, H., Cressler, D. L. *Community life for the mentally ill: An alternative to institutional care.* Chicago: Aldine, 1969.

Farber, M. L. Prison research: Techniques and methods. *Journal of Social Psychology,* 1941, *14*, 295–310.

Ferster, C., Nurnberger, J., & Levitt, E. The control of eating. *Journal of Mathematics,* 1962, *1*, 87–109.

Fishbein, M. *Readings in attitude theory and measurement.* New York: Wiley, 1967.

Fite, M. Aggressive behavior in young children and children's attitudes toward aggression. *Genetic Psychological Monographs,* 1940, *22,* 151–319.

Fixsen, D. L., Phillips, E. L., & Wolf, M. M. Achievement place: The reliability of self-reporting and peer-reporting and their effects on behavior. *Journal of Applied Behavior analysis,* 1972, *5,* 19–30.

Freud, S. *Beyond the pleasure principle.* London: International Psychoanalytic Press, 1922.

Freud, S. *New introductory lectures on psychoanalysis,* trans. J. H. Sprott. New York: Norton, 1933.

Friedman, P. R. Legal regulation of applied behavior analysis in mental institutions and prisons. *Arizona Law Review,* 1975, *17,* 39–104.

Fry, P. S. Effects of desensitization treatment on core-condition training. *Journal of Counciling Psychology,* 1973, *20,* 214–219.

Glass, G. V., Wilson, V. L. & Gottman, J. M. *Design and analysis of time-series experiments.* Boulder, Colo.: Colorado Associated University Press, 1973.

Goldfried, M. R., & Davison, G. C. *Clinical behavior therapy.* New York: Holt, 1976.

Goldfried, M. R., & D'Zurilla, T. J. A behavioral-analytic model for assessing competence. In C. D. Spielberger (Ed.), *Current topics in clinical and community psychology* (Vol. 1). New York: Academic Press, 1969.

Goldfried, M. R., & Kent, R. N. Traditional versus behavioral personality assessment: A comparison of methodological and theoretical assumptions. *Psychological Bulletin,* 1972, *77,* 409–420.

Goldfried, M. R., & Sprafkin, J. N. Behavioral personality assessment. In J. T. Spence, R. C. Carson, & J. W. Thibaut (Eds.), *Behavioral approaches to therapy.* Morristown, N. J.: General Learning Press, 1976.

Goldfried, M. R., & Trier, C. S. Effectiveness of relaxation as an active coping skill. *Journal of Abnormal Psychology,* 1974, *83,* 348–355.

Goldiamond, I. Self-control procedures in personal behavior problems. *Psychological Reports,* 1965, *17,* 851–868.

Goldstein, A. P. *Structured learning therapy: Toward a psychotherapy for the poor.* New York: Academic Press, 1973.

Goldstein, A. P. Relationship-enhancement methods. In F. H. Kanfer & A. P. Goldstein (Eds.), *Helping people change.* New York: Pergamon, 1975.

Goldstein, A. P., Martens, J., Hubben, J., Van Belle, H.A., Schaaf, W., Wiersma, H., & Goedhart, A. The use of modeling to increase indepdendent behavior. *Behaviour Research and Therapy,* 1973, *11,* 31–42.

Goldstein, I. B. Electromyography: A measure of skeletal muscle response. In N. S. Greenfield & R. A. Sternbach (Eds.), *Handbook of psychophysiology.* New York: Holt, 1972.

Gottman, J. M., & McFall, R. M. Self-monitoring effects in a program for potential high school dropouts: A time-series analysis. *Journal of Consulting and Clinical Psychology,* 1972, *39,* 273–281.

Gottman, J. M., McFall, R. M.; Barnett, J. T. Design and analysis of research using time series. *Psychological bulletin,* 1969, Vol. 72, 299–306.

Gough, H.G. Predicting social participation. *Journal of Social Psychology,* 1952, *35,* 227–243.

Gough, H. G., Wenk, E. A., & Rozynko, V. V. Parole outcome as predicted from the CPI, the MMPI, and a base expectancy table. *Journal of Abnormal Psychology,* 1965, *70,* 432–441.

Grant, R. L. The Problem-Oriented Record: A critique from a believer. *New England Journal of Medicine*, 1972, *288*, 606–608.

Grant, R. L. Enthusiasm no substitute for hard work. *International Journal of Psychiatry*, 1973, *11*, 366–373.

Grant, R. L., & Maletzky, B. M. A scientific approach to psychiatric record keeping. *Psychiatry in Medicine*, 1972, *3*, 119–129.

Green, E. E., Walters, E. D., Green, A. M., & Murphy, G. Feedback technique for deep relaxation. *Psychophysiology*, 1969, 371–377.

Greenfield, N. S., & Sternbach, R. A. *Handbook of psychophysiology*. New York: Holt, 1972.

Grossman, S. P. *Essentials of Physiological Psychology*. New York: Wiley, 1973.

Gruzelier, J., & Venables, P. Skin conductance orienting activity in a heterogeneous sample of schizophrenics. *Journal of Nervous and Mental Disease*, 1972, *155*, 277–287.

Guilford, J. P. *Psychometric methods* (rev. ed.). New York: McGraw-Hill, 1954.

Gulliksen, H. *Theory of mental tests*. New York: Wiley, 1950.

Gunn, C. G., Wolf, S., Block, R. T., & Person, R. J. Psychophysiology of the cardiovascular system. In N. S. Greenfield & R. A. Sternbach (Eds.), *Handbook of psychophysiology*. New York,: Holt, 1972.

Hagen, R. L., Craighead, W. E., & Paul, G. L. Staff reactivity to evauative behavioral observations. *Behavior Therapy*, 1975, *6*, 201–205.

Haley, J. *Strategies of psychotherapy*. New York: Grune & Stratton, 1963.

Hayley, J. *Problem-solving therapy*. San Francisco: Jossey-Bass, 1976.

Hall, R. V. *Behavior modification, Vol. 1: The measurement of behavior*. Lawrence, Kansas: H & H Enterprises, 1971.

Hall, R. V., Lund, D., & Jackson, D. Effects of teacher attention on study behavior. *Journal of Applied Behavior Analysis*, 1968, *1*, 1–12.

Hall, R., Panyan, M., Rabon, D., & Broden, M. Instructing beginning teachers in reinforcement procedures which improve classroom control. *Journal of Applied Behavior Analysis*, 1968, *1*, 315–322.

Hanley, J., Rickles, W., Crandall, P., & Walters, R. Automatic recognition of EEG correlates of behavior in a chronic schizophrenic patient. *American Journal of Psychiatry*, 1972, *128*, 1524–1528.

Hansen, J. C., Stevic, R. R., & Warner, Jr., R. W. *Counseling: Theory and process*. Boston: Allyn & Bacon, 1972.

Hartman, D. P. Considerations in the choice of interobserver reliability estimates. *Journal of Applied Behavior Analysis*, 1977, *10*, 103–116.

Hartmann, D. P., & Hall, R. V. The changing criterion design. *Journal of Applied Behavior Analysis*, 1976, *9*, 527–532.

Hathaway, S. R., & McKinley, J. C. Minnesota Multiphasic personality inventory: *Manual for administration and scoring*. New York: Psychological Corp., 1967.

Hawkins, R. P., Axelrod, S., & Hall, R. V. Teachers as behavior analysts: Precisely monitoring student performance. In J. A. Brigham, R. P. Hawkins, J. Scott, & J. F. McLaughlin (Eds.), *Behavior analysis in education: Self-control and reading*. Dubuque, Iowa: Kendall-Hunt, 1976.

Hawkins, R. P., & Dotson, V. A. Reliability scores that delude: An Alice in Wonderland trip through the misleading characteristics of inter-observer agreement scores in interval recording. In E. Ramp & G. Semb (Eds.), *Behavioral analysis: Areas of research and application*. Englewood Cliffs, N. J.: Prentice-Hall, 1975.

Hayes, S. C., & Cavior, N. Multiple tracking and the reactivity of self-monitoring: I. Negative behaviors. *Behavior Therapy*, 1977, *8*, 819–831.

Herbert, E. W., & Baer, D. M. Training parents as behavior modifiers. *Journal of Applied Behavior Analysis*, 1972, *5*, 139–149.

Herbert, E. W., Pinkston, E. M., Hayden, M. L., Sajwaj, T. E., Pinkston, S., Cordua, G., & Jackson, C. Adverse effects of differential parental attention. *Journal of Applied Behavior Analysis*, 1973, *6*, 15–30.

Hersen, M., & Barlow, D. H. *Single case experiemntal designs: Strategies for studying behavior change.* New York: Pergamon, 1976.

Hersen, M., & Bellack, A. *The behavior therapy handbook.* New York: Pergamon, 1976.

Hersen, M., & Eisler, R. M. Behavioral approaches to study and treatment of psychogenic ties. *Genetic Psychology Monographs*, 1973, *87*, 289–312.

Hersen, M., Eisler, R. M., & Miller, P. M. An experimental analysis of generalization in assertive training. *Behaviour Research and Therapy*, 1974, *12*, 295–310.

Hoats, D. L. A pair of electronic devices for detecting restricted-band audio and ultrasonic frequencies. *Behavior Research Methods and Instrumentation*, 1975, *7*, 542–544.

Holt, R. P. Clinical and statistical prediction: A reformulation and some new data. *Journal of Abnormal Psychology*, 1958, *56*, 1–12.

Houck, J. E., & Hansen, J. C. Diagnostic interviewing. In R. H. Woody & J. D. Woody (Eds.), *Clinical assessment in counseling and psychotherapy.* Englewood Cliffs, N. J.: Prentice-Hall, 1972.

Itill, T., Saletu, B., & Davis, S. EEG findings in chronic schizophrenics based on digital computer period analysis and analog power spectra. *Biological Psychiatry*, 1972, *5*, 1–13.

Ivey, A. E. *Microcounseling: Innovations in interviewing training.* Springfield, Ill.: Thomas, 1971.

Jackson, B. Treatment of depression by self-reinforcement. *Behavior Therapy*, 1972, *3*, 298–307.

Jacobson, E. *Progressive relaxation* (2nd ed.). Chicago: University of Chicago Press, 1938.

Jersild, A., & Fite, M. *The influence of nursery school experience on children's social adjustment.* New York: Colombia University Press, 1939.

Johnson, S. M., & Bolstad, O. D. Methodological issues in naturalistic observation: Some problems and solutions for field research. In L. A. Hamerlynck, L. C. Handy, & E. J. Mash (Eds.), *Behavior change: Methodology, concepts and practice.* Champaign, Ill.: Research Press, 1973.

Johnson, S. M., & Bolstad, O. D. Reactivity to home observations: A comparison of audio recorded behavior with observers present or absent. *Journal of Applied Behavior Analysis*, 1975, *8*, 181–185.

Johnson, S. M., Bolstad, O. D., & Lobitz, G. K. Generalization and contrast phenomena in behavior modification with children. In L. A. Hamerlynck, L. C. Handy, & E. J. Mash (Eds.), *Behavior modification and families. Vol. 1. Theory and research. Vol. 2. Applications and developments.* New York: Brunner/Mazel, 1976.

Johnson, S. M., Christensen, A., & Bellamy, G. T. Evaluation of family intervention through unobtrusive audio recordings: Experiences in "bugging" children. *Journal of Applied Behavior Analysis*, 1976, *9*, 213–219.

Johnson, S. M., & Lobitz, G. K. Parental manipulations of child behavior in home observations. *Journal of Applied Behavior Analysis*, 1974, *7*, 23–31.

Johnson, S. M., & White, G. Self-observation as an agent of behavioral change. *Behavior Therapy*, 1971, *2*, 488–497.

Jones, R. R. Intraindividual stability of behavior observations: Implications for evaluating behavior modification treatment programs. Paper presented at the meeting of the Western Psychological Association, Portland, Oregon, April, 1972.

Jones, R. R. "Observation" by telephone: An economical behavior sampling technique. *Oregon Research Institute Technical Report*, 1974, *14*, 1–15.

Jones, R. R., Reid, J. B., & Patterson, G. R. Naturalistic observation in clinical assessment. In P. McReynolds (Ed.), *Advances in psychological assessment* (Vol. 3). San Francisco: Jossey-Bass, 1975.

Kallman, W. M., & Feuerstein, M. Psychophysiological procedures. In A. R. Ciminero, K. S. Calhoun, & H. E. Adams (Eds.), *Handbook of behavioral assessment*. New York: Wiley, 1977.

Kamp, A., Schryer, C., & Van Leeuwen, W. Occurrence of "beta bursts" in human frontal cortex related to psychological parameters. *Electroencephalography and Clinical Neurophysiology*, 1972, *33*, 257–267.

Kanfer, F. H. Self-monitoring: Methodological limitations and clinical application. *Journal of Consulting and Clinical Psychology*, 1970, *35*, 148–152.

Kanfer, F. H. Self-management methods. In F. H. Kanfer & A. P. Goldstein, (Eds.), *Helping people change*. New York: Pergamon, 1975.

Kanfer, F. H. & Goldstein, A. P. (Eds.). *Helping people change*. New York: Pergamon, 1975.

Kanfer, F. H. and Marston, A. R. Determinants of self-reinforcement in human learning. *Journal of Experimental Psychology*, 1963, *66*, 245–254.

Kanfer, F. H., & Phillips, J. S. *Learning foundations of behavior therapy*. New York: Wiley, 1970.

Kanfer, F. H., & Saslow, G. Behavioral diagnosis. In C. M. Franks (Ed.), *Behavior therapy: Appraisal and status*. New York: McGraw-Hill, 1969.

Kass, R., & O'Leary, K. The effects of observer bias in field-experimental settings. Paper presented at symposium, University of Kansas, Lawrence, Kansas, 1970.

Katz, M. M., & Lyerly, S. B. Methods for measuring adjustment and social behavior in the community: I. Rationale, description, descriminative validity and scale development. *Psychological Reports*, 1963, *13*, 503–535.

Katz, R. C. A procedure for concurrently measuring elapsed time and response frequency. *Journal of Applied Behavior Analysis*, 1973, *6*, 719–720.

Katz, R. C., & Wooley, F. R. Improving patients' records through problem orientation. *Behavior Therapy*, 1975, *6*, 119–124.

Kazdin, A. E. Self-monitoring and behavior change. In M. J. Mahoney & C. E. Thoresen (Eds.), *Self-control: Power to the person*. Monterey, Calif.: Brooks-Cole, 1974a.

Kazdin, A. E. Reactive self-monitoring: The effects of response desirability, goal setting, and feedback. *Journal of Consulting and Clinical Psychology*, 1974, *42*, 704–716b.

Kazdin, A. E. Methodology of applied behavior analysis. In T. Brigham & A. C. Catania (Eds.), *Handbook of applied behavior research: Social and instructional processes*. New York: Irvington Press/Halsted Press, 1978.

Kazdin, A. E., & Kopel, S. A. On resolving ambiguities of the multiple-baseline design: Problems and recommendations. *Behavior Therapy*, 1975, *6*, 601–608.

Kelly, E. L. Alternate criteria in medical education and their correlates. In A. Anastasi (Ed.), *Testing problems in perspective*. Washington, D. C.: American Council on Education, 1966.

Kelly, E. L., & Fisher, D. W. *Prediction of performance in clinical psychology.* Ann Arbor,; University of Michigan Press, 1951.

Kelly, G. A. *The psychology of personal constructs.* New York: Norton, 1955.

Kendall, M. G., & Buckland, W. R. *Dictionary of statistical terms.* Edinburgh: Oliver and Boyd, 1957.

Kendall, P. C., & Finch, A. J., Jr. A cognitive-beahvioral treatment for impulse control: A case study. *Journal of Consulting and Clinical Psychology,* 1976, *44,* 852–857.

Kent, R. Comment: A methodological critique of "interventions for boys with conduct problems." *Journal of Consulting and Clinical Psychology,* 1976, *44,* 297–302.

Kent, R. N., & Foster, S. L. Direct observational procedures: Methodological issues in naturalistic settings. In A. R. Ciminero, K. S. Calhoun, & H. E. Adams (Eds.), *Handbook of behavioral assessment.* New York: Wiley, 1977.

Kent, R. N., O'Leary, K. D., Diament, C., & Dietz, A. expectation biases in observational evaluation of therpaeutic change. *Journal of Consulting and Clinical Psychology,* 1974, *42,* 774–781.

Kiesler, D. J. Experimental designs in psychotherapy research. In A. E. Bergen & S. L. Garfield (Eds.), *Handbook of psychotherapy and behavior change.* New York: Wiley, 1971.

Kipp, J. J. An investigation of sixth grade students' opinions and interests in school science. *Dissertation Abstracts International,* 1971, *32,* 1983.

Kiresuk, T., & Sherman, R. Goal attainment scaling: A general method for evaluating comprehensive community mental health programs. Community *Mental Health Journal,* 1968, *4,* 443–453.

Knapp, T. J., & Loveless, S. E. Instrumentation and techniques: A simple procedure for determining reliability scores in interval recording. *Behavior Therapy,* 1976, *7,* 557–558.

Kraepelin, E. *Lehrbuch der psychiatrie* (5th ed.). Leipzig: Barth, 1896.

Kubany, E. S., & Sloggett, B. B. Coding procedure for teachers. *Journal of Applied Behavior Analysis,* 1973, *6,* 339–344.

Kuypers, D. S., Becker, W. C., & O'Leary, K. D. How to make a token system fail. *Exceptional Children,* 1968, *35,* 101–109.

Lacey, J. I., Bateman, D. E., & Van Lehn, R. Autonomic response specificity: An experimental study. *Psychosomatic Medicine,* 1953, *15,* 8–21.

Lacey, J. I., & Lacey, B. C. The relationship of resting autonomic activity to motor impulsivity. In H. C. Solomon, S. Cobb, & W. Penfield (Eds.), *The brain and human behavior* (Vol. 36). Baltimore: Williams, & Wilkins, 1958.

Lacey, J. I., & Lacey, B. C. Some autonomic-CNS interrelationships. In P. Black (Ed.), *Physiological correlates of emotion.* New York: Academic Press, 1970.

Lacey, J., & Smith, R. Conditioning and generalization of unconscious anxiety. *Science,* 1954, *120,* 1045–1052.

Lang, P. J. Fear reduction and fear behavior: Problems in treating a construct. In J. M. Shlien (Ed.), *Research in psychotherapy* (Vol. 3). Washington, D. C.: American Psychological Association, 1968.

Lang, P. J. The application of psychophysiological methods to the study of psychotherapy and behavior modification. In A. E. Bergin & S. L. Garfield (Eds.), *Handbook of psychotherapy and behavior change.* New York: Wiley, 1971.

Lang, P. J., & Lazovik, A. D. Experimental desensitization of a phobia. *Journal of Abnormal and Social Psychology,* 1963, *66,* 519–525.

Lang, P. J., Rice, D. G., & Sternbach, R. A. The psychophysiology of emotion. In N. S. Greenfield & R. A. Sternbach (Eds.), *Handbook of psychophysiology*. New York: Holt, 1972.

Lasky, J. J., Hover, G. L., Bostian, D. W., Duffendack, S. C., & Nord, C. L. Post-hospital adjustment as predicted by psychiatric patients and by their staff. *Journal of Consulting Psychology*, 1959, *23*, 213–218.

Lawlis, G. F. A psychological view of the chronically unemployed: Personality and motivation. *Psychological Reports*, 1971, *28*, 838.

Lazarus, A. A. *Behavior therapy and beyond*. New York: McGraw-Hill, 1971.

Lazarus, A. A. *Clinical behavior therapy*. New York: Brunner/Mazel, 1972.

Lazarus, A. A. *Multimodal behavior therapy*. New York: Springer, 1976.

Lazarus, A. A., & Fay, A. *I can if I want to*. New York: Morrow, 1975.

Levine, F., & Grinspoon, L. Telemetered heart rate and skin potential of a chronic patient especially during periods of hallucinations and periods of talking. *Journal of Consulting and Clinical Psychology*, 1971, *37*, 345–350.

Levy, R., Issacs, A., & Behrman, J. Neurophysiological correlates of senile dementia: The sematosensory evoked response. *Psychological Medicine*, 1971, *1*, 159–165.

Lewin, K. *A dynamic theory of personality*. New York: McGraw-Hill, 1935.

Lewinsohn, P. M. Clinical and theoretical aspects of depression. In K. S. Calhoun, H. E. Adams, & K. M. Mitchell (Eds.), *Innovative treatment methods in psychopathology*. New York: Wiley, 1974.

Lewinsohn, P. M., & Atwood, G. E. Depression: A clinical research approach, the case of Mrs. G. *Psychotherapy: Theory, Research, and Practice*, 1969, *6*, 166–171.

Libet, J. M., & Lewinsohn, P. M. Concept of social skill with special reference to the behavior of depressed persons. *Journal of Consulting and Clinical Psychology*, 1973, *40*, 304–312.

Lichstein, K. L., & Wahler, R.G. The ecological assessment of an autistic child. *Journal of Abnormal Child Psychology*, 1976, *4*, 31–54.

Lifshitz, K., & Gradizan, J. Relationship between measures of the coefficient of variation of the mean absolute EEG voltage and spectial intensities in schizophrenics and control subjects. *Biological Psychiatry*, 1972, *5*, 149–163.

Lindsley, O. R. A reliable wrist counter for recording behavior rates. *Journal of Applied Behavior Analysis*, 1968, *1*, 77–78.

Lipinski, D. P., Black, J. L., Nelson, R. O., & Ciminero, A. R. The influence of motivational variables on the reactivity and reliability of self-recoding. *Journal of Consulting and Clinical Psychology*, 1975, *43*, 637–646.

Lipinski, D., & Nelson, R. O. Problems in the use of naturalistic observation as a means of behavioral assessment. *Behavior Therapy*, 1974, *5*, 341–351.

Lira, F., Nay, W. R., McCullough, J. P., & Etkin, M. The relative effects of modeling and roleplaying in reducing avoidance behaviors. *Journal of Consulting and Clinical Psychology*, 1975, *43*, 608–618.

Lobitz, G. K., & Johnson, S. M. Normal versus deviant children: A multimethod comparison. *Journal of Abnormal Child Psychology*, 1975, *3*, 353–374.

Locke, E. A., Cartledge, N., & Koeppel, J. Motivational effects of knowledge of results: A goal setting phenomenon? *Psychological Bulletin*, 1968, *70*, 474–485.

Lorei, T. W. Prediction of community stay and employment for released psychiatric patients. *Journal of Consulting Psychology*, 1967, *31*, 349–357.

Lovaas, O. I., Freitag, G., Gold, V. J., & Kassorla, I. C. Recording apparatus and procedure for observation of behaviors of children in free play settings. *Journal of Experimental Child Psychology*, 1965, *2*, 108–120.

Lubin, B. Adjective checklists for the measurement of depression. *Archives of General Psychiatry*, 1965, *12*, 57–62.

Lyman, R. D., Rickard, H. C., & Elder, I. R. Contingency management of self-report and cleaning behavior. *Journal of Abnormal Child Psychology*, 1975, *3*, 155–162.

Lytton, H. Observation studies of parent-child interaction: A methodological review. *Child Development*, 1971, *42*, 651–684.

Mahoney, M. J. The self-management of covert behavior: A case study. *Behavior Therapy*, 1971, *2*, 575–578.

Mahoney, M. J. Fat fiction. *Behavior Therapy*, 1975, *6*, 416–418.

Mahoney, M. J. Reflections on the cognitive-learning trend in psychotherapy. *American Psychologist*, 1977, *32*, 5–13.

Mahoney, M. J., Moore, B. S., Wade, T. C., & Moura, N. G. M. The effects of continuous and intermittent self-monitoring on academic behavior. *Journal of Consulting and Clinical Psychology*, 1973, *41*, 65–69.

Mahoney, M. J., Moura, N. G. M., & Wade, T. C. Relative efficacy of self-reward, self-punishment, and self-monitoring techniques for weight loss. *Journal of Consulting and Clinical Psychology*, 1973, *40*, 404–407.

Mahoney, M. J., & Thoreson, C. E. *Self-control: Power to the person.* Belmont, Calif.: Brooks/Cole, 1974.

Mahoney, K., Van Wagenen, R. K., & Meyerson, L. Toilet training of normal and retarded children. *Journal of Applied Behavior Analysis*, 1971, *4*, 173–181.

Malmo, R., & Shagass, C. Physiological studies of reaction to stress in anxiety and early schizophrenia. *Psyhosomatic Medicine*, 1949, *11*, 25.

Malmo, R., Smith, A., & Kohlmeyer, W. Motor manifestation of conflict in interview: A case study. *Journal of Abnormal and Social Psychology*, 1956, *52*, 268–271.

Marholin II, D., Siegel, L. J., & Phillips, D. Transfer and treatment: A search for empirical procedures. In M. Hersen, R. M. Eisler, & P. M. Miller (Eds.), *Progress in behavior modifcation* (Vol. 3). New York: Academic Press, 1976.

Mariotto, M. J., Paul, G. L. A multimethod validation of the inpatient multidimensional psychiatric scale with chronically institutionalized patients. *Journal of Consulting and Clinical Psychology*, 1974, *42*, 497–508.

Martin, P. J., & Lindsey, C. J. Irregular discharge as an unobtrusive measure of . . . something: Some additional thoughts. *Psychological Reports*, 1976, *38*, 627–630.

Martin, R. *Legal challenges to behavior modification.* Champaign, Ill.: Research Press, 1975.

Mash, E. J., & Terdal, L. G. (Eds.). *Behavior therapy assessment: Diagnosis, design, and evaluation.* New York: Springer, 1976.

McArthur, M., & Hawkins, R. The modification of several classroom behaviors of an emotionally disturbed child in a regular classroom. In R. Ulrich, T. Stachnik, & J. Mabrey (Eds.), *Control of human behavior: Behavior modification in education.* Glenview, Ill.: Scott, Foresman, 1974.

McCullough, J. P. Procedural-evaluational manual for the VCU psychological services center. Unpublished manuscript, September, 1973.

McCullough, J. P., Cornell, J. E., McDaniel, M. H., & Mueller, R. K. Utilization of the simultaneous treatment design to improve student behavior in a first-grade classroom. *Journal of Consulting and Clinical Psychology*, 1974, *42*, 471–481.

McFall, R. Effects of self-monitoring on normal smoking behavior. *Journal of Consulting and Clinical Psychology*, 1970, *35*, 135–142.

McFall, R. M. Analogue methods in behavioral assessment: Issues and prospects. In J. D. Cone & R. P. Hawkins (Eds)., *Behavioral assessment: New directions in clinical psychology*. New York: Brunner/Mazel, 1977.

McFall, R., & Hammen, E. Motivation, structure and self-monitoring: Role of non-specific factors in smoking reduction. *Journal of Consulting and Clinical Psychology*, 1971, *37*, 80–86.

McFall, R. M., & Lillesand, D. B. Behavior rehearsal with modeling and coaching in assertion training. *Journal of Abnormal Psychology*, 1971, *77*, 313–323.

McFarland, M. *Relationships between young sisters as revealed in their overt responses*. New York: Columbia University Press, 1938.

McGee, R. K. *Crisis prevention in the community*. Baltimore; University Park Press, 1974.

McGuigan, F., & Pavek, G. On the psychophysiological identification of covert nonoral language processes. *Journal of Experimental Psychology*, 1972, *92*, 237–245.

McLaughlin, J. G., & Nay, W. R. Treatment of trichotillomania with positive coverants and response cost. *Behavior Therapy*, 1975, *6*, 87–91.

McNamera, J. Teacher and students as sources for behavior modification in the classroom. *Behavior Therapy*, 1971, *2*, 205–213.

McNamera, J. The use of self-monitoring techniques to treat nailbiting. *Behaviour Research and Therapy*, 1972, *10*, 193–194.

Meehl, P. E. *Clinical versus statistical prediction: A theoretical analysis and a review of the evidence*. Minneapolis: University of Minnesota Press, 1954.

Meichenbaum, D. Self-instructional methods. In F. H. Kanfer & A. P. Goldstein (Eds.), *Helping people change*. New York: Pergamon, 1975.

Melbin, M. An interaction recording device for participant observers. *Human Organization*, 1954, *13*, 29–33.

Mercatoris, M., Hahn, L. G., & Craighead, W. E. Mentally retarded residents as paraprofessionals in modifying mealtime behavior. *Journal of Abnormal Psychology*, 1975, *84*, 299–302.

Miller, L. C., Hampe, E., Barrett, C. L., & Noble, H. Children's deviant behavior within the general population. *Journal of Consulting and Clinical Psychology*, 1971, *37*, 16–22.

Mischel, W. *Personality and assessment*. New York: Wiley, 1968.

Mischel, W., & Liebert, R. Effects of discrepancies between observed and imposed reward criteria on their acquisition and transmission. *Journal of Personality and Social Psychology*, 1966, *3*, 45–53.

Morales v. Turman, 383 F. Supp. 53 (E. D. Tex. 1974).

Morganstern, K. P. Behavioral interviewing: The initial stages of assessment. In M. Hersen & A. Bellack (Eds.), *Behavioral assessment: A practical handbook*. New York: Pergamon, 1976.

Nay, W. comprehensive behavioral treatment in a training school for delinquents. In K. Calhoun, H. Adams, & K. Mitchell (Eds.), *Innovative treatment methods in psychopathology*. New York: Wiley, 1974.

Nay, W. R. A systematic comparison of instructional techniques for parents. *Behavior Therapy*, 1975, *6*, 14–21.

Nay, W. R. *Behavioral intervention: Contemporary strategies*. New York: Gardner Press, 1976.

Nay, W. R. Analogue measures. In A. R. Ciminero, K. S. Calhoun, & H. E. Adams (Eds.), *Handbook of behavioral assessment*. New York: Wiley, 1977.

Nay, W., & Kerkoff, T. Informational feedback in training behavioral coders. *Psychological Reports*, 1974, *35*, 1175–1181.

Nelson, R. O., Lipinski, D. P., & Black, J. L. The reactivity of adult retardates' self-monitoring: A comparison among behaviors of different valences, and a comparison with token reinforcement. *Psychological Record*, 1976, *26*, 189–201.

Nelson, C. M., & McReynolds, W. T. Self-recording and control of behavior: A reply to Simkins. *Behavior Therapy*, 1971, *2*, 594–597.

Noble, P., & Lader, M. An electromyographic study of depressed patients. *Journal of Psychosomatic Research*, 1971, *15*, 233–239.

Norman, A. Biotelemetry and developmental psychology: Preliminary observations of heart rate change during unrestrained activity. *Proceedings of the Annual Convention of the American Psychological Association*, 1970, *5*, 313–314.

Notterman, J. Schoenfeld, W., & Bersh, P. Conditioned heart rate responses in human beings during experimental anxiety. *Journal of Comparative Physiological Psychology*, 1952, *45*, 1–8.

Ober, D. C. Modification of smoking behavior. *Journal of Consulting and Clinical Psychology*, 1968, Vol. 32, 543–549.

O'Brien, F., Azrin, N. H., & Bugle, C. Training profoundly retarded children to stop crawling. *Journal of Applied Behavior Analysis*, 1972, *5*, 131–137.

O'Leary, K. D., & Drabman, R. Token reinforcement programs in the classroom: A review. *Psychological Bulletin*, 1971, *75*, 379–398.

O'Leary, K., & Kent, R. Behavior modification for social action: Research tactics and problems. In L. A. Hamerlynck, L. C. Handy, & E. J. Mash (Eds.), *Behavior change: Methodology, concepts, and practice*. Champaign: Ill.: Research Press, 1973.

O'Leary, K. D., Kent, R. N., & Kanowitz, J. Shaping data collection congruent with experimental hypotheses. *Journal of Applied Behavior Analysis*, 1975, *8*, 43–51.

O'Leary, K. D., Romanczyk, R. G., Kass, R. E., Dietz, A., & Santogrossi, D. Procedures for classroom observation of teachers and children. Unpublished manuscript, State University of New York at Stony Brook, 1971.

Orne, M. T. Demand characteristics and the concept of quasi-controls. In R. Rosenthal & R. Rosnow (Eds.), *Artifact in behavioral research*. New York: Academic Press, 1969.

Osgood, C. E., Suci, G. J., & Tannenbaum, P. H. *The measurement of meaning*. Urbana: University of Illinois Press, 1957.

Paden, R. C., Himelstein, H. C., & Paul, G. L. Videotape vs. verbal feedback in the modification of meal behavior of chronic mental patients. *Journal of Consulting and Clinical Psychology*, 1974, *42*, 623.

Palmer, J., & McGuire, F. The use of unobtrusive measures in mental health research. *Journal of Consulting and Clinical Psychology*, 1973, *40*, 431–436.

Patterson, G. R. Interventions for boys with conduct problems: Multiple settings, treatments, and criteria. *Journal of Consulting and Clinical Psychology*, 1974, *42*, 471–481.

Patterson, G. R., Cobb, J. A., & Ray, R. S. Direct intervention in the classroom: A set of procedures for the aggressive child. In F. W. Clark, D. R. Evans, & L. A. Hamerlynck (Eds.), *Implementing behavioral programs for schools and clinics*. Champaign, Ill.: Research Press, 1972.

Patterson, G. R., Cobb, J. A., & Ray, R. S. A social engineering technology for retraining the families of aggressive boys. In H. E. Adams, & I. P. Unikel (Eds.), *Issues and trends in behavior therapy*. Springfield, Ill.: Thomas, 1973.

Patterson, G. R., & Harris, A. Some methodological considerations for observation procedures. Paper presented at the meeting of the American Psychological Association, San Francisco, September, 1968.

Patterson, G. R., Ray, R. S., Shaw, D. A., & Cobb, J. A. *A manual for coding of family interactions.* New York: Microfiche Publications, 1969.

Paul, G., & Lentz, R. J. *A comparative study of milieu versus social learning programs.* Cambridge, Mass.: Harvard University Press, 1977.

Pfeiffer, J., & Heslin, R. *Instrumentation in human relations training.* Iowa City: Univsersity Associates, 1975.

Porter, R., Wolf, A., & Penry, J. Human electroencephalographic telemetry: A review of systems and their applications and a new receiving system. *American Journal of EEG Technology,* 1971, *11,* 145–149.

Powell, J. Martindale, A., & Kulp, S. An evaluation of time-sample measures of behavior. *Journal of Applied Behavior Analysis,* 1975, *8,* 463–469.

Purcell, K., & Brady, K. *Assessment of interpersonal behavior in natural settings: A research technique and manual.* Denver, Colo.: Children's Asthma Research Institute, 1965.

Putnam, D. G., Kiesler, D. J., Bent, R. J., & Stewart, A. Goal attainment scaling manual. Unpublished manuscript, 1972, rev. 1973.

Rappaport, J. *Community psychology: Values, research and action.* New York: Holt, 1977.

Raush, H. L. On the locus of behavior: Observations in multiple settings within residential treatment. Symposium on "Observation research with emotionally disturbed children: Session 1," 1958.

Raush, H. L., & Bordin, E. S. Warmth in personality development and in psychotherapy. *Psychiatry,* 1957, *20,* 351–363.

Redfield, J., & Paul, G. L. Bias in behavioral observation as a function of observer familiarity with subjects and typicality of behavior. *Journal of Consulting and Clinical Psychology,* 1976, *44,* 156.

Reid, J. B. Reliability assessment of observation data: A possible methodological problem. *Child Development,* 1970, *41,* 1143–1150.

Reid, J. B., & DeMaster, B. The efficacy of the spot-check procedure in maintaining the reliability of data collected by observers in quasi-natural settings: Two pilot studies. *Oregon Research Institute Bulletin,* 1972, *12.*

Reid, J. B., & Hendriks, A. F. A preliminary analysis of the effectiveness of direct home intervention for treatment of predelinquent boys who steal. In L. A. Hamerlynck, L. C. Handy, & E. J. Mash (Eds.), *Behavior change: Methodology, concepts, and practice.* Champaign, Ill.: Research Press, 1973.

Reid, J. B., & Patterson, G. R. Follow-up analyses of a behavioral treatment program for boys with conduct problems: A reply to Kent. *Journal of Consulting and Clinical Psychology,* 1976, *44,* 297–302.

Reid, J. B., Skindrud, K. D., Taplin, P. S., & Jones, R. R. The role of complexity in the collection and evaluation of observation data. Paper presented at the meeting of the American Psychological Association, Montreal, Canada, August, 1973.

Repp, A. C., Dietz, D. E., Boles, S. M., Dietz, S. M., & Repp, C. F. Differences among common methods for calculating interobserver agreement. *Journal of Applied Behavior Analysis,* 1976, *9,* 109–113.

Rimm, D., & Masters, J. *Behavior therapy.* New York: Academic Press, 1974.

Risley, T. R., & Hart, B. M. Developing correspondence between the non-verbal and verbal behavior of preschool children. *Journal of Applied Behavior Analysis,* 1968, *1,* 267–281.

Roberts, R., & Renzaglia, G. The influence of tape recording on counseling. *Journal of Counseling Psychology*, 1965, *12*, 10–16.

Rogers, C. *Client-centered therapy*. Boston: Houghton Mifflin, 1951.

Rogers, C. Client-centered psychotherapy. *Scientific American*, 1952, *187*, 66–74.

Romanczyk, R. G. Self-monitoring in the treatment of obesity: Parameters of reactivity. *Behavior Therapy*, 1974, *5*, 531–540.

Romanczyk, R. G., Kent, R. N., Diament, C., & O'Leary, K. D. Measuring the reliability of observational data: A reactive process. *Journal of Applied Behavior Analysis*, 1973, *6*, 175–184.

Romanoff, B. D., Lewittes, D. J., & Simmons, W. L. Accuracy of "significant others" judgments of behavior change. *Journal of Counseling Psychology*, 1976, *23*, 409–413.

Rosenhan, D. On being sane in insane places. *Science*, 1973, *179*, 250–258.

Rosenthal, R. *Experimental effects in behavioral research*. New York: Appleton-Century-Crofts, 1966.

Rosenthal, R., & Fode, K. L. The effect of experimental bias on the performance of the albino rat. *Behavior Science*, 1963, *8*, 183–189.

Rosenthal, R., & Jacobson, L. Teachers' expectancies: Determinants of pupils' IQ gains. *Psychological Reports*, 1966, *19*, 115–118.

Rosenthal, R., & Jacobson, L. *Pygmalion in the classroom: Teacher expectation and pupils' intellectual development*. New York: Holt, 1968.

Rubin, S. E., Lawlis, G. F., Tasto, D. L., & Namenek, T. Factor analysis of the 122-item fear survey schedule. *Behaviour Research and Therapy*, 1969, *7*, 381–386.

Rugh, J. D., & Schwitzgebel, R. L. Instrumentation for behavioral assessment. In A. R. Ciminero, K. S. Calhoun, & H. E. Adams (Eds.), *Handbook of behavioral assessment*. New York: Wiley, 1977.

Rutner, I. T., & Bugle, C. An experimental procedure for the modification of psychotic behavior. *Journal of Consulting and Clinical Psychology*, 1969, *33*, 651–653.

Sandifer, M. G., Jr., Pettus, C., & Quade, D. A study of psychiatric diagnosis. *Journal of Nervous and Mental Disease*, 1964, *139*, 350–356.

Sands, W. L. Psychiatric history and mental status. In A. M. Freedman, H. I. Kaplan, & H. S. Kaplan (Eds.), *Comprehensive textbook of psychiatry*. Baltimore: Williams & Wilkins, 1967.

Santogrossi, D., O'Leary, K., Romanczyk, R., & Kaufman, K. Self-evaluation by adolescents in a psychiatric hospital school token program. *Journal of Applied Behavior Analysis*, 1973, *6*, 277–287.

Sarason, I. G., & Ganzer, V. J. Modeling and group discussion in the rehabilitation of juvenile delinquents. *Journal of Consulting Psychology*, 1973, *20*, 442–449.

Schachter, J. Pain, fear, and anger in hypertensives and normotensives: A psychophysiological study. *Psychosomatic Medicine*, 1957, *19*, 17–29.

Schmidt, H. O., & Fonda, C.P. The reliability of psychiatric diagnosis: A new look. *Journal of Abnormal and Social Psychology*, 1956, *52*, 262–267.

Schwitzgebel, R. L., & Schwitzgebel, R. K. (Eds.), *Psychotechnology: Electronic control of mind and behavior*. New York: Holt, 1973.

Sechrest, L. B. Personality. *Annual Review of Psychology* (vol. 27). Palo Alto, CA: Annual Reviews, 1976.

Sellitz, C., Johoda, M., Deutch, M., & Cook, S. *Research methods in social relations*. New York: Holt, 1959.

Serber, M. Teaching nonverbal components of assertive training. *Journal of Behavior Therapy and Experimental Psychiatry*, 1972, *3*, 179–183.

Shagass, C., & Malmo, R. Psychodynamic themes and localized muscular tension during psychotherapy. *Psychosomatic Medicine*, 1954, *16*, 295–313.

Shaw, D. A. Family maintenance schedules for deviant behavior. Doctoral dissertation, University of Oregon, 1971.

Sidman, M. *Tactics of scientific research.* New York: Basic Books, 1960.

Sidowski, J. B. *Experimental methods and instrumentation in psychology.* New York: McGraw-Hill, 1966.

Simkins, L. The reliability of self-recorded behaviors. *Behavior Therapy*, 1971, *2*, 83–87, (a).

Simkins, L. A. rejoinder to Nelson and McReynolds on the self-recording of behavior. *Behavior Therapy*, 1971, Vol. 2, 598–601, (b).

Skindrud, K. D. An evaluation of observer bias in experimental-field studies of social interaction. Unpublished doctoral dissertation, University of Oregon, 1972.

Skinner, B. F. The operational analysis of psychological terms. In H. Feigl & M. Brodbeck (Eds.), *Readings in the philosophy of science.* New York: Appleton-Century-Crofts, 1953.

Skinner, B. F. *Verbal behavior.* New York: Appleton-Century-Crofts, 1957.

Sklar, B., Hanley, J., & Simmons, W. An EEG experiment aimed toward identifying dyslexic children. *Nature*, 1972, *240*, 414–416.

Smith, R. E., Diener, E., & Beaman, A. L. Demand characteristics and the behavioral avoidance measure of fear in behavior therapy analogue research. *Behavior Therapy*, 1974, *5*, 172–182.

Snyder, M. The self-monitoring of expressive behavior. *Journal of Personality and Social Psychology*, 1974, *30*, 526–537.

Sobell, M. B., & Sobell, L. C. Individualized behavior therapy for alcoholics: Rationale, procedures, preliminary results and appendix. *California Mental Health Research Monographs*, 1972, *13*, 1–81.

Sommer, R. G. Guide to scientific instruments. *Science*, 1974, *186*, 9–162.

Soskin, W., & John, V. The study of spontaneous talk. In R. G. Barker (Ed.), *The stream of behavior.* New York: Appleton-Century-Crofts, 1963.

Stallings, W. M., & Gillmore, G. M. A note on "accuracy" and "precision." *Journal of Educational Measurement*, 1971, *8*, 127–129.

Sterman, M., & Friar, L. Suppression of seizures in an epileptic following sensorimotor EEG feedback training. *Electroencephalography and Clinical Neurophysiology*, 1972, *33*, 89–95.

Sternbach, R. A. A comparative analysis of autonomic responses in startle. *Psychosomatic Medicine*, 1960, *22*, 204–210.

Sternbach, R. A. *Pain: A psychophysiological analysis.* New York: Academic Press, 1968.

Stevens, J., Lonsburg, B., & Cole, S. Electroencephalic spectra and reaction time in disorders of higher nervous functions. *Science*, 1972, *176*, 1346–1349.

Stone, L. J. Experiments in group play and readiness for destruction In E. Lerner & L. B. Murphy (Eds.), Methods for the study of personality of young children. *Monographs of the Society for Research in Child Development*, 1941, *23*, 227–233.

Stuart, R. B. A three-dimensional program for the treatment of obesity. *Behaviour Research and Therapy*, 1971, *9*, 177–186.

Stuart, R., & Davis, B. *Slim chance in a fat world.* Champaign, Ill.: Research Press, 1972.

Sullivan, H. S. *The interpersonal theory of psychiatry*. New York: Norton, 1953.

Sullivan, H. S. *The psychiatric interview* (1st ed.). New York: Norton, 1954.

Suratt, P. E., Ulrich, R., & Hawkins, R. An elementary student as a behavioral engineer. *Journal of Applied Behavior Analysis*, 1969, *2*, 85–92.

Tallent, N. *Psychological report writing*. Englewood Cliffs, N. J.: Prentice-Hall, 1976.

Taplin, P. S., & Reid, J. B. Effects of instructional set and experimenter influence on observer reliability. *Child Development*, 1973, *44*, 547–554.

Tasto, D. L. Self-report schedules and inventories. In A. R. Ciminero, K. S. Calhoun, & H. E. Adams (Eds.), *Handbook of behavioral assessment*. New York: Wiley, 1977.

Tasto, D. L., & Hickson, R. Standardization item analysis and scaling of the 122-item Fear Survey Schedule. *Behavior Therapy*, 1970, *1*, 473–484.

Terman, L. M., & Merrill, M. *Measuring intelligence: A guide to the administration of the new revised Stanford-Binet tests of intelligence*. Boston: Houghton Mifflin, 1960.

Thomas, D. R., Becker, W. C., & Armstrong, M. Production and elimination of disruptive classroom behavior by systematically varying teacher's behavior. *Journal of Applied Behavior Analysis*, 1968, *1*, 35–45.

Thompson, R. F. *Foundations of Physiological Psychology*. New York: Harper & Row, 1967.

Thompson, R. F., Lindsley, D. B., & Eason, R. G. Physiological psychology. In J. B. Sidowski (Ed.), *Experimental methods and instrumentation in psychology*, New York: McGraw-Hill, 1966.

Thorne, F. C. *Principles of psychological examining: A systematic textbook of applied integrative psychology*. Brandon, Vermont: *Journal of Clinical Psychology*, 1955.

Toepfer, C., Reuter, J., & Maurer, C. Design and evaluation of an obedience training program for mothers of preschool children. *Journal of Consulting and Clinical Psychology*, 1972, *39*, 194–198.

Truax, C. B., & Carkhuff, R. R. *Toward effective counseling and psychotherapy*. Chicago: Aldine, 1967.

Ullmann, L. P., & Gruel, L. Validity of symptom rating from psychiatric records. *Archives of General Psychiatry*, 1962, *7*, 130–134.

Ullmann, L. P., & Hunrichs, W. A. The role of anxiety of psychodiagnosis: Replication and extension. *Journal of Clinical Psychology*, 1958, *14*, 276–279.

Ulrich, R. E., Stachnik, T. J., & Stainton, W. R. Student acceptance of generalized personality interpretations. *Psychological Reports*, 1963, *13*, 831–834.

Venables, P. H., & Martin, I. The relation of palmar sweat gland activity to level of skin potential and conductance. *Psychophysiology*, 1967, *3*, 302–311.

Voas, R. B. Generalization and consistency of muscle tension level. Unpublished doctoral dissertation, University of California, Los Angeles, 1952.

Wahler, R. G., House, A. E., & Stambaugh, E. E. *Ecological assessment of child problem behavior: A clinical package for home, school, and institutional settings*. New York: Pergamon, 1976.

Wahler, R. G., & Leske, G. Accurate and inaccurate observer summary reports, *The Journal of Nervous and Mental Disease*, 1973, *15*, 386–394.

Walker, H. M. *Walker problem behavior identification checklist*. Los Angeles: Western Psychological Services, 1970.

Wallen, R. W. *Clinical psychology: The study of persons*. New York: McGraw-Hill, 1956.

Walter, H. I., & Gilmore, S. K. Placebo versus social learning effect in parent training procedures designed to alter the behavior of aggressive boys. *Behavior Therapy*, 1973, *4*, 361–377.

Ward, C. H., Beck, A. T., Mendelson, M., Mock, J. E., & Erbaugh, J. K. The psychiatric nomenclature: Reasons for diagnostic disagreement. *Archives of General Psychiatry*, 1962, *7*, 198–205.

Watson, D., & Friend, R. Measurement of social-evaluative anxiety. *Journal of Consulting and Clinical Psychology*, 1969, *33*, 448–551.

Watson, D., & Tharp, R. *Self-directed behavior: Self-modification for personal adjustment*. Monterey, Calif.: Brooks/Cole, 1972.

Watzawick, P., Beavin, J. H., & Jackson, D. D. *Pragmatics of human communication: A study of interactional patterns pathologies, and paradoxes.* New York: Norton, 1967.

Webb, E. J., Campbell, D. T. Schwartz, R. D., & Sechrest, L. *Unobtrusive measures: A survey of nonreactive research in the social sciences.* Chicago: Rand McNally, 1966.

Wechsler, D. *Wechsler Intelligence Scale for Children: Manual.* New York: Psychological Corp., 1949.

Wechsler, D. *The Wechsler Intelligence Scale for Children* (Rev. ed.). New York: Psychological Corp., 1958.

Weed, L. L. *Medical records, medical evaluation and patient care.* Cleveland: Case Western Reserve University, 1970.

Weick, K. E. Systematic observational methods. In G. Lindzey & E. Aronson (Eds.), *The handbook of social psychology* (Vol. 2), 2nd ed. Reading, Mass.: Addison-Wesley, 1968.

White, G. The effects of observer presence on mother and child behavior. Doctoral dissertation, University of Oregon, 1972.

Wiggins, J. S. *Personality and prediction: Principles of personality assessment.* Reading, Mass.: Addison-Wesley, 1973.

Wiggins, N., Blackburn, M., & Hackan, J. R. Prediction of first-year graduate success in psychology. *Journal of Educational Research*, 1969, *63*, 81–85.

Williams, R. J., & Brown, R. A. Differences in baseline drinking behavior between New Zealand alcoholics and normal drinkers. *Behaviour Research and Therapy*, 1974, *12*, 287–294.

Winer, B. J. *Statistical principles in experimental design.* New York: McGraw-Hill, 1962.

Wolach, A. H., Roccaforte, P., & Breuning, S. E. Converting an electronic calculator into a counter. *Behavior Research Methods and Instrumentation*, 1975, *7*, 365–367.

Wolach, A. H., Roccaforte, P., & Van Berschot, S. N. Converting an electronic calculator into a combination stopwatch-calculator. *Behavior Research Methods and Instrumentation*, 1975, *7*, 549–551.

Wolf, M. M., & Risley, T. R. Reinforcement: Applied research. In R. Glaser (ed.), *The nature of reinforcement.* New York: Academic Press, 1971.

Wolpe, J. *The practice of behavior therapy.* New York: Pergamon, 1973.

Wolpe, J., & Lang, P. J. *Fear Survey Schedule.* San Diego,: Educational and Industrial Testing Service, 1969.

Woodworth, R. S., & Schlosberg, H. *Experimental psychology* (Rev. ed.). New York: Holt, 1954.

Wright, H. Observational child study. In P. H. Mussen (Ed.), *Handbook of research methods in child development.* New York: Wiley, 1960.

Wyatt, V. Stickney, 344 F. Supp. 373, 380 (M. D. Ala. 1972).

Zigler, E., & Phillips, L. Psychiatric diagnosis: A critique. *Journal of Abnormal and Social Psychology*, 1961, *63*, 607–618.

Zimet, C. N., & Brackbill, G. A. The role of anxiety in psychodiagnosis. *Journal of Nervous and Mental Disease*, 1956, *12*, 173–177.

Zubin, J. A cross-cultural approach to pshchopathology and its implications for diagnostic classification. In L. D. Eron (Ed.), *The classification of behavior disorders*. Chicago: Aldine, 1966.

Author Index

Adams, H., 13, 255, 283
Adkins, D., 176
Agras, S., 200
Alban, L., 145
Alexander, J., 200
Allen, K., 220
Allport, G., 157
Arkowitz, H., 198
Arrington, R., 204, 218
Atwood, G., 127
Ault, M., 30
Ax, A., 263
Axelrod, S., 145, 151
Azrin, N., 204, 205

Baer, D., 139
Bailey, K., 146, 199
Balaban, 188
Bandura, A., 30, 33, 34, 35, 103
Barker, R., 155, 181, 189, 190
Barlow, D., 316
Barnett, J., 318
Barrett, D., 98
Barrish, H., 163
Basmajian, J., 266
Bateman, D., 263
Beaman, 257
Beavin, J., 30
Beck, A., 9
Becker, W., 112, 114, 184
Behrman, J., 267
Bell, R., 148
Bellack, A., 13, 255
Bellamy, G., 145, 146, 185, 216
Benjamin, A., 60, 61, 62, 63, 67, 329
Bent, R., 106
Bernal, M., 146
Bernstein, D., 200
Bersh, P., 262
Bertalanfly, L., 22
Bijou, S., 30, 220, 223, 224
Binet, 7
Black, J., 119, 136, 140
Blackburn, M., 186
Blanchard, E., 35, 103, 266

Bleuler, 7
Black, R., 262
Blunden, D., 111, 112
Boles, S., 204, 223
Bolstad, O., 112, 145, 146, 183, 184, 185, 235, 241, 242, 250
Bordin, E., 59
Boren, J., 140
Borkovec, T., 114, 200, 201
Bostian, D., 37 (see Lasky et al.)
Boyd, R., 204
Brackbill, G., 9, 10
Brady, K., 146
Brammer, L., 81, 90
Breuning, S., 145, 216
Brock, G., 78
Broden, M., 163
Brown, C., 256, 257, 258, 259, 260, 261, 262
Brown, R., 200
Browning, R., 314, 316, 328
Buckland, 219
Bugental, D., 176
Bugle, C., 138, 204, 205
Burgess, E., 100
Buss, A., 107
Butler, N., 98

Calhoun, K., 13, 255, 283
Campbell, D., 113, 125, 149, 150, 151, 177, 178, 317, 318, 327
Cannell, C., 49, 50, 69, 71
Caputo, J., 114
Carkhuff, R., 49, 58, 59, 67
Carter, R., 200
Cartledge, N., 120
Cartwright, R., 266
Cautela, J., 111
Cavior, N., 136, 137, 139
Chapman, R., 119, 124
Christensen, A., 145, 146, 185, 216
Ciminero, A., 13, 119, 124, 133
Clark, R., 163
Cobb, J., 100, 103, 158, 163, 164, 167, 171, 174, 176, 181, 184, 212, 213, 237
Cohen, J., 225

Cole, S., 267
Cone, J., 13
Cook, S., 188
Cordua, G., 200
Cornell, J., 328
Craighead, W., 42, 183, 184
Crandall, P., 267
Cressler, D., 11, 37
    (*see* Fairweather et al.)
Cronbach, L., 2, 95, 108, 110, 119, 220, 231,
    232, 235
Crowne, D., 115
Cureton, E., 192
Cureton, L., 192

Danish, S., 78
D'Augelli, A., 78
Davie, R., 98
Davis, B., 127
Davis, S., 267
Davison, G., 13, 58, 80
Dawe, H., 206
Deanne, G., 263
Deifenderfer, A., 255
De Master, B., 242, 244
Depue, R., 269
Deutch, M., 188
De Vault, M., 204
Diament, C, 139, 237, 242
Diener, E., 257
Dietz, A., 173, 237
Dietz, D., 204, 223
Dietz, S., 204, 223, 330
Doster, 255, 283
Dotson, V., 220, 224
Drabman, R., 138, 320, 321
Duffendack, S., 37 (*see* Lasky et al.)
Dunlap, A., 163
Dunnette, M., 226, 231
Durfee, R., 192
D' Zurilla, T., 169

Eason, R., 259
Edelberg, R., 267
Edwards, A., 115
Eisler, R., 146, 200, 201
Elder, I., 140, 151
Ellis, A., 16
Epstein, L., 266
Erbuagh, J., 9
Etkin, M., 103
Eyberg, S., 147, 165, 182, 241

Fairweather, G., 11, 37
Farber, M., 52
Fay, A., 16

Ferster, C., 28
Feuerstein, M., 255
Fishbein, M., 170
Fisher, D., 97
Fiske, D., 113, 177, 178
Fixsen, D., 120, 134, 140
Fleischmann, D., 114
Fode, K., 246
Fonda, C., 8, 9
Foster, S., 182, 220, 225, 226
Fowles, D., 269
Freitag, G., 145
Freud, S., 7, 79
Friar, L., 267
Friedman, P., 306, 319
Friend, R., 114
Fry, P., 188, 189

Ganzer, V., 39
Gibson, D., 146
Gilmore, S., 166
Gillmore, 219
Glass, G., 318
Glesser, G., 108, 220
Goldhart, A., 197
Gold, V., 145
Goldfried, M., 13, 58, 80, 111, 168, 169, 201,
    220
Goldiamond, I., 28
Goldstein, A., 39, 58, 64, 67, 197
Goldstein, H., 98
Goldstein, I., 264, 265
Gottman, J., 120, 133, 135, 318
Gough, H., 37, 115
Gradizan, J., 267
Green, A., 266
Grant, R., 300, 304, 305
Green, E., 266
Greenberg, L., 111, 112
Greenfield, N., 256
Grinspoon, L., 262
Gruel, L., 9
Gruzelier, J., 268
Guilford, J., 101
Gunn, C., 262
Gurman, 24

Hackman, J., 186
Hagen, R., 183, 184
Haley, J., 24, 30
Hall, R., 145, 151, 163, 330, 331, 332
Hammen, E., 119, 123, 133
Hampe, E., 98
Hanley, J., 267
Hansen, J., 56, 57, 74, 81, 86
Harris, A., 145, 180, 183, 184, 220

Harris, F., 220
Hart, B., 140
Hartmann, D., 226, 330, 331, 332
Hathaway, S., 115
Hawkins, R., 13, 145, 151, 163, 184, 220, 224
Hayden, M., 200
Hayes, S., 137, 139
Hendricks, A., 176
Herbert, E., 139, 200
Hersen, M., 13, 146, 200, 201, 255, 316
Heslin, R., 99, 109, 110
Hickson, R., 102
Himelstein, H., 176
Hines, P., 198
Hippocrates, 6
Hoats, D., 147
Holt, R., 108
Houck, J., 56, 57, 74, 86
Hover, G., 37 (*see* Lasky et al.)
Hubben, J., 197
Hunrichs, W., 9

Issacs, A., 267
Itill, T., 267
Ivey, A., 60, 61, 67, 78

Jackson, B., 120
Jackson, C., 200
Jackson, D., 30
Jacobson, E., 265
Jacobsen, L., 10, 246
Jagodzinski, M., 140
John, V., 146
Johnson, M., 220
Johnson, S., 112, 114, 120, 133, 145, 146, 147, 165, 176, 182, 183, 184, 185, 216, 235, 241, 242, 250
Johoda, M., 188
Jones, R., 148, 168, 172, 181, 220, 228, 229, 230, 231, 233, 234, 235, 245
Jones, 262

Kahn, R., 49, 50, 69, 71
Kallman, W., 255
Kamp, A., 267
Kanfer, F., 11, 17, 18, 19, 20, 21, 22, 23, 33, 34, 38, 80, 120, 121, 126, 133, 135, 137, 138, 140
Kanowitz, J., 248
Kass, R., 173, 247
Kassorla, J., 145
Kastenbaum, R., 111
Kaswan, J., 176
Katz, M., 186
Katz, R., 124, 306
Kaufman, K., 120, 138

Kazdin, A., 42, 120, 124, 126, 133, 134, 136, 137, 138, 317, 321, 327, 332
Kelly, E., 37, 97
Kelly, G., 11
Kendall, 219
Kent, R., 111, 139, 148, 168, 169, 182, 183, 220, 225, 226, 238, 240, 242, 244, 248
Kerkoff, T., 237, 238, 239
Kiesler, D., 106, 317
Kipp, J., 145
Kiresuk, T., 104, 106, 299
Knapp, T., 224
Kriskern, 24
Koeppel, J., 120, 327
Kohlmeyer, W., 265
Kraepelin, E., 7
Kubany, E., 209, 210
Kulp, S., 204, 212, 213, 214, 215
Kupers, C., 33
Kuypers, D., 184

Lacey, B., 255, 263
Lacey, J., 255, 262, 263
Lader, M., 265
Lang, P., 13, 102, 200, 257, 263, 283
Lasky, J., 37
Lawlis, G., 102
Layden, T., 119
Lazarus, A., 14, 15, 16, 17, 18, 22, 38, 41, 80, 255, 274, 283
Lazovik, A., 200
Lentz, R., 183, 201, 212, 213, 214
Leske, G., 238
Levine, F., 262
Levitt, E., 28
Levy, R., 267
Lervin, K., 189
Lewinsohn, P., 127, 212, 213
Lewittes, D., 186
Libet, J., 213
Lichstein, K., 191, 193, 198
Liebert, R., 33
Lifshitz, K., 267
Lillesand, D., 39
Lindsey, C., 151
Lindsley, D., 259
Lindsley, O., 145
Lipinski, D., 119, 124, 133, 136, 139, 140, 220
Lira, F., 103
Lobitz, G., 112, 114, 145, 147, 176, 182, 242
Locke, E., 120
Locke, J., 100
Lansburg, B., 267
Lorei, T., 37
Lovaas, O., 145
Love, I., 176

Loveless, S., 224
Lubin, B., 127
Lyerly, S., 186
Lyman, R., 140, 151
Lytton, H., 149

Mahoney, M., 11, 42, 119, 120, 121, 124, 133, 141, 205
Maletzky, B., 300
Malmo, R., 265
Marabotto, C., 136
Marholin, D., 193
Mariotto, M., 177, 212, 213, 214
Marlowe, D., 115
Martens, J., 197
Martin, I., 256
Martin, P., 151
Martin, R., 42, 55, 147, 306, 319
Martindale, A., 204, 212, 213, 214, 215
Marston, A., 33
Mash, E., 67, 165, 255
Masters, J., 80
Maurer, C., 200
Maynard, H., 11, 37 (*see* Fairweather et al.)
McArthur, M., 163
McCullough, J., 103, 106, 328
McDaniel, M., 328
McFall, R., 39, 119, 120, 123, 133, 134, 135, 195, 318
McGee, R., 11
McGovern, K., 198
McGuigon, F., 266
McGuire, F., 151
McKinley, J., 115
McLaughlin, J., 120, 125, 129
McNamara, J., 120, 126, 133
McReynolds, W., 26, 126, 141
Meehl, P., 108, 169, 309
Meichenbaum, D., 11, 26, 35
Melbin, M., 161
Mendelson, M., 9
Mercatoris, M., 184
Merrill, M., 38, 77
Meyerson, L., 205
Miller, L., 98
Miller, P., 201
Mischel, W., 33, 37, 38
Mock, J., 9
Morganstern, K., 37, 41, 42, 58, 67, 72
Moura, N., 119, 133
Mueller, R., 328
Murphy, G., 266

Namenek, T., 102
Nanda, H., 108, 220
Nay, W., 23, 32, 36, 42, 67, 78, 97, 103, 120,
125, 129, 139, 140, 145, 150, 182, 195, 196, 198, 201, 237, 238, 239, 241, 323
Nelson, C., 26, 126, 141, 220
Nelson, R., 119, 124, 133, 136, 139, 140
Nietzel, M., 200
Noble, H., 98
Noble, P., 265
Nord, C., 37 (*see* Lasky et al.)
Norman, A., 262
Notterman, J., 262
Nurnberger, J., 28

O'Brien, F., 204, 205
Odbert, H., 157
Odder, 262
O'Leary, K., 120, 138, 139, 148, 173, 184, 212, 215, 236, 237, 238, 240, 242, 244, 247, 248, 322, 323
Orne, M., 141
Osgood, C., 102

Paden, R., 176
Palmer, J., 151
Panyon, M., 163
Pasteur, L., 7
Patterson, G., 100, 103, 145, 163, 164, 166, 167, 168, 171, 174, 176, 180, 181, 183, 184, 193, 212, 213, 215, 220, 228, 230, 237, 245
Paul, G., 176, 177, 183, 184, 201, 212, 213, 214, 238, 249, 250
Pavek, G., 266
Penry, J., 267
Perloff, B., 33
Person, R., 262
Pesses, D., 146
Peterson, R., 30, 220
Pettus, C., 9
Pfeiffer, J., 99, 109, 110
Phillips, D., 193
Phillips, E., 120, 134, 140
Phillips, J., 34
Phillips, L., 9, 37
Pinkston, E., 200
Porter, R., 267
Powell, J., 204, 212, 213, 214, 215
Purcell, K., 146
Putnam, D., 106

Quade, D., 9

Rabon, D., 163
Rajaratnam, N., 108, 220
Rappaport, J., 11
Raush, H., 59, 189, 190, 191
Ray, R., 100, 103, 158, 163, 164, 167, 171, 174, 176, 181, 184, 212, 213, 237

Redfield, J., 213, 214, 238, 249
Reid, J., 166, 168, 175, 176, 181, 183, 220, 228, 230, 238, 242, 243, 244, 245, 246
Renzaglia, G., 146, 148, 184
Repp, A., 204, 223, 330
Repp, C., 204, 223
Reuter, J., 200
Rice, D., 263
Rickard, H., 140, 151
Rickles, W., 267
Rimm, D., 80
Risley, T., 140, 316
Ritter, B., 35, 103
Roberts, R., 146, 148, 184
Roccaforte, P., 145, 216
Rogers, C., 49, 61
Romanoff, B., 186
Romanczyk, R., 120, 135, 138, 139, 184, 242
Rosenhan, D., 10
Rosenthal, R., 10, 246, 250
Rozynko, V., 37
Rubin, S., 102
Rugh, J., 269
Rutner, I., 138

Sajwaj, T., 200
Saletu, B., 267
Sandifer, M., 9
Sands, W., 77
Sanders, D., 11, 37 (*see* Fairweather et al.)
Santogrossi, D., 120, 138, 173
Sarason, I., 39
Saslow, G., 17, 18, 19, 20, 21, 22, 23, 38, 80
Saunders, M., 163
Schaaf, W., 197
Schachter, S., 263
Schmidt, H., 8, 9
Schoenfeld, W., 262
Scholsberg, H., 268
Schryer, C., 267
Schwartz, R., 125, 149, 150, 151
Schwitzgebel, R., 269
Sechrest, L., 125, 149, 150, 151, 155
Selltiz, C., 188
Serber, M., 201
Shagass, C., 265
Shaw, D., 100, 103, 158, 163, 164, 167, 171, 174, 176, 184, 212, 213
Sherman, R., 104, 106, 299
Shostrum, L., 81, 90
Sidman, M., 132, 317
Sidowski, J., 255, 270
Siegel, L., 193
Simkins, L., 26, 138, 140, 141
Simmons, W., 186, 267
Skindrud, K., 236, 242, 244, 245, 246, 247

Skinner, B., 31, 120, 121
Sklar, B., 267
Sloggett, B., 209, 210
Smith, A., 265
Smith, J., 119, 123
Smith, R., 257, 262
Snyder, M., 309
Sobell, L., 120
Sobell, M., 120
Sommer, R., 270
Soskin, W., 146
Sowder, T., 146, 199
Spitalnik, R., 138
Sprafkin, J., 111
Spring, C., 111, 112
Stachnick, T., 309
Stainton, W., 309
Stallings, 219
Stanley, J., 317, 318, 327
Sterman, M., 267
Sternbach, R., 256, 263
Stevens, J., 267
Stevic, R., 81
Stewart, A., 106
Stone, N., 201
Stover, D., 314, 316
Stuart, R., 119, 123, 125, 127, 133
Suchman, 188
Suci, G., 102
Sullivan, H., 57, 79, 80, 91
Suratt, P., 184

Tallent, N., 282, 300, 308, 309
Tannenbaum, P., 102
Taplin, P., 175, 238, 242, 243, 245, 246, 250
Tasto, D., 102
Terdal, L., 67, 165, 255
Terman, L., 38, 77
Tharp, R., 127
Thomas, E., 200
Thomas, M., 100
Thompson, R., 259
Thoreson, C., 120, 121, 124
Thorne, F., 83, 84, 87
Toepfer, C., 200
Trier, C., 201
Truax, C., 58, 59

Ullmann, L., 9
Ulrich, R., 184, 309

Van Belle, H., 197
Van Berschot, S., 145
Van Leeuwen, W., 267
Van Lehn, R., 263
Van Wagenen, R., 205

Venables, P., 256, 268
Voas, R., 265

Wade, T., 119, 133
Wahler, R., 191, 193, 238
Walker, H., 112
Wall, R., 201
Wallen, R., 52, 53, 54, 71, 72, 74
Walter, H., 166
Walters, E., 266
Walters, R., 30, 34, 35
Walters, R., 267
Ward, C., 9
Warner, R., 81
Watson, D., 114, 127
Watzlawick, P., 30
Webb, E., 125, 149, 150, 151
Wechsler, D., 77
Weed, L., 300
Weerts, T., 200
Weick, K., 158, 162, 180, 220, 226, 227
Wellman, 262

Wenk, E., 37
White, G., 120, 133, 145, 183, 184
Wiersma, H., 197
Wiggins, J., 2, 95, 115, 178, 220, 232
Wiggins, N., 186
William, D., 146
Williams, R., 200
Wilson, V., 318
Winer, B., 226
Wolach, A., 145, 216
Wolf, A., 267
Wolf, M., 120, 134, 140, 316
Wolf, S., 262
Wolpe, J., 38, 80, 84, 102, 104
Woodworth, R., 268
Wooley, F., 306
Wright, H., 155, 156, 157, 172, 181, 189, 190,
    203, 204, 206, 207, 212, 217, 218, 220

Zigler, E., 9
Zimet, C., 9, 10
Zubin, J., 9

Subject Index

The A-B Design, 316–320; continuation affect, 317; history, 317; instrument decay, 318; maturation, 317; regression, 318; transient physical status, 318

ABA or ABAB Design, 321–323

The ABACA/Successive Treatments Design, 323

Analogue assessment, 125–202; (*see also* Clinical contrived setting); validations of, 202

Assessment problems, demand characteristics, 96, 135; method variance, 101, 110, 178; response sets, 115–116

The B Design, 316

B-C Design, 320–321

Baseline, 131, 227

Baserates, 228

Behavior v. constructs, 113, 168, 177

Behavior change, goals of, incorporate new behavior, 23; increase behavior frequency, 23; reduce behavior frequency, 23

Behavior Coding System (BCS), 100, 103, 145, 163, 164, 167, 171, 174, 176, 181, 212, 228

Behavioral Approach Test, 200, 201

Behavioral Assertiveness Test, 201–202

Behavioral Checklist, 213

Behavioral deficit, 18

Behavioral diagnosis, 18–21; definition, 18, 19; functional relationships, 30, 18, 21; motivation, 18, 19, 135; past behavior, 18; physical-biological resources, 18, 20; self-control, 18, 20, 121; social relationships, 18, 21; sociocultural mileu, 18, 20; sociocultural-physical environment, 21

Bipolar Adjective Checklist, 114

"Calibrating" observer, 241; (*see also* Observer drift)

Card-sorting, 170

Case history, 79; information categories, 82–87; issues, 87–88; organization of, 88–89; questions, 81; questioning strategies, 89–90; reconnaissance, 79

Case history organization, 88–89; developmental unit approach, 88; open-ended approach, 88; within category approach, 88–89

Chance agreements, 225–226; (*see also* Reliability assessment); chance correspondence agreement, 225–226; Kappa agreement, 225

Changing-Criterion Design, 330–332

Checklists, computer scoring, 98; Louisville Behavior Checklist, 98

Classical Psychometric Theory, 108, 168–169, 220

Classroom Behavior Inventory, 112

Client motivation, 41, 135; ethical/legal issues, 42; "homework" assignments, 42; preintervention motivation, 42; "resistance," 42

Client resources, 38–41; ability/deficit, 38; cognitive-intellectual, 38; financial resources, 41; information, 39; person support, 40; physical abilities, 39; physical surroundings, 40; social skills, 39

Clinical assessment, causality, 12; description, 6; evaluation, 12; methods, 12

Clinical assessment errors, 278–284; detection, 278, 279–280; integration-interpretations, 278, 280–282; multimethod approach recommendation, 283–284; selection, 278, 282–283

Clinical contrived setting, 195–203; analogue assessments, 125–202; audiotape analogues, 195, 197–198; enactments, 195, 200–201; paper-and pencil, 195–196; role-play, 195, 201–203; videotape analogues, 195, 198–200

Clinical decision making, assessment errors, 278–283; communicating findings, 299–309; modality matrix, 273–277; multimethod assessment examples, (a) child behavior problem, 285–295; (b) adult male, 295–299

Clinical natural setting, 193–195; advantages, 194–195; assumptions of approach, 194

Communicating assessment findings, 299–309; example outline, 302–304; formats, 301, (a) intake report, 301; (b) progress report, 301; (c) termination summary, 301; (d)

359

specific assessment results, 301; potential pitfalls, 308-309; (a) Barnum report, 309; written record keeping, 300-301

Comprehensive clinical assessment, 5; behavioral assessment, 13; (a) observation—in situ, 13; (b) self-report, 13; ecological assessment, 24, 189-193; interview, 17; (a) significant others, 17; (b) self-report, 17; outline, 42-45; psychological testing, 12; psychometric instruments, 13; systems-level assessment, 24, 30

Conditions, 27-30, 167; activities, 29; antecedents, 30; consequences, 30; location, 27; stimulus control, 28; times, 29

Confidentiality, 54; (*see also* Ethical/legal issues); audio/video tape, 55; consent, 55; court decisions, 55; privacy, 55

Consequences of behavior, activity, 33; intrinsic, 33; material, 32; social, 32

Construct, 113, 168, 177-179, 282

Continuous sampling, 211

Covert events, 33, 119, 126, 135, 141, 201

"Criterion observers," 238; (*see also* Observer drift)

"Criterion protocol," 238; (*see also* Observer drift)

Cueing devices, advantages, 216-217; construction of, 216; for interval recording, 216-218; limitations, 217-218

Current behavior assessment, (*see also* Reliability assessment); cognitive/imaginal referents, 26; duration, 26; frequency, 26; intensity, 43; physical referents, 26; physical sensations, 26; referents of phenomena, 25; temporal features, 26; verbal/motor component, 25; d^2 statistic, 228

Decision making, (*see* Clinical decision making)

Description of target, conditions, 43; definition of, 172; nature of target, 134; referents, (a) overt, 43; (b) covert, 43; self-statement of concern, 5, 42; selection, choice of, 135, 166-167; valence of, 135, 136

Detection errors, 277-278; inadequate methods choice, 279; inadequate modality choice, 279; method error, 279, 280; sources of bias, 280

Diagnosis and classification, 7

DSM, 7, 8; criticisms of, (a) general, 8; (b) homogenity of classification, 9; (c) labeling, 9; (d) reliability, 9; (e) utility, 12

Domains of behavior, (*see* Response systems)

Ecological assessment, 189, 193; inter-

dependence in, 190; multivariate statistics, 191

Electroencephalography (EEG), 266-267; biofeedback and, 266; biotelemetry of, 267; computer analysis of, 267; dreaming and, 266; frequencies of, 266

Electrocardiograph (EKG), 261-264; artifactual data, 262; biotelemetry data, 262; cognitive set and, 263-264; relation to emotion, 263; response stereotype, 263

Electromyogram (EMG), 264-266; action potential, 264; integration of, 264; motor unit, 264; relation to anxiety, 265-266

Employee Aptitude Survey, 236

Errors, in clinical assessment, 278-284; in detection, 279-280; in integration/interpretation, 280-282; in testing, 96, 101, 110, 115-116, 135, 178

Ethical/legal issues, 54-55, 147, 195, 305-306, 318, 319, 322-323

Evaluation of treatment, (*see* Treatment evaluation)

Event sampling, 203, 204-207, 224-225; advantages, limitations, 207; example, 205

Fear Survey Schedule, 102

Free response measures, 96-97; paper-and-pencil analogue, 97; sentence-completion, 97

Functional analysis, 30; (*see also* Behavioral diagnosis, 18-21, and Situational analysis, 169)

Generalizability, 108, 231-235; factor analysis of variance, 232; "D" study, 233; "G" study, 232; generalizability coefficients, 235; three facet design, 233; (a) observers, 233; (b) occasions, 233; (c) subjects, 233; (d) interaction, 233; universe of conditions, 232

Goal-attainment scaling, 104-107, 299

Group vs. Single-Subject Designs, 315-316

Historical-developmental information, 81; description of birth, 82; developmental history, 82; educational history, 85; family characteristics, 84; family history, 84; interpersonal skills, 84; medical history, 83; occupational history, 87; sexual development, 86

Historical information, 36

Idiosyncratic rating schemes, GAS Scale, 104, 105, 106, 107, 299; (a) goal attainment, 104; SUDS Scale, 104; (b) subjective units discomfort, 104

Independent observations, instrument construction, 167; methods options, 144; (a) mechanical approaches, 144–149; (b) product-related, 149–155; (c) written methods, 155–165; target selection, 166–167

Independent observation methods, 144; mechanical approaches, 144–149; product-related measures, 149–155; written methods, 155-165

Intake-orientation interview, 51; introduction, 52; (a) BCA as "threat," 52; (b) BCA as "accomplice," 54; (c) BCA as "omnipotent," 53; (d) expectations, 52; (e) rapport, 52

Integration-interpretation errors, 280–282; error of congruence, 281; inadequate conceptualization, 282; overgeneralization, 281; theoretical bias constructs, 282

Interindividual stability, 231

Interobserver agreement, complexity as predictor, 247–248; computation of, 222–226; correlation coefficient, 221, 226; empty intervals problem, 223; expectations and biases, 246–250; overall agreement, 222, 223; percentage of observation intervals, 221; sample size, 223

Interview, categories of, 49–51; case history, 51; intake-orientation, 51; pinpointing, 51; (a) research, 49; (b) therapeutic, 49; confidentiality of, 54; setting for, 55

Interview questioning, 69–73; clear statements, 70; embedded questioning, 72; frame of reference, 69; held-over question, 72; narrowing, 72; open v. closed, 70; pre-programmed responses, 69; progressive questioning, 71

Interviewer responses, interpretation, 62; minimal verbal response, 60; pre-programmed, 69; questioning, 69–73; reflection, 62; restatement, 61; silence, 60; summarization, 61

Interviewing techniques, 69–73

Intraindividual stability, 228

Marriage Adjustment Schedule, 100

Mechanical devices, audio/video recording, 145–148; cueing devices, 216–218; electronic filters, 147; ethical limitations on, 54–55, 147; for recording behavior, 144–149; frequency counter, 145; telephone, 148–149

Minnesota Clerical Test, 236, 296

Minnesota Multiphasic Personality Inventory, 115

Modality-method matrix, 277; facet, defined, 274, 275; matrix, 276–277; methods categories, 275; modality, defined, 273–274

Modeling, 30; inhibitory/disinhibitory effects, 35; observational learning, 34; social facilitation effects, 35

Multidimensional reliability assessment, error sources, (a) chance response tendencies, 227; (b) environment changes, 227; (c) inadequate content sampling, 226

Multimodal assessment, Basic Id., 14; (a) affect, 14, 15; (b) behavior, 14, 15; (c) cognition, 14, 16; (d) def., 14; (e) drugs, 14, 17; (f) imagery, 14, 15; (g) interdependency, 17; (h) interpersonal, 14, 16; (i) sensation, 14, 15

Multimethod assessment approach, basic assumptions, 283–284; examples, (a) child behavior problem, 285–295; (b) young adult male, 295–299

Multiple baseline design, 324–328; different persons, 324; different settings, 324; different targets, 324; methodological issues, 326–328

Multi-trait multimethod validation, 113, 177–179

Multivariate coding systems, 165, 191; cluster analysis, 192

Natural setting, 181–193; control of, 182; ecological validity of, 181; issues, (a) artificiality, 182; (b) base-rate problems, 185; (c) extraneous variables, 185–186; (d) observer presence, 183; (e) reactivity, 182; (f) recommendations for, 184–185

Nonspecific written records, advantages, 157; disadvantages, 158; instructions for, 156; specimen record keeping, 155

Nonverbal behavior, eye contact, 78; facial expressions, 78; motor behavior, 77; posture, 77

Observational methods, independent observations, 144–165; self-observations, 119–142

Observer-collected v. mechanical data, 183

Observer drift, definition of, 240; issues of, 240–245; recommendations for reducing, 249–250

Observer expectations and biases, 246–250; evaluative feedback and, 248; familiarity, 249; recommendations, 249–250

Observer selection and training, 236–245; feedback to observers, 239; observer drift, 240–245; outline of manual, 237; videotape training, 238

Overdetection errors, 224

Overt-covert assessment, 242

Participant observation, 186–189; advantages/disadvantages, 187; observation by significant others, 186
Physical appearance, 74
Problem definition, 57; focusing with questions, 68; (a) frame of reference, 69; orientation, 57; statement of problem, 57; (a) reconnaissance, 57, 79; (b) questionnaire, 57; "tracking," 58
Problem Oriented Record, 300, 301, 304–308; example, 306–308
Procedures for classroom observation, 236
Psychophysiological methods, 255–270; major modalities, 261–270; (a) EEG, 266–267; (b) EKG, 261, 264; (c) EMG, 264–266; (d) others, 269–270; (e) skin responses, 267–269
Psychophysiological responses, 257–259; amplitude, 259; bioelectrical signals, 258; characteristics, 257–258; counterprinter, 260; electrode, 259; FM analogue tape recorder, 261; frequency, 259; measurement methods, 259–260; oscilloscope, 260; period, 259; physical-biological phenomena, 259; transduced bioelectrical signals, 258–259; waveform, 259, 260

Rapport, commitment, 59; empathy, 64–67; spontaneity, 60; therapist warmth, 59
Rating scales, Continuous Scale, 101, 163; Fear Survey Schedule, 102; Graphic Rating Scale, 101; Likert Scale, 99; Marriage-Adjustment Schedule, 100; Symptom Check List, 100
Reinforcement Survey Schedule, 110
Reliability, computation of, 222–226; classical psychometric theory, 108, 220; generalizability, 108, 231–235; internal consistency, 108, 109, 220; of observational method, 175–179; of paper-and-pencil tests, 108; of self-observations, 138–142; of self-report, 108–110; sources of error, 226–227; stability, 108, 109, 227; test-retest, 220, 227
Reliability assessment, definition and methodology, 220–221; interobserver agreement, 221; training of observers, 236
Reporting assessment results, 299–309
Representativeness of data, with partial interval sampling, 214–215; with whole interval sampling, 214–215
Response sets, acquiescence, 115; social desirability, 115
Response systems/domains, affective domain, 22; imagery, 22; motoric, 13; multiple domains, 256; physiological, 13; verbal-cog-

nitive, 13

Scored-interval agreement, 224
Selection errors, goals for intervention, 282–283
Selection of self-report, 107; norms, 107; reliability, 108
Self-control, 18, 20, 120, 121; (*see also* Self regulation)
Self monitoring, definition of problem, 122; mechanical devices, 124–125; (a) advantages, 124; (b) disadvantages, 124; product-related methods, 125–126; (a) advantages, 125; (b) disadvantages, 125; recording procedures, 123; sampling of, 130; (a) event sampling, 130; (b) time sampling, 130–131; setting of, 130; written records, 126–130; (a) advantages, 129
Self observation, issues, 133–142; feedback, 120, 137; methods and issues, 119–122; reactivity, 120, 133–138, 182; recommendations, 139–142; self-monitoring methods, 122–132; self-regulation, 121; reliability of information, 138–142
Self-regulation, 120–121, 137; self control, 18, 20, 120–121; self evaluation, 121, 137; self monitoring, 26, 28, 133, 120–142; self reinforcement, 33, 137
Semantic differential, 102–103
Setting, clinical contrived, 195–202; clinical natural, 193–195; natural, 181–193
Skin responses, 267–269; baseline assessment of, 268; conductance (SC), 267; GSR, 267, 268; impedence (SI), 267; Ohm's law, 267; relation to emotion, 268–269; skin resistences (SR), 267
Significance, clinical vs. statistical, 314–315
Simultaneous Treatment Design, 328–330; counterbalanced, 328; Latin-square, 328–329
Single Subject Designs, 315–316
Situational analysis, 169
Social avoidance and Distress Scale, 114
"Source" videotapes, 238
Specific written records, advantages, 165; continuous record, 163; field-format, 162; limitations, 165; on-off approaches, 158; on-off example, 160
Specimen recording, 155, 172
"Spot-check" reliability assessment, 242; problems with, 242
Subjective units of discomfort, 104
Systems level assessment, 24, 30–31, 189–193

Target behavior, attributions about, 42; definition of, 172; nature of, 134; overt/covert

referents, 43; selection of, 135, 166–167; self-statements about, 5, 42; surrounding conditions, 43; valence of, 135, 136
Therapeutic contracts, 140
Time-behavior, behavior-behavior relations, 145
Time-out procedure, 196
Time Sample Behavioral Checklist, 176–177
Time sampling, 203, 207–218; cueing devices, 216–218; generalizability of findings, 208; interoccasion interval, 209; methodology, 211–216; observational interval, 208; random sampling, 209; recording interval, 208
Time sampling methodology, nonspecific recording, 212; specific recording, 211
Time-Series Designs, 318
Treatment evaluation strategies, A-B Design, 316–320; A-B-A or A-B-A-B Design, 321–323; A-B-A-C-A or successive treatments, 323; B Design, 316; B-C Design, 320–321; changing-criterion, 330–332; clinical vs. statistical significance, 314–315; Group vs. Single-Subject Designs, 315–316; multiple baseline, 324–328; simultaneous treatment, 328–330

Underinclusiveness errors, 224
Unobtrusive measures, 146, 149–155; archive, 151–155; erosion, 149–150; related issues, 182–186; reliability and, 244; trace, 150–151
Unscored-interval agreement, 224

Valence, 135, 136
Validity, concurrent, 111; construct, 113, 168, 177–179; content/face validity, 110, 169; convergent, 112, 177–178; discriminant, 112, 178; ecological, 181; of observational method, 175–179
Variable interval, 210–211; momentary time sampling, 212, 213; partial interval sampling, 212; representativeness of data, 214; whole interval sampling, 212
Voice and speech, 74; deviations, 76; ease, 75; intensity, 75; manner, 76; organization, 76; pitch, 75; reaction time, 75; relevance, 75; speed, 75; spontaneity, 75; vocabulary, 76

Written records, general, 123, 126–130; nonspecific, 126–130, 155–158; specific, 126–130, 158–165
Written self report, checklists, 98; free response measures, 96–97; idiosyncratic rating schemes, 104; rating scales, 99–102; selection criteria, 107; semantic differential, 102–103